T0344435

Clinical Principles of Transfusion Medicine

Clinical Principles of Transfusion Medicine

ROBERT W. MAITTA, MD, PhD
Department of Pathology,
University Hospitals Cleveland Medical Center,
Case Western Reserve University School of Medicine,
Cleveland, OH, United States

ELSEVIER

ELSEVIER

3251 Riverport Lane
St. Louis, Missouri 63043

Content Strategist: Kayla Wolfe
Content Development Manager: Taylor Ball
Content Development Specialist: Kristen Helm
Publishing Services Manager: Deepthi Unni
Project Manager: Janish Ashwin Paul
Designer: Gopalakrishnan Venkatraman

Working together
to grow libraries in
developing countries

Printed in United States of America

Last digit is the print number: 9   8   7   6   5   4   3   2   1

www.elsevier.com • www.bookaid.org

List of Contributors

Editor

Robert W. Maitta, MD, PhD
Department of Pathology
University Hospitals Cleveland Medical Center
Case Western Reserve University School of Medicine
Cleveland, OH, United States

Authors

Ian Baine, MD, PhD
Department of Laboratory Medicine
Yale University School of Medicine
New Haven, CT, United States

Jacquelyn D. Choate, MD
Blood Bank Medical Director
Department of Pathology and Laboratory Medicine
Avera McKennan Hospital and University Health
    Center
Sioux Falls, SD, United States

Robert A. DeSimone, MD
Transfusion Medicine Fellow
Weill Cornell Medical College
New York Presbyterian Hospital-Weill Cornell
    Medicine
New York, NY, United States

Michelle L. Erickson, MD, MBA
Medical Director
Transfusion Medicine
WellSpan Health System
York, PA, United States
Pathology Department
WellSpan York Hospital
York, PA, United States

Ruchika Goel, MD, MPH
Assistant Professor of Pathology and Laboratory
    Medicine
Weill Cornell Medical College
New York Presbyterian Hospital-Weill Cornell Medicine
New York, NY, United States

Amit Gokhale, MD
Department of Laboratory Medicine
Yale University School of Medicine
New Haven, CT, United States

Jeanne E. Hendrickson, MD
Department of Laboratory Medicine
Department of Pediatrics
Yale University School of Medicine
New Haven, CT, United States

Hong Hong, MD, PhD
Assistant Attending Physician
Department of Laboratory Medicine
Memorial Sloan Kettering Cancer Center
New York, NY, United States

Robert W. Maitta, MD, PhD
Department of Pathology
University Hospitals Cleveland Medical Center
Case Western Reserve University School of
    Medicine
Cleveland, OH, United States

Faisal Mukhtar, MD
Associate Medical Director Transfusion Services
Assistant Clinical Professor
Department of Pathology, Immunology and
    Laboratory Medicine
University Florida Health
Gainesville, FL, United States
Department of Pathology, Immunology and
    Laboratory Medicine
UF Health Shands Hospital
Gainesville, FL, United States

Joseph Peter R. Pelletier, MD
Clinical Associate Professor
Medical Director Transfusion Services
Department of Pathology, Immunology and
    Laboratory Medicine
University of Florida
Gainesville, FL, United States

Huy P. Pham, MD, MPH
Division of Laboratory Medicine
Department of Pathology
University of Alabama at Birmingham
Birmingham, AL, United States
Department of Pathology
Keck School of Medicine of the University of
    Southern California
Los Angeles, CA, United States

Hollie M. Reeves, DO
Assistant Medical Director of Transfusion Medicine,
    Blood Bank, and Apheresis Center
Department of Pathology
University Hospitals Cleveland Medical Center
Cleveland, OH, United States
Assistant Professor of Pathology
Case Western Reserve University School of Medicine
Cleveland, OH, United States

Ronit Reich-Slotky, PhD, MSc
Supervisor
Cellular Therapy Laboratory
New York Presbyterian Hospital-Weill Cornell
    Medicine
New York, NY, United States

Sara Rutter, MD
Department of Laboratory Medicine
Yale University School of Medicine
New Haven, CT, United States

Sierra C. Simmons, MD, MPH
Division of Laboratory Medicine
Department of Pathology
University of Alabama at Birmingham
Birmingham, AL, United States

**Judith A. Sullivan, MS, MT(ASCP)SBB,
CQA(ASQ)**
Independent Quality Consultant
Silver Spring, MD, United States

Christopher A. Tormey, MD
Department of Laboratory Medicine
Yale University School of Medicine
New Haven, CT, United States
Pathology & Laboratory Medicine Service
VA Connecticut Healthcare System
West Haven, CT, United States

Ljiljana V. Vasovic, MD
Assistant Professor of Pathology and Laboratory
    Medicine
Weill Cornell Medical College
New York Presbyterian Hospital-Weill Cornell
    Medicine
New York, NY, United States

Lance A. Williams III, MD
Division of Laboratory Medicine
Department of Pathology
University of Alabama at Birmingham
Birmingham, AL, United States

Chisa Yamada, MD
Associate Professor of Pathology
Department of Pathology
University of Michigan
Medical Director of Apheresis Services
Associate Medical Director of Transfusion Medicine
Michigan Medicine
Ann Harbor, MI, United States

Preface

Transfusion medicine has not been idle but has metamorphosed into a medical discipline that has become more complex over the years since transfusions were performed for the first time centuries ago. All medical practitioners are well aware of the usefulness of blood components in the treatment of patients. However, in many instances, these practices have not been fully aware of the many complexities that we now know and others that are brought about by transfusion of blood components that we are yet to find out. New evidence becomes available at such fast pace that it is challenging to remain abreast of the new data. In this setting, practitioners in disciplines that depend on transfusion support for their patients have slowly but steadily moved toward a more comprehensive review of their approach to transfusions. Furthermore, in light of current declines in blood collections and increase in cost, it is imperative that these practice reviews occur in the midst of this new reality because fewer donors are added to existing donor pools. For those of us in the transfusion medicine field it has become clear that the approach to saving blood and preserving the available inventory for those who need it the most cannot occur without firm involvement of an entire institution. Yet, to do this we must look at the past, understand the principles of transfusion of a specific blood component, understand the principles of testing, understand the non-infrequent transfusion-related adverse events, and realize that at times patient-specific requirements, as in pediatric patients, need to be considered when reviewing practices. This book has gone back to the basics to reintroduce historical biological aspects of red cell antigenic typing, red cell and human leukocyte antigen alloimmunization, and complications of hematopoietic stem cell transplantation, to mention a few of the topics being covered. Transfusion recommendations in obstetric patients, pediatric patients, stem cell recipients, and blood component dosage and indications in those in critical need of massive transfusions of blood components are described in the context of new data in different patient populations.

We hope that the reader will use this book to get an understanding of transfusions, their usefulness, and the challenges in understanding the potential adverse events brought about by them. "Primum non nocere" is engraved in all physicians' psyche from their first day of training when they first vow to do no harm to a patient. Transfusion practices are an extension of this solemn oath we took early in our careers. Blood components help us treat patients who at times are in very fragile clinical presentations, but this does not justify the indiscriminate use of this valuable resource without thinking of the potential complications when utilized. As we confront a changing landscape in blood availability, this vow should come to the forefront and help us establish new dialogs across disciplines to rethink blood transfusion appropriateness.

Robert W. Maitta, M.D., Ph.D.
Department of Pathology
University Hospitals Cleveland Medical Center
Case Western Reserve University School of Medicine
Cleveland, OH, United States

Contents

CHAPTER 1

Quality Concepts in Transfusion Medicine

JUDITH A. SULLIVAN, MS, MT(ASCP)SBB, CQA(ASQ)

Until 1997, "quality" in transfusion medicine was a concept that related to quality control, that is, testing performed to ensure that reagents and equipment functioned as expected. Transfusion medicine (indeed, most of healthcare) lagged behind other industries in introducing the concepts of quality assurance and quality systems. In 1997, AABB (formerly known as the American Association of Blood Banks) introduced the concept of quality systems to the blood banking community for the first time in its 18th edition of *Standards for Blood Banks and Transfusion Services*. Since then, transfusion services and blood banks have embraced quality concepts and, especially, quality systems as a means of providing superior patient care.

What is a quality system? The AABB defines a quality system as "the organizational structure, responsibilities, policies, processes, procedures, and resources established by executive management to achieve quality."[1] In essence, it is the support structure put in place by those in authority to ensure that a quality product or service can be provided to a customer on a consistent basis.

One could question the applicability of a quality systems approach in the transfusion medicine arena. After all, we collect and transfuse blood components, not manufacture automobiles. We do not provide a product that can be reproduced within certain tolerance limits. However, the inherent variability of the components that we provide to patients necessitates the implementation of a quality system. The provision of the best possible component in any reproducible manner demands a quality framework including:
- Management knowledgeable in, and committed to, quality concepts
- Well-developed policies, processes, and procedures
- Staff who are trained and competent, and who follow processes and procedures as written
- Equipment that is selected with care, qualified before use, and well maintained
- Quality supplies from qualified vendors

- Processes to make changes in a controlled manner and to manage documents and records
- Means to identify and correct errors so that they do not recur
- Methods to assess effectiveness and continuously improve
- Safe environment for personnel and patients

Accrediting organizations such as the AABB, the College of American Pathologists, and The Joint Commission have established requirements for the implementation of quality functions that support operations. The AABB defines 10 Quality System Essentials (QSEs) that form the framework for a quality system (see Table 1.1). Each of these elements, integrated into the day-to-day activities of transfusion service, provides the structure that allows the provision of the right component to the right patient on a consistent basis.

ORGANIZATION

An effective quality system is not simply a vague notion that is discussed at periodic meetings. It must be defined and documented, implemented, and maintained. The development, implementation, and maintenance of a quality system rests with executive management: the personnel within the organization having the authority to establish or change quality policy. For a quality system to be truly effective, the oversight and responsibility must reside at the highest possible level within the organization. "Executive management" may be one individual or a group of individuals. In either case, the organization must clearly define its executive management. However, the quality system cannot exist with executive management alone. All personnel must be trained so that they:
1. know what the quality system is;
2. understand its importance; and
3. recognize and act on their role in the system.

Other important elements under the QSE organization are as follows.

TABLE 1.1 Quality System Essentials	
1	Organization
2	Resources
3	Equipment
4	Supplier and customer issues
5	Process control
6	Documents and records
7	Deviations, nonconformances, and adverse events
8	Assessments: internal and external
9	Process improvement
10	Facilities and safety

Data from American Association of Blood Banks (AABB). *Committee Quality System Essentials (QSEs)*; August 2017. Available at: http://www.aabb.org/membership/governance/committees/Documents/AABB-Committee-QSEs.pdf.

Defined Structure

The transfusion service of the blood bank must identify the individuals responsible for providing products and services, the individuals responsible for key quality functions, and the relationship among personnel. Organizational charts are often used to visually define personnel and relationships.

Medical Director Responsibilities

The medical director has the ultimate responsibility for the establishment of policies, processes, and procedures of the transfusion service of the blood bank.

Management Review of the Quality System

A quality system must be evaluated periodically if it is to provide any lasting benefit to the organization. The executive management is responsible for evaluating the effectiveness of the quality system on an ongoing basis and to make changes to the system based on the results of the review. The effectiveness of the quality system may be evaluated through such reviews as:
- Findings from internal and external assessments and subsequent follow-up actions
- Error reports, root cause analysis, and corrective action
- Customer surveys and complaints
- Process improvement activities

Reviews must be documented, along with any changes to the quality system resulting from the review.

Policies, Processes, and Procedures

Written policies, processes, and procedures form the backbone of any quality system, providing consistent practice within the transfusion service or the blood bank. Personnel perform their functions based, not upon hearsay, but upon clear written instructions. Processes are well defined, so they can be followed by everyone in the same way. When new personnel are trained they are given accurate information. Consistent execution of policies, processes, and procedures leads to consistent products and services.

The AABB standards define *policy* as, "a documented general principle that guides present and future decisions." They express the commitment and the intent of the organization with regard to a quality element. A *process* is "a set of related tasks and activities that accomplish a work goal." It usually involves more than one person or one group within a program. Processes are often depicted by flowcharts. A *procedure* is "a series of tasks usually performed by one person according to instructions." Procedures are to the transfusion service or blood bank what recipes are to cooks. See Table 1.2 for an example of a policy, process, and procedure as it relates to equipment.

A final word about policies, processes, and procedures: They must be in writing, and they must be followed as written. Personnel must be trained not to deviate from written processes and procedures. Conversely, processes and procedures must be written in such a way that they are easy to understand and easy to follow.

Exceptions to Policies, Processes, and Procedures

Given a particular clinical situation or patient, the medical director can justify and approve exceptions to policies, processes, and procedures. This approval must occur before the event's occurrence and must be in writing. Exceptions must be monitored, and if recurring, should be evaluated for incorporation into existing policies, processes, and procedures.

RESOURCES

The primary "resource" in a transfusion service or blood bank is the personnel. All personnel must be qualified, trained, and competent.

Qualifications

The blood bank or transfusion service must define in writing the qualifications needed for an individual to be hired for a specific position. Usually, these qualifications are included as part of a job description. Each

TABLE 1.2 Policy, Process, Procedure	
Policy: Equipment *Rule*	Transfusion at XYZ hospital identifies equipment that is critical to the provision of services and ensures that the calibration, maintenance, and monitoring of equipment conforms to specified require- ments
Process: Equipment Selection *What we do*	1. Establish equipment need 2. Determine if the item is in budget 3. Identify vendors 4. Perform site visits to evaluate 5. Others
Procedure: Use of a Cell Washer *How we do things*	1. Place tubes in cell washer 2. Latch lid 3. Select number of washes 4. Select "Start"

organization must define the level of education, training, and/or experience needed to qualify for each position.

Training

Once qualified personnel are hired, the transfusion service or blood bank must have a written process for training each individual according to its policies, processes, and procedures. Simply because a newly hired personnel has 5 years' experience in performing testing, it does not mean that he or she is ready to perform that function in *my* department using *my* equipment and procedures. Training to specific policies, processes, and procedures ensures common understanding among staff and consistent implementation. When new processes or procedures are introduced, or existing ones are changed, there must also be a process for identifying and assessing the training needs and providing additional training as necessary.

Competency

Because an individual has been trained in a specific task, it does not necessarily guarantee that he or she is competent, that is, capable of independently performing the task according to the procedure. Therefore the transfusion service or blood bank must have a process for assessing competency before releasing an individual to work independently. Methods of competency assessment may include a combination of:
- Direct observation of task performance
- Monitoring the recording and reporting of test results

- Review of worksheets, quality control records, and preventive maintenance records
- Direct observation of performance of instrument maintenance and function checks
- Assessment of test performance via "unknown" specimens
- Assessment of problem-solving skills[2]

The competency assessment of testing personnel is regulated under the Clinical Laboratory Improvement Amendments, and all transfusion services and blood banks must adhere to these regulations. However, nontesting personnel should also have their competency assessed before independently performing critical tasks. To ensure that individuals remain competent in assigned tasks, competency must be assessed at least annually. Written records of the assessment must be maintained. If assessment indicates that an individual is not competent, documentation of follow-up actions must also be maintained.

EQUIPMENT

Personnel can only be as good as the equipment they operate. Equipment that is not carefully selected, qualified, calibrated, and maintained is incapable of providing a consistent, quality component or service, regardless of the skills of the individual operating it.

Selection

The transfusion service must define a process that is used to select equipment. The process should allow for a deliberate consideration of all elements necessary for selection, for example:
- What is my budget?
- How will this equipment be used?
- What specifications must the equipment meet?
- Who will operate it?
- How often will it be used?
- What kind of support will the manufacturer provide in installation and ongoing maintenance?
- What types of disposables will be needed and how easy is to acquire them?
- What experiences (positive and negative) have other users had with this equipment?
- How reliable is the manufacturer?

A defined process ensures that the best selection is made taking into account all the critical parameters, especially for those times when the equipment must be purchased on an emergency basis.

Qualification

Once the equipment is purchased, it must be qualified, that is, it must be evaluated to ensure that it will work as expected *before* it is placed in use. A qualification plan must be developed, approved, implemented, and evaluated before equipment use. Qualification involves three stages:

- Installation qualification: This process ensures that the equipment is installed according to the requirements (operator's manual, applicable standards and regulations, fire code, etc.).
- Operational qualification: This process ensures that the equipment does what the manufacturer says it can do. Do all the buttons have the desired effect when pushed? Does the centrifuge spin? Does the refrigerator cool to the required temperature? Does the platelet agitator indeed move as expected?
- Performance qualification: This process answers the question, "Does this equipment perform as expected in *my* environment, using *my* procedures and *my* personnel?" It may involve testing various scenarios to determine if the equipment will function as expected under different circumstances.

Once the qualification is complete, the plan is reviewed to ensure that it was followed as written, expected results were achieved, any discrepancies were identified and addressed, and documentation is complete.

Calibration

If a piece of equipment requires calibration, a process must be defined to ensure that the calibration occurs before use, after activities that may affect calibration, and at specified intervals. Safeguards must be in place to ensure that calibration settings cannot be inadvertently changed. If it is discovered that a piece of equipment is out of calibration, it must be removed from service and a process to assess the effect of the calibration change on any product that may have been produced or testing that was performed must be followed.

Preventive Maintenance

To ensure that the equipment continues to work as expected, the transfusion service or blood bank must define a process and schedule for preventive maintenance. At a minimum, manufacturer's recommendations for the type and frequency of maintenance must be followed. Records of preventive maintenance must be maintained.

SUPPLIER AND CUSTOMER ISSUES

As with the equipment, the final product or service will only be as good as the critical materials used in its manufacture. When the transfusion service or blood bank qualifies its suppliers of equipment, materials, and services; defines agreed-upon expectations; and verifies the acceptability of the supplies before use, it has taken steps to ensure a consistent supply of quality critical materials and services.

Supplier Qualification

Critical materials are defined as those that can affect the quality of products or services. The transfusion service or blood bank is responsible for identifying materials that it considers to be critical and to qualify the suppliers of the materials. "Qualify" in this situation means to determine, before entering into a contract, that a supplier can consistently provide materials that meet requirements.

Some factors to consider in supplier qualification:

- Licensure, certification, or accreditation by a reputable organization
- Product requirements
- Review of a supplier's relevant quality documents
- Review of the transfusion service's or blood bank's experience with the supplier
- Cost of products or services
- Delivery arrangements
- Financial security, market position, and customer satisfaction
- Postsales support

The transfusion service or blood bank must define a process for qualifying new suppliers, maintain a current list of qualified suppliers, and ensure through policy that only qualified suppliers are used. Ongoing monitoring of a supplier's performance is documented and feedback provided, including complaints and quality issues. In situations in which the transfusion service or blood bank does not have direct authority for purchasing decisions, it is essential that it provides input regarding its requirements and feedback regarding the ability of suppliers to meet the requirements of those with contracting authority.

Agreements

Once a supplier of equipment, materials, or services has been qualified, agreements are established between the transfusion service or blood bank and the supplier to define the expectations and reflect that both parties have accepted the terms. Agreements can be as formal as legal contracts or as informal as oral commitments.

In any case the agreement must be reviewed periodically and any changes incorporated as needed.

Receipt, Inspection, and Testing of Materials

Upon delivery and before use, materials must be inspected to ensure that they are acceptable and will function as expected. Depending upon the material, the inspection may involve visual examination, testing, or receipt of documentation from the supplier that the material has been tested and meets the requirements (e.g., certificate of analysis). The method of inspection must be defined and the documentation of inspection should be maintained.

PROCESS CONTROL

As mentioned previously, written policies, processes, and procedures form the backbone of the quality system. Process control is the management of these processes and procedures to ensure that they are performed uniformly and, as intended, result in the provision of a consistent, predictable product or service. Elements of process control are as follows.

Validation

Once a process or procedure has been written, and before it is put into use, the following questions must be asked and answered:

- Is it understandable to those who will use it?
- Is it complete?
- Is it easy to use?
- Does it provide the expected outcome on a consistent basis?

Answering these questions is the purpose of validation. Before a new process or procedure is implemented, a validation plan is developed and carried out. Elements of a validation plan may include:

- Purpose of the validation
- Scope of the plan
- Definition of the responsibilities of the individuals involved
- Type and extent of activities
- Method of validation
- Needed resources
- Expected outcomes
- Review and approval

Once the validation has been conducted and documented, the results are reviewed. If the expected outcomes were not achieved, changes are made to the process or procedure and then revalidated. Upon successful validation, the process or procedure can be approved, the staff can be trained and evaluated for competency, and then the process or procedure can be implemented.

Change Control

When a new process or procedure is implemented, what effect might it have on other parts of the transfusion service or blood bank, or even other departments? When changes are made to the existing processes or procedures, how does the transfusion service or blood bank know whether these changes will affect the quality of the component or service related to this process or procedure? How can the transfusion service or blood bank prevent unauthorized changes to the processes and procedures? Answering these questions is the purpose of change control.

Change does not occur in a vacuum, and often, change has unexpected consequences. To anticipate and minimize these consequences, change must be planned and controlled and a change control process must be defined and consistently used. As with new processes and procedures, changes to the existing processes and procedures must be validated; the scope of the validation plan should correspond to the significance of the proposed change. For both new and changed processes and procedures, the anticipated effect on other processes, procedures, equipment, and personnel within the transfusion service or blood bank and other departments must be defined, evaluated, and communicated to all affected parties *before* the process or procedure is implemented. A change control plan must also include how the effectiveness of any change will be evaluated, and over what time period. Unanticipated consequences of the change must be documented and addressed.

Quality Control

The purpose of quality control is to ensure that ensure that the reagents, equipment, and processes function as expected and that a product or service of consistent quality is provided. Each blood bank or transfusion service must define a quality control program based on the products and services it provides to ensure that the reagents, equipment, and methods perform as expected. Both the frequency and the type of quality control must be defined. At a minimum, quality control must meet the manufacturer's instructions.

Use of Materials

When the transfusion service or blood bank qualifies its suppliers, it specifies its requirements for equipment, supplies, and services. It is then the responsibility of the transfusion service or blood bank to use materials in accordance with the manufacturer's written instructions so that the materials will perform as expected.

Identification and Traceability

To allow for the investigation of errors, discrepancies, adverse outcomes, and other problems, the transfusion service or blood bank must define and utilize a process to identify who performed each step in a process and when it was performed. Blood components, critical materials, laboratory samples, and patient and donor records must be identified and traceable. All blood products must be labeled according to the requirements, and blood products issued for transfusion must be labeled to ensure proper recipient identification.

Inspection

To ensure that a nonconforming product is detected as early in the process as possible and before administration to the recipient, the transfusion service or blood bank must define the stages in the process at which inspection and testing of the product will occur and have a process to ensure that the final component is acceptable before being issued for transfusion. In addition, the transfusion service or blood bank must have a means to ensure that if a nonconforming component is identified, it is removed in a controlled manner from the process so that it is not inadvertently administered.

Handling, Storage, and Administration

Having used validated procedures performed by trained and competent individuals with qualified, calibrated equipment and acceptable supplies to produce a component of high quality, the transfusion service or blood bank must now have a process in place to ensure that this component is handled, stored, and administered in a manner that will prevent damage and limit deterioration, providing maximum benefit for the intended recipient. Standards defining appropriate storage and expiration for both red cell and non–red cell components have been established.[1]

DOCUMENTS AND RECORDS

As mentioned previously, quality system documents include policies, processes, and procedures. To capture the outcome of a process or procedure, the transfusion service or blood bank designs forms. A form, once completed, becomes a record (see Fig. 1.1).[3] All documents including policies, processes, procedures, forms, and labels must be identified, and they must be approved before their use and again after modification. They must also be controlled, that is, the transfusion service or blood bank must have a process to ensure that only current documents are available, and that obsolete versions cannot be used. Elements of document control are the following.

Master List of Documents

The master list is "document control at-a-glance." It contains a listing of all policies, processes, procedures, forms, and labels. The following information may be incorporated into the master list:

- Title of the document
- Current version number
- Date of implementation
- Locations of all copies
- Date of retirement of the document

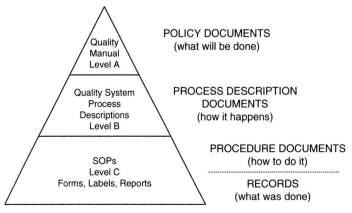

FIG. 1.1 Quality system document hierarchy. *SOP*, standard operating procedure.

The master list should be a living document: as a new process is written and implemented, it should be added to the list, and the former version noted as archived.

Standardized Formats for Documents

For ease of development as well as for ease of use, policies, processes, and procedures should be written in standard formats. The transfusion service or blood bank must define and utilize its standard format (often called the "SOP for SOPs"). The standard format should include a means to uniquely identify each document (e.g., document control number or version number) and a means to capture the dates the document was created, approved, implemented, and reviewed, as well as to review signatures.

Review and Approval of New and Revised Documents Before Use

Before a document is placed in use, it must be reviewed and approved. Validation, change control, and training must also occur as appropriate.

Biannual Review

An authorized individual must review all the policies, processes, and procedures at least every 2 years to ensure that these documents remain relevant to the transfusion service or blood bank. Documentation of review must be maintained.

Use of Only Current and Valid Documents

Policies, processes, and procedures are of little use if they are not current and if the individuals using them do not have easy access to them. The transfusion service or blood bank should have a process for the distribution of new or changed documents. In addition, staff should be trained not to add additional information to the copies of the documents they use, as this information has not been authorized and is not controlled.

Identification and Archival of Obsolete Documents

When a new version of a document is to be implemented, there must be a process to locate and retrieve all copies of the former version. Documents must be archived in accordance with all applicable standards and federal, state, or local laws.

The documentation that an activity has been performed is a record. Records prove that a product or service conforms to specified requirements and that each step of the process is performed. Policies, processes, and procedures must be in place for the management of records, including how the records will be:

- Identified (i.e., what records will be maintained)
- Collected
- Indexed for easy retrieval
- Accessed in a timely manner by only authorized personnel
- Filed
- Stored to ensure confidentiality and protection from damage
- Retained according to record retention policies
- Disposed of when appropriate to do so

In addition, the record system must make it possible to trace a component from the source to final disposition, to review the records related to that component, and to investigate any adverse events that a patient receiving the component may have experienced.

DEVIATIONS, NONCONFORMANCES, AND ADVERSE EVENTS

In spite of the best efforts, events will occur that deviate from requirements. A process must be defined as one that can capture adverse events. Staff should be encouraged to report events, assured that they will not be punished if they do so. In this way, problems can be identified and used as opportunities for improvement. Once an event is identified, processes must be in place to:

- Assess any components or critical materials involved in establishing whether they are in conformance with defined acceptance criteria
- Determine disposition of the component or critical material
- Prevent any nonconforming component or critical material from unintentional distribution or use
- Quarantine, retrieve, and recall nonconforming components or critical materials
- Report any nonconforming component or critical material that was released to the patient's physician, customer, and/or supplier as applicable
- Investigate the cause of the adverse event
- Institute corrective action as appropriate
- Monitor adverse events to identify trends

The transfusion service must have a process to evaluate any complications arising from blood product administration. The fact that such complications occur rarely only emphasizes the need for an established process so that when the administration is interrupted, the evaluation can be performed effectively so that proper clinical management of the patient is not delayed. Of particular concern is the occurrence of a suspected hemolytic reaction. The process for managing such an event must include:

- Discontinuation of administration
- Comparison of the blood container label and other records to the patient identification at the patient's bedside
- Notification of the patient's physician and the transfusion service
- Transport of the implicated unit and tubing and posttransfusion specimens to the transfusion service
- Clerical check in the transfusion service
- Evaluation of posttransfusion specimens for hemolysis
- Laboratory testing (ABO, Rh, direct antiglobulin test)
- Evaluation of results and further testing that may be required
- Documentation and reporting of the event and the investigation

ASSESSMENTS

To ensure that both operations and the quality system are operating effectively, the transfusion service or blood bank must have processes to assess both of these elements on a routine basis. External inspections by accrediting organizations do not excuse the need to develop processes to perform internal operational and quality assessments. Those responsible for performing internal assessments should be knowledgeable of quality principles, trained in auditing principles and communication, and should not assess areas for which they have direct responsibility. A schedule for assessments must be defined, and appropriate tools and forms must be developed.

Upon completion of an internal assessment, the results should be communicated to those responsible for the area under assessment. If problems were identified, investigation and corrective action must be instituted. For assessments to be of use, results of assessments and any resulting actions must be reviewed by the executive management.

A peer review program must be developed to monitor and address transfusion practices. Policies and expected utilization should be defined and overseen by a committee responsible for reviewing blood utilization for the organization. Examples of review may include:

- Ordering practices and appropriateness of use
- Significant adverse events, deviations, and near miss events
- Ability of services to meet patient needs
- Usage and discard

PROCESS IMPROVEMENT

The transfusion service or blood bank must have processes in place to implement corrective and preventive actions to prevent nonconformances from recurring and to collect and analyze quality indicator data. Opportunities for process improvement may arise as a result of planned and unplanned deviations, nonconformances, adverse events, internal and external assessments, and customer complaints.

Corrective action is taken in response to problems that have been identified. Processes and procedures for corrective action include:

- Documentation of the problem
- Investigation of the cause of the problem
- Determination of the action to be taken to correct the problem
- Identification of the individual(s) responsible for implementation
- Establishment of a time frame for implementation
- Evaluation of the effectiveness of the action
- Reevaluation if the action was not effective

It is important that the extent of investigation and corrective action be in proportion to the importance of the problem so that the resources are used effectively. It is equally important that efforts are made to identify the root cause of the problem, and that the investigation does not stop at the first, obvious answer, which may simply be a symptom of an underlying cause. Although it is easy to lay the cause at the feet of the individuals involved in a problem, the majority of problems are a result of process and system issues, and unless these issues are investigated and addressed, the problem will tend to resurface.

Preventive action is active anticipation of potential problems. It involves monitoring data and identifying trends that may signal a problem is about to occur. For example, quality control data may be monitored over time. Although data are within acceptable limits, it may be noted that a downward trend has developed, which, if left unaddressed, will eventually lead to a nonconforming product. Viewing the data for trends allows for investigation and resolution even before a problem has occurred. Once a potential problem has been identified, follow-up uses the same processes and procedures described earlier for corrective action.

The documentation of corrective and preventive actions should be reviewed by executive management in a timely manner. In addition, executive management should actively participate in process improvement by defining quality objectives on an ongoing basis. Quality indicator data must be defined, collected, and evaluated on a scheduled basis, and the results communicated to all affected parties.

SAFETY

It is the responsibility of the transfusion service or blood bank to provide a safe environment and to develop policies, processes, and procedures that minimize risks to the health and safety of employees, donors, volunteers, patients, and third-party providers. Suitable quarters, environment, and equipment must be available to maintain safe operations. All applicable local, state, and federal regulations must be followed. In addition, there must be monitoring of adherence to biological, chemical, and radiation safety standards and regulations where applicable. Processes for handling and discarding blood components must be defined and implemented to prevent human exposure to infectious agents, and documentation of disposal must be maintained.

CONCLUSION

The provision of the right component to the right patient, at the right dose, and at the right time is the ultimate goal of any transfusion service or blood bank. The proper design and implementation of a quality system provides the support and framework needed by personnel to perform their functions effectively on a day-to-day basis. Trained and competent staff who follow validated, current procedures with qualified equipment and supplies and who know how to recognize and resolve problems and improve processes are able to provide quality components to patients who need them. A quality system is not only in the best interest of the transfusion service or blood bank but also in the best interest of the patient.

REFERENCES

1. Ooley PW, ed. *Standards for Blood Banks and Transfusion Service*. 30th ed. Bethesda, MD: AABB; 2015.
2. Code of federal regulations. *Title 42 CFR Part 493.1451(b) (8)*. Washington, CD: US Government Printing office; 2005.
3. Nevalainen DE, Berte LM, Callery MF. *Quality Systems in the Blood Bank Environment*. Bethesda, MD: AABB; 1998.

CHAPTER 2

Regulatory Oversight and Accreditation

JUDITH A. SULLIVAN, MS, MT(ASCP)SBB, CQA(ASQ)

Although the first blood bank was established in the United States in 1937 at the Cook County Hospital in Chicago, Illinois,[1] federal regulatory oversight of blood banks did not begin until the 1970s. Today, transfusion services and blood banks are regulated by a number of federal agencies as well as state agencies. Failure to comply with regulations can not only carry severe penalties but also endanger patient safety.

FOOD AND DRUG ADMINISTRATION

The Food and Drug Administration (FDA) considers blood to be both a biologic and a drug. As a result, blood donor centers, blood banks (hospital-based services that collect blood and/or manufacture blood components and transfuse them), and transfusion services must comply with all the FDA regulations that address both biologics (21 CFR 600) and drugs (21 CFR 200).[2] In particular, blood banks are required to follow Current Good Manufacturing Practices (cGMPs), a set of requirements that, when followed by manufacturers of blood and blood components, help ensure that products manufactured will have the required quality (Box 2.1). Although transfusion services do not collect blood or manufacture blood components, they are required to follow cGMPs, because the FDA lists compatibility testing under its umbrella of "manufacturing."

In addition to regulations, the FDA periodically publishes guidance, which reflects the current thinking of the agency on a particular topic. Many of these start in draft form to allow comments from interested individuals and then are issued as final guidance. Although each guidance states that an "alternative approach" may be used, blood banks, in general, follow guidance as written.

The FDA inspections of blood establishments began in the 1970s. In 1976, the Federal Food, Drug, and Cosmetic Act was amended to strengthen the FDA's authority to regulate medical devices. It also required blood banks to register their establishments with the FDA and to list the components that they prepared. The FDA was charged with inspection of all transfusion services, blood banks, and blood centers in the United States.

To carry out this mandate, the FDA field offices staffed with investigators became involved in the inspection process. Today, the FDA routinely inspects blood banks and blood centers every 2 years. Inspections of transfusion services became the responsibility of the Centers for Medicare and Medicaid Services (CMS) in 1980 as a result of a Memorandum of Understanding with the FDA. However, the FDA still retains the right to inspect transfusion services in the event of egregious noncompliance or if a transfusion-related fatality occurs.

CENTERS FOR MEDICARE AND MEDICAID SERVICES

When the Congress passed the Clinical Laboratory Improvement Amendments (CLIA) in 1988, it charged the CMS with enforcement of regulations. The CLIA regulations can be found in 42 CFR 493.[3] They apply to all laboratory testing (except research) performed on humans and currently cover about 254,000 laboratory entities. All testing performed on blood donors and patients requiring transfusion is regulated under the CLIA.

Some of the highlights of the CLIA regulations include:

Personnel requirements: The CLIA specifies the levels of education and experience required for individuals holding positions of laboratory director, technical supervisor, clinical consultant, general supervisor, and testing personnel. It also specifies responsibilities for each of these positions. During an inspection, it is expected that documentation can be provided to show that each individual filling these positions has the necessary qualifications and has indeed fulfilled his or her mandated responsibilities. Of particular note is the technical supervisor position. In specialties such as microbiology, hematology, immunology, and chemistry, the minimum educational requirement for the technical specialist is a bachelor's degree in a chemical, physical, or biological science. However, for the specialty of immunohematology, the technical supervisor must be a doctor of medicine or a doctor of osteopathy.

Proficiency testing (PT): Laboratories must enroll in an approved PT program for each regulated analyte they test. For blood banks, this includes ABO/Rh, antibody screen, antibody identification, and cross-match. Three times a year, five specimens are received from the PT provider. They must be tested, and the results should be reported back to the provider. Testing must be rotated among all testing personnel, and if unsatisfactory results are obtained, there must be evidence of training and remedial action. If a laboratory demonstrates continued unsuccessful performance, the CMS may impose sanctions that include monetary penalties or suspension, limitation, or revocation of the facility's CLIA certificate.

Competency assessment: The CLIA requires that all testing personnel have competence to perform testing independently, assessed after training, twice in the first year they perform testing, and annually thereafter. Methods used to perform competency assessment are clearly specified in the regulations (Box 2.2). If an individual is deemed not to be competent, he or she must be removed from testing, retrained, and his or her competency reassessed. Individuals in other CLIA roles (technical supervisor, clinical consultant, general supervisor) must also be assessed for competency in their mandated responsibilities. All documentation must be maintained.

Quality system: The CLIA regulations include specific requirements for preanalytic systems (test requests and specimen handling), analytic systems (procedure manual, equipment and supplies, quality control, specimen testing), and postanalytic systems (results reporting).

The CLIA requires that laboratories be inspected every 2 years. However the, CMS does not have a sufficient number of surveyors to perform all inspections. As a result, the CMS uses accreditation organizations (AOs) to perform its inspections (Box 2.3). These organizations must demonstrate to the CMS that their standards or requirements are at least as stringent as the CLIA regulations to receive "deemed" status. The laboratory inspection by one of these organizations takes the place of the federally mandated CLIA inspection. The organizations' deemed status must be renewed no less frequently than every 6 years. The CMS uses validation surveys to ensure the quality of the AO's inspection. Either concurrent with or shortly after the AO inspection, a CMS surveyor inspects the laboratory. The findings are compared with the AO's findings. Major discrepancies in the two sets of findings are considered during the process of renewing the AO's deemed status. The CMS may also send its surveyors to a laboratory for an inspection at any time if a complaint is received against that laboratory.

Two states, Washington and New York, have state licensure programs that have received exemption from

CLIA program requirements. Thus an inspection by one of these two states takes the place of a CLIA-mandated inspection.

ACCREDITATION

As mentioned earlier, the CMS recognizes a number of accrediting organizations whose standards or requirements meet or exceed the CLIA regulations. Accreditation is a voluntary process that blood banks use to ensure that their processes operate at the highest level of quality to ensure safety for their donors and patients. The accrediting agencies most familiar to blood banks are the AABB (formerly the American Association of Blood Banks) and the College of American Pathologists (CAP).

AMERICAN ASSOCIATION OF BLOOD BANKS

Established in 1947, the AABB began its accreditation program in 1957 and accredits almost all the blood donor centers in the United States and many transfusion services and blood banks. Its first *Standards for Blood Banks and Transfusion Services* (at that time named *Standards for a Blood Transfusion Service*) was published in 1958 and is now in its 30th edition.[4]

AABB Standards are based on a quality systems approach similar to the International Organization for Standardization and are divided into 10 quality system essentials (Box 2.4). Its accreditation program utilizes both paid and volunteer individuals to assess a blood bank's compliance to these standards. Blood banks are assigned a yearly quarter (for example, the first quarter of every odd numbered year) as an assessment window, and the assessments are unannounced.

The AABB assessors receive both initial and ongoing training to ensure competence. During an assessment, they use interviews, direct observation of procedures, and record reviews to verify compliance. A single discrepancy (for example, one quality control record was not reviewed) may not be the cause for a nonconformance. However, a pattern of discrepancies signals a system problem that must be addressed.

At the end of the assessment, a summary report detailing any nonconformances is presented to the blood bank. The blood bank is expected to perform a root cause analysis and present a corrective action plan that includes the immediate action taken, any corrective action that will be taken, and process control checks for monitoring effectiveness. When that corrective action plan is approved by the AABB, a certificate

---

> **BOX 2.4**
> **AABB Quality System Essentials**
>
> 1. Organization
> 2. Resources
> 3. Equipment
> 4. Supplier and customer issues
> 5. Process control
> 6. Documents and records
> 7. Deviations, nonconformances, and adverse events
> 8. Assessments: internal and external
> 9. Process improvement through corrective and preventive action
> 10. Facilities and safety

Data from Ooley PW, ed. *Standards for Blood Banks and Transfusion Services.* 30th ed. Bethesda: AABB; 2016; with permission.

---

of accreditation is issued to the blood bank. At the next assessment, the implementation of the corrective action plan is verified. However, if the nonconformance is deemed to threaten patient safety, evidence of implementation is required before the certificate of accreditation is issued.

The AABB may choose to withhold accreditation and require a reassessment if serious quality system issues are identified, or if the corrective action plan submitted for the prior assessment has not been completed.

COLLEGE OF AMERICAN PATHOLOGISTS

Established in 1946, the CAP began its accreditation program in 1964. The CAP accredits a wide variety of laboratory disciplines, including transfusion medicine. Facilities are assigned a 3-month inspection window based on their anniversary date, and the inspections are unannounced.

The CAP utilizes a peer review approach to inspections. One CAP-accredited laboratory is assigned to perform the inspection of another CAP laboratory. The team is composed of a pathologist and laboratorians. The requirements are listed as detailed checklists, one for each area of the laboratory, a checklist with common requirements across disciplines (for example, PT), and leadership and general laboratory checklists. Compliance is measured against each checklist item.[5]

At the end of the inspection, a report listing deficiencies is presented to the laboratory. The team may also list recommendations. The laboratory is expected to submit a plan of corrective action for the deficiencies, but it is not required to respond to recommendations. The action plan must include evidence that the deficiency has been corrected. Upon approval of the corrective action plan, the CAP issues a certificate of accreditation.

The AABB and CAP have developed an agreement so that hospital-based blood banks and transfusion services that are accredited by both organizations do not have to manage inspections by both organizations. Upon request by the blood bank for an AABB-CAP coordinated assessment, the team assigned by the AABB uses both the AABB Standards and the CAP checklists to perform a single assessment. The findings of the assessment are reported based on both sets of requirements, and the blood bank submits a plan of corrective action to both the AABB and CAP. This assessment not only limits the number of inspections a blood bank must face but also serves as a CLIA inspection.

REFERENCES

1. *Highlights of Transfusion Medicine History*. AABB.org. http://www.aabb.org/tm/Pages/highlights.aspx.
2. Code of federal regulations. *Title 21, CFR Parts 210, 211, 606, 610, 630, and 640*. Washington, DC: US Government Printing Office; 2014 (Revised annually).
3. Code of federal regulations. *Title 42, CFR Part 493*. Washington, DC: US Government Printing Office; 2014 (Revised annually).
4. Ooley PW, ed. *Standards for Blood Banks and Transfusion Services*. 30th ed. Bethesda, MD: AABB; 2015.
5. College of American Pathologists. *Laboratory Accreditation Program Checklists*. Chicago: CAP; 2017.

CHAPTER 3

ABO and Rh Blood Groups

JACQUELYN D. CHOATE, MD

ABO HISTORY

The ABO blood group was discovered by Dr. Karl Landsteiner in 1901. He was awarded the 1930 Nobel Prize for Physiology and Medicine for his landmark work in the discovery of what is still one of the most important antigen systems. In experimentation with blood from himself and his staff, he noted different patterns of agglutination between plasma and red cells. He identified these as types, which he designated as "A," "B," and "C" (later to be known as "O"). In 1902, his colleagues discovered the fourth main type as "AB." His observations led to what has become known as the "Landsteiner law": for whichever ABO antigens that are lacking on the red blood cell (RBC) surface, the corresponding antibody will be present in the serum. Therefore type A individuals have anti-B in their serum, type B individuals have anti-A, and type O individuals have anti-A and anti-B (Table 3.1). The rare Bombay phenotype individuals who lack the H-antigen have anti-A, anti-B, and anti-H. An anti-A,B antibody has also been identified, present only in group O individuals, which recognizes an epitope presumed to be common to the A and B antigens, which has yet to be identified.[1] These ABO antibodies are "naturally" occurring, or "expected," in contrast to antibodies to other blood group antigens, which are unexpected and usually stimulated by exposure through transfusion or pregnancy. They are stimulated in all immunocompetent individuals by environmental antigens, particularly bacteria. The normal intestinal flora carry polysaccharides similar to the A and B antigens, providing the stimulus for the formation of anti-A and anti-B.[2] ABO antibodies are usually high titer and predominantly IgM with some IgG and IgA. They are capable of binding complement and causing intravascular hemolysis, thus starting off the dangerous cascade of an acute hemolytic transfusion reaction (HTR), which could lead to shock, renal failure, disseminated intravascular coagulation, and even death. IgM is not capable of crossing the placenta, but the smaller amounts of IgG and IgA that are present can, and are capable of causing hemolytic disease of the fetus and newborn (HDFN), which is usually mild. This is most common in group O mothers with non–group O infants. The anti-A, anti-B,

and anti-A,B present in group O individuals can have significant amounts of IgG; however, the HDFN is still typically mild because the ABO antigens, although present, are not fully developed on the RBCs. Also, the ABO tissue antigens provide additional targets for absorbing these antibodies.

The ABO genes are inherited in a codominant manner, with one allele inherited from each parent and both being expressed. The resulting prevalence of ABO blood groups differs in various populations (Table 3.2). This becomes important in transfusion requirements and for procuring blood, as well as in solid organ transplant.

ABO ANTIGENS AND GENETICS

The ABO antigens are carbohydrate structures carried on large oligosaccharide molecules, which are attached to glycoproteins and glycolipids in the RBC membrane. The RBC membranes have over 2 million ABO antigens. The antigens are synthesized by glycosyltransferase enzymes, which sequentially add the terminal monosaccharide sugars to the backbone carbohydrate chain, which is termed the H antigen. The A glycosyltransferase adds N-acetylgalactosamine in α-1,3 linkage to the H antigen, and the B glycosyltransferase adds galactose in α-1,3 linkage to the H antigen. Group O individuals lack the A and B glycosyltransferases and therefore only have H antigen present on the surface of the RBCs (Fig. 3.1). Rare individuals also lack the H antigen and are designated as the "Bombay" phenotype (group O_h). They make potent anti-H in addition to anti-A and anti-B and must be transfused blood only from other individuals with the Bombay phenotype.

ABO antigens are also expressed in other tissues including endothelial and epithelial cells of the lung, digestive system, and urinary and reproductive tracts. Hence these antigens are very important in solid organ transplant, with an ABO match considered to be more important than a human leukocyte antigen match. ABO antibodies in the recipient are capable of binding antigens in the transplanted organ, causing complement activation and acute rejection. However, ABO barriers

TABLE 3.1
ABO Blood Group Reactions

| REACTION WITH RBCs TESTED WITH | | REACTION WITH PLASMA TESTED WITH | | INTERPRETATION |
Anti-A	Anti-B	A_1 Cells	B Cells	ABO Group
0	0	+	+	O
+	0	0	+	A
0	+	+	0	B
+	+	0	0	AB

RBC, red blood cell.

TABLE 3.2
ABO Blood Groups and Incidence

ABO Group	White	African American	Asian
O	45	49	43
A	40	27	27
B	11	20	25
AB	4	4	5

Adapted from Westhoff CM, Shaz BH. ABO and H blood group system. In: Shaz BH, Hillyer CD, Abrams CS, Roshal M, eds. *Transfusion Medicine and Hemostasis: Clinical and Laboratory Aspects*. 2nd ed. San Diego: Elsevier; 2013; with permission.

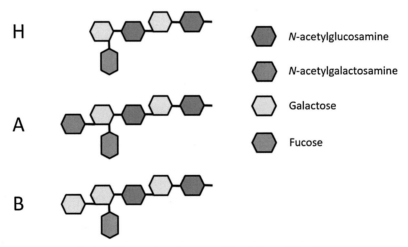

FIG. 3.1 Biochemical structure of the A, B, and H antigens.

are being crossed with immunosuppression and conditioning regimens and have even been carried out in emergent situations such as fulminant hepatic failure.[3]

ABO antigens are also found in secretions (saliva) and fluids (milk and urine) in individuals who carry the *Se(FUT2)* gene, about 80% of the population. This gene encodes a fucosyltransferase enzyme similar to the *H(FUT1)* gene product and allows formation of the H antigen on type 1 glycoproteins (vs. type 2 glycoproteins), which are present in secretions produced by epithelial cells. Subsequently, individuals who have the appropriate genes for the A and B glycosyltransferases can secrete ABO antigens and are called secretors.

The gene for the ABO antigens was cloned in 1990,[4] and it actually encodes the enzymes responsible for the addition of the carbohydrate subunits. The ABO locus has been mapped to chromosome 9q34 and encodes the A and B glycosyltransferases.[5] The gene contains seven exons and is over 18 kb.[6] It encodes a 354-amino acid transferase enzyme, differing by only four amino acids between the A and B transferases. Mutations in the gene may result in loss of glycosyltransferase activity, thus resulting in group O RBCs. The most common group O phenotype (O_1) is due to single nucleotide deletion (guanine-258) that results in a truncated product with no enzyme activity. A variety of other mutations of these transferase genes result in reduced expression of the antigens, or in variability of the antigen structure. This leads to the subgroups of A and B that are observed to react weakly, or not at all, with the standard anti-A or anti-B sera. There are more than 100 known alleles of the ABO gene consisting of not only mutations but also insertions, deletions, and gene rearrangements, and there is more information about them at the NCBI Blood Group Antigen Gene Mutation Database website (https://www.ncbi.nlm.nih.gov/projects/gv/mhc/xslcgi.cgi?cmd=bgmut/summary).

Subgroup A or B individuals have weaker expression of these antigens. These subgroups may be inherited or acquired. When inherited, they are due to variability in the ABO genes, which may result in quantitative or qualitative changes.[7] A1 is the most common A gene variant, accounting for approximately 80% of A individuals. A2 is the most common subgroup of A, with A1 and A2 together accounting for about 99% of group A individuals. The difference between A1 and A2 is both quantitative and qualitative. The number of A antigens is reduced on A2 compared with A1 RBCs. Also, the A2 antigen is structurally different, due to the substitution of leucine at position 156 with a frameshift at the 3'-end.[8] This makes the enzyme product less efficient in converting H-antigen to A. Importantly, because of the structural differences, A subgroup individuals are capable of making anti-A1. This antibody does not usually cause hemolysis, but rare hemolytic anti-A1 has been reported. These individuals, therefore, should be transfused with group O RBCs or with compatible A subgroup RBCs. The *Dolichos biflorus* lectin can be used to distinguish A1 from A2 and other A subgroups, as it will cause agglutination of A1 and A1B, but not A2 or A2B RBCs. B subgroups also exist but are very rare, and they result in weakened expression of the B antigen.

ABO TESTING

The type of the infamous type and screen blood bank test consists of the ABO and Rh determination of the patient. Since ABO antibodies are naturally occurring, it is possible to do both a forward typing (or front type or cell grouping) and a reverse typing (or back type or plasma grouping). Rh and other alloantibodies would not be expected to be present in most patients, unless they have been previously transfused or they are pregnant. This is why only anti-D is used to detect the D antigen and other alloantibodies are detected with the antibody screen. The forward typing is performed by setting up serologic reactions, mixing the patient's RBCs with anti-A and anti-B; the reverse typing is performed by mixing the patient's plasma with A1 and B RBCs. These reactions may be performed using tube, gel, and solid phases. The serologic reactions are incubated, centrifuged, and interpreted based on the degree of agglutination. The reaction is graded from 0 (no reaction) to 4+ (strongest agglutination with one solid clump). Because ABO antibodies are predominantly IgM, they can be detected at immediate spin phase. These antisera and reagent RBCs are commercially available and are licensed by the Food and Drug Administration. The antibodies are usually monoclonal reagents, having been produced as polyclonal reagents from human sera in the past. The reaction pattern must be interpreted and should be congruent (see Table 3.1); if not there is a typing discrepancy that must be resolved before transfusion takes place. Group O RBCs can be provided in the meantime.

ABO DISCREPANCIES

Typing discrepancies can occur for several reasons, both inherited and acquired, as well as due to technical error, which may need to be excluded (Table 3.3). The first steps in resolving a discrepancy include repeating the test with washed patient and reagent cells and obtaining a patient history, for example, previous transfusion or stem cell transplant. Discrepancies can occur secondary to the vast allelic diversity of the ABO locus resulting in altered antigens, which cause unexpected reactions with standard reagents, for example, A2 or A2B subgroup individuals with an anti-A1 antibody. Acquired B phenotype is observed as a false-positive discrepancy with the forward type, showing reactions of both anti-A and anti-B reagents with the patient's red cells, usually with the anti-B reaction being weaker. However, the back typing shows the normal expected reactions between the patient serum and A1 and B reagent red cells (0 and +, respectively). Acquired B phenotype can arise only in A patients, usually A1, who are bacteremic. This bacteremia is usually the result of intestinal obstruction, gram-negative infections of the gut, or colorectal or gastric malignancy. It is useful to research the patient record to correlate this clinical history when acquired B phenotype is suspected; however, this phenotype may be the first indication that one of these serious issues has developed. The microbial deacetylating enzyme can remove an acetyl group from the N-acetyl-galactosamine at the terminus of the A antigen resulting in galactosamine, and thus causing it to resemble the sugar galactose at the terminus of the B antigen. This modification into a B-like antigen is at the expense of the A antigen, which becomes decreased on the RBC membrane. However, this effect is transient, with modification occurring only during the presence of the bacterial enzyme. Newly synthesized RBCs after the period of bacteremia will have normal A antigen expression. Anti-B reagents can cross-react with the resulting modified antigen; usually they are weak, but they may also be strong. This is often seen with the monoclonal anti-B reagent ES-4. However, the patient's own anti-B does not behave in this same way and does not recognize the modified antigen as a true B antigen, explaining why massive hemolysis is not seen in this situation. This information can be used to help resolve the discrepancy by incubating the patient's own RBCs with their serum. There will be no agglutination because the patient's anti-B does not react with the acquired B antigen. It can also be helpful to try a different anti-B reagent that does not recognize the acquired B antigen, which is usually specified in the package insert. Also, treatment with acetic anhydride or acidification of the reaction mixture can eliminate the anti-B reactivity and confirm the

suspicion of an acquired B phenotype. Other false-positive forward typing discrepancies can result from heavy protein coating of the RBCs, coating of the RBCs with Wharton jelly, or antibodies to the dyes coloring anti-A or anti-B reagents. False-negative forward type reactions, in addition to being inherited as weak subgroups of A or B (discussed previously) can also be acquired. A common scenario is due to weakened A or B antigen expression in hematologic disease, including acute leukemia or other conditions such as stress hematopoiesis. Chromosomal deletions of the ABO locus can result in loss of the transferase enzymes and therefore antigen expression.[9] Other scenarios include when A, B, or AB patients have been transfused massive amounts of type O blood; the presence of inhibitor substances that neutralize the anti-A or anti-B reagents; or when patients have received ABO nonidentical stem cell transplants. Detection of weakly expressed RBC antigens may be enhanced by a variety of methods such as 30-min incubation at room temperature with washed RBCs, treatment with proteolytic enzymes, or testing the saliva (if the patient is a secretor) for the presence of ABO substances. False-positive reverse typing reactions are due to the presence of unexpected antibodies, such as anti-A1 in A2 individuals (discussed previously). Cold agglutinins are another common cause of false-positive reverse type reactions. This can be resolved by allowing the reagents to come to room temperature, incubating the RBCs at 37°, and washing them with warm saline. Dithiothreitol can also be used to remove IgM antibodies. False-negative reverse typing reactions result from the absence of expected antibodies due to a variety of conditions affecting antibody production. Infants do not produce their own ABO antibodies until about 3–6 months of age. Therefore forward typing only is performed on cord blood specimens, as ABO antigens are fully developed at birth. Immunodeficient patients may not be able to produce significant levels of anti-A and anti-B. Expression of ABO antibodies can be weak in the elderly. Large amounts of intravenous (IV) fluid can dilute antibodies, if administered during treatment or resuscitation or if present in the sample because of drawing blood above an IV.

GENETIC ABO TESTING

The ABO group was the first blood group to be molecularly defined[9]; however, ABO genotyping is not currently widely used clinically. ABO serologic testing is an established, reliable, and inexpensive way to determine blood type. It can be performed in less than 10 minutes to quickly provide type-specific

TABLE 3.3
ABO Typing Discrepancies

Technical Error	Acquired B Phenotype
A2 subgroup with anti-A1	Protein- or IgG-coated RBCs
B(A) phenotype	Wharton jelly–coated RBCs
Weakened antigen expression	Antibodies to reagent dyes
Weakened antibody production	Cold agglutinins
Massive transfusion of type O blood	ABO-incompatible stem cell transplant

RBC, red blood cells.

blood in emergency situations. Molecular methods must be capable of detecting the multiple ABO alleles, and gene expression and epigenetic mechanisms must be considered.[10] However, ABO genotyping can be useful in resolving typing discrepancies in patient settings. It can also be used to properly label a donor unit, as well as to distinguish acquired weakened agglutination from weak reactions due to subgroup alleles.

Rh BLOOD GROUP HISTORY

The Rh system, which includes the D, C, c, E, and e antigens, differs from the ABO system in several ways, and is second only to the ABO system in importance in transfusion medicine. The Rh antigens are highly immunogenic, especially the D antigen. These antigens are membrane-spanning proteins, in contrast to polysaccharide moieties. The antibodies to these antigens are not naturally occurring like the ABO antibodies; however, when stimulated they are capable of causing severe acute HTRs and HDFN, which can be fatal. Hemolytic disease of the newborn was first described in 1609 in a set of stillborn twins with jaundice and hydrops.[11] Levine and Stetson in 1939,[12] discovered in a postpartum woman who had just delivered a stillborn fetus what they termed unexpected intragroup agglutination. She required postpartum blood transfusion, and as a group O patient, she was transfused whole blood from her group O husband. She had a severe HTR, and it was discovered that her serum agglutinated her husband's red cells, as well as that of the majority of type O donors. She was able to be further transfused with "carefully selected" compatible RBCs. Levine and colleagues later correctly concluded that the patient had been immunized by the fetus who carried an antigen inherited from its father. However, they did not name this antigen. At the same time, Landsteiner and Wiener were performing research on blood group antigens by injecting rhesus monkey RBCs into rabbits and guinea pigs. The resulting antiserum agglutinated not only rhesus monkey cells but also 85% of a group of white research subjects from New York, dubbed "Rh positive," the remaining 15% were called "Rh negative"[2]; thus the antigen was named. These antibodies appeared to have the same specificity as what was named the "Rhesus factor"; however, much later it was discovered that the rabbit antiserum was reacting to a different antigen, named LW for Landsteiner and Wiener. The initially discovered human specificity was what we now know as anti-D. Additional important antigens of the system (C, c, and E) were named by Fisher in 1941, and e was identified in 1945.[13]

ANTIGENS AND NOMENCLATURE

The Rh blood group is complex because of the number of antigens that have been reported, but the most important of the group are D, C, c, E, and e. These main antigens of the group, and their variants, are carried on the RhD protein, encoded by the *RHD* gene, and the RhCE protein, encoded by the *RHCE* gene. This, however, was not known at the time that the two commonly used nomenclature systems were proposed. The Fisher-Race nomenclature was based on the belief that there were three closely linked genes (D, C/c, and E/e). The Wiener nomenclature was based on the belief that there was only one "agglutinogen" that carried several blood group factors. Neither theory was correct; the presence of two genes was not proposed until 1986 by Tippet.[14] In the meantime, both the naming systems had been adopted. In the Fisher-Race designation "D" indicates the presence of the RhD antigen and "d" indicates, when used, the lack of the D antigen. Since there is no actual "d" antigen, this is often dropped to avoid confusion. The RhCE protein may carry different combinations of the four antigens C, c, E, or e. Therefore there are eight haplotypes based on the antigens present (Table 3.4), and the Fisher-Race designation uses three letters (DCE) changing from uppercase to lowercase according to which antigens are present on that haplotype. The Wiener nomenclature is preferred for spoken communication. In this system, "R" indicates that the D antigen is present and "r" (little "r") indicates that it is not. The C, c, E, and e antigens, when carried with D, are indicated by subscripts: R_1 for Ce, R_2 for cE, R_0 for ce, and R_Z for CE. When carried without D, they are represented by superscripts: "prime" (r') for Ce, "double prime" (r") for cE, "y" for CE (r^y), and no superscript for ce (r). The Rh genotypes and their phenotypes and frequencies are presented in Table 3.5.

TABLE 3.4 Rh Antigen Nomenclature	
WEINER AND FISHER-RACE NOMENCLATURE	
D-positive Haplotypes	**D-negative Haplotypes**
R_1: DCe	r': dCe
R_2: DcE	r": dcE
R_0: Dce	r: dce
R_Z: DCE	r^y: dCE

TABLE 3.5
Rh Genotypes and Phenotypes

| Phenotype Expressed on Cell | GENOTYPE EXPRESSED IN DNA | | Prevalence (%)[†] |
	Fisher-Race Notation	Wiener Notation	
D+ C+ E+ c+ e+ (RhD+)	Dce/DCE	R_0R_Z	0.0125
	Dce/dCE	R_0r_Y	0.0003
	DCe/DcE	R_1R_2	11.8648
	DCe/dcE	R_1r''	0.9992
	DcE/dCe	R_2r'	0.2775
	DCE/dce	R_Zr	0.1893
D+ C+ E+ c+ e− (RhD+)	DcE/DCE	R_2R_Z	0.0687
	DcE/dCE	R_2r_Y	0.0014
	DCE/dcE	R_Zr''	0.0058
D+ C+ E+ c− e+ (RhD+)	DCe/dCE	R_1r_Y	0.0042
	DCE/dCe	R_Zr'	0.0048
	DCe/DCE	R_1R_Z	0.2048
D+ C+ E+ c− e− (RhD+)	DCE/DCE	R_ZR_Z	0.0006
	DCE/dCE	R_Zr_Y	<0.0001
D+ C+ E− c+ e+ (RhD+)	Dce/dCe	R_0r'	0.0505
	DCe/dce	R_1r	32.6808
	DCe/Dce	R_1R_0	2.1586
D+ C+ E− c− e+ (RhD+)	DCe/DCe	R_1R_1	17.6803
	DCe/dCe	R_1r'	0.8270
D+ C− E+ c+ e+ (RhD+)	DcE/Dce	R_2R_0	0.7243
	Dce/dcE	R_0r''	0.0610
	DcE/dce	R_2r	10.9657
D+ C− E+ c+ e− (RhD+)	DcE/DcE	R_2R_2	1.9906
	DcE/dcE	R_2r''	0.3353
D+ C− E− c+ e+ (RhD+)	Dce/Dce	R_0R_0	0.0659
	Dce/dce	R_0r	1.9950
D− C+ E+ c+ e+ (RhD−)	dce/dCE	rr_Y	0.0039
	dCe/dcE	$r'r''$	0.0234
D− C+ E+ c+ e− (RhD−)	dcE/dCE	$r''r_Y$	0.0001
D− C+ E+ c− e+ (RhD−)	dCe/dCE	$r'r_Y$	0.0001
D− C+ E+ c− e− (RhD−)	dCE/dCE	r_Yr_Y	<0.0001
D− C+ E− c+ e+ (RhD−)	dce/dCe	rr'	0.7644
D− C+ E− c− e+ (RhD−)	dCe/dCe	$r'r'$	0.0097
D− C− E+ c+ e+ (RhD−)	dce/dcE	rr''	0.9235
D− C− E+ c+ e− (RhD−)	dcE/dcE	$r''r''$	0.0141
D− C− E− c+ e+ (RhD−)	dce/dce	rr	15.1020

Adapted from Race RR, Mourant AE, Lawler SD, et al. The Rh chromosome frequencies in England. *Blood*. 1948;3(6):689–695; with permission.

D ANTIGEN

The presence of the D antigen is designated as "Rh positive," and the absence is indicated as "Rh negative". The presence or absence of the D antigen varies according to ethnicity (Table 3.6). Most of the individuals of the 15% of European descent who are Rh negative have a complete deletion the *RHD* gene, resulting from an unequal crossover event between the Rhesus boxes upstream and downstream from the gene.[15] This deletion probably occurred on a Dce haplotype, as *ce* is the most common allele carried with the deletion. The D-negative phenotype can also occur due to mutations resulting in an inactive or silent *RHD* gene, including insertions, premature stop codons, and hybrids of the *RHD/RHCE* gene. Only 1% of Asians are D negative, and most have a mutant *RHD* gene associated with Ce. About 8% of African Americans are D negative, and although they may have the same deletion as the Caucasian population, two other mechanisms are common as well. One is inheriting a 37-bp internal duplication that introduces a premature stop codon resulting in an *RHD* pseudogene. The other is inheriting a hybrid *RHD-CE-D* gene, which contains nucleotide sequences from the *RHCE* gene and produces no D antigen and abnormal C antigen.[16] The important point is that genetic events responsible for the D-negative phenotype vary by population, and this must be considered when performing molecular methods to determine the D status.

WEAK D

Weak D (formerly D[U]) is a serologic phenotype that may be the result of several mutations, giving no or weak (≤2+) reactivity in initial testing using direct agglutination with anti-D reagents at room temperature but reacting moderately to strongly with antihuman globulin.[17] The molecular basis for the weak D phenotype is heterogeneous, consisting of over 50 possible point mutations leading to amino acid substitutions in the predicted intracellular and transmembrane portions, rather than the outer surface, of the antigen.[18] It is theorized that these mutations may affect the insertion of the protein into the membrane, resulting in decreased quantity of the antigen on the surface of the red cells, but the D epitopes are still intact. This explains the serologic reactions that are weak but still present and also explains why weak D individuals can receive D-positive RBCs without making anti-D. Most Caucasian individuals with weak D phenotypes are weak D type 1, 2, or 3, and they can be managed as D positive individuals for the purposes of transfusion and pregnancy (no RhIg required), as recommended by the Interorganizational Work Group on RHD Genotyping.[17] There are several other weak D types in which anti-D alloimmunization has been observed, and these patients are best treated as D negative. Although the weak D antigen is less immunogenic, it is still capable of alloimmunizing D-negative recipients and certain other weak mutant D antigens including partial D (see later). This is important in the labeling of donor units for transfusion, as it important that a D-negative labeled unit is truly D negative, to avoid an HTR. For this reason, donor testing must include a method sensitive enough to detect the presence of weak D, such as using the antihuman globulin phase. Still, this serologic method may not detect a very weak form of weak D_{el}, which is still capable of sensitization of the D-negative recipient,[19] and these donors will have to be removed from the D-negative donor pool when discovered.

PARTIAL D

The partial D phenotype, which has also been known as D mosaic or D variant, was first described when it was observed that some individuals who were typed

TABLE 3.6 Frequency of Rh Antigens			
	Caucasians	**Blacks**	**Asians**
D	85%	92%	99%
C	68%	27%	93%
E	29%	22%	39%
c	80%	96%	47%
e	98%	98%	96%

Data from Reid M, Lomas-Francis C, Olsson M. *The Blood Group Antigen Facts Book*. 3rd ed. New York: Elsevier Academic Press; 2012.

as Rh positive and transfused with Rh-positive blood would make anti-D. Typing of partial D with common current D typing reagents can lead to strong, variable, or weak reactions. This leads to problems on both the patient and donor sides of testing, as it is important that these individuals should be transfused with Rh-negative blood and pregnant females should receive RhIg. Unfortunately though, these individuals are usually discovered only after they have already made anti-D. It was predicted that these individuals were missing a portion of the D antigen, not enough to eliminate its detection by anti-D reagents, but enough to allow alloantibody production to the missing portion. This theory was correct, but what was not expected was that these missing portions are replaced by portions of the *RHCE* gene in most cases.[20] This is the result of a gene conversion, and leaves the donor *RHCE* gene unchanged. These exchanges may consist of single amino acid changes, short stretches of amino acids, or single or multiple exons. The mutations are predicted to be located in the extracellular protein loops, in contrast to the weak D mutations, which are expected to be cytoplasmic or transmembrane in location. This explains why these mutations are able to alter the epitope expression of the molecule and why these individuals recognize the normal D antigen as foreign. Partial D type IV is the most common form in Caucasians[21] and can be the result of replacement of two, three, or four exons of the RHD gene by the corresponding exons of the RHCE gene.[22]

C/c AND E/e ANTIGENS

The situation with the C and E antigens is unique in that although they are referred to as separate antigens, they are carried on the same protein, RhCE. The four major allelic forms encode four different possible major proteins (ce, cE, Ce, and CE). There are four amino acids responsible for the difference between C and c, Cys16Trp, He60Leu, Ser68Asn, and Ser103Pro,[23] but with only the Ser103Pro being extracellular, it is responsible for the polymorphism. Only one extracellular amino acid change is responsible for the difference between E and e, Pro226Ala. The amino acids of exon 2 of RHC are identical to those of exon 2 of RHD and are thought to have formed by the transfer of exon 2 of RHD into the *Rhce* gene.[24] This explains the presence of the G antigen on red cells that are D or C positive, or both.[25] This can cause serologic difficulties when an antibody forms to one or more of these antigens, which must be resolved for clinical management, as discussed later.

There are several altered forms of RhCE resulting from single amino acid changes (for example, C^W and C^X) or gene conversions or replacements. V and VS antigens are low-frequency antigens that are seen in up to 30% of black individuals and result from a Leu245Val substitution in the Rhce protein.[26] Variation in the e antigen is more frequently seen than E and c variants, which are rare, but do exist. An e variant, D^{HAR} (R_O^{HAR}), is found in individuals of German descent and has variable typing with anti-D reagents, typing Rh positive with monoclonal anti-D containing IgM and Rh negative with polyclonal anti-D, including weak D. These individuals do not carry *RHD*, but exon 5 of *Rhce* has been replaced by exon 5 of *RHD*.[27] Importantly, even though they are sometimes typed as Rh positive, it is important that they be treated as Rh negative for transfusion, and receive RhIg during pregnancy, because they are capable of being alloimmunized and making anti-D. Many other e variants exist and are common in individuals of African descent, who have an increased incidence of sickle cell disease. Interestingly, these patients phenotype as e positive but form alloantibodies with e-like specificity following transfusion. The alleles responsible include DHar, ceSL, R^N, ceAR, ceEK, ce^S, and ceMO.[28]

Rh$_{null}$

Individuals who are Rh$_{null}$ lack the expression of all Rh antigens. They have variable degrees of anemia, with spherocytosis and stomatocytosis and increased osmotic fragility.[29] Two different types have arisen on two different genetic backgrounds. The regulator type is more common and is caused by mutations in, or lack of, the *RHAG* gene, and resulting no expression of Rh and RhAG proteins. RhAG does not carry Rh antigens but is important in targeting the Rh proteins to the RBC membrane. The amorph type is due to mutations of the *RHCE* gene in the absence of the *RHD* gene, and they express no Rh proteins with reduced amounts of RhAG.[30]

GENES AND PROTEINS

The genes *RHD* and *RHCE* encode the RhD and RhCE proteins, are 97% identical, and are located on chromosome 1p34-p36.[31] Each has 10 exons, and they are the result of a gene duplication. The Rh proteins are 417-amino acid proteins that migrate in sodium dodecyl sulfate-polyacrylamide gel electrophoresis gels with an approximate molecular weight ratio of 30–32 kD, and therefore they are sometimes referred to as Rh30 proteins.[32] They are predicted to have 12 membrane-spanning regions and be linked to fatty acids in the lipid bilayer.[33] They differ by only 32–35 amino acids, depending on the version of RhCE that is present. The complex intron-exon structure of RHD and RHCE is discussed and illustrated in the review by Avent and Reid.[34]

The single gene *RHAG* is 47% identical to the *RH* genes, and the RhAG protein is a 409-amino acid protein that shares 37% amino acid identity with the RhD/RhCE proteins.[35] It is also a glycosylated trans-membrane-spanning protein and coprecipitates with the Rh30 proteins, although it is referred to as Rh50 to reflect its apparent molecular weight. The *RHAG* gene is located at chromosome 6p11-21.1[35]; the RhAG protein is not polymorphic and does not have Rh antigens. The RhAG protein is important in association with the Rh proteins in the membrane, thought to form a tetramer composed of 2 RhAG molecules with 2 RhCE or RhD molecules, forming a core complex.[36]

ANTIBODIES

Because of the high immunogenicity of the D antigen, up to 85% of exposed D-negative persons will make high-titer, high-affinity anti-D antibodies that will persist for the rest of their life. The lack of response of the other 15% may be due to dose, other alleles, or other yet unknown reasons. The antibodies are mostly IgG, usually subclasses IgG1 and IgG3 (although some do have an IgM component). They bind optimally at 37°C. Rh antibodies do not typically activate complement, thought to be due to low copy number of the Rh antigens on the cell surface; however, they can still cause severe transfusion reactions, with hemolysis of the incompatible RBCs being mostly extravascular. Because anti-D is IgG, it can easily cross the placenta and cause severe HDFN, with fetal anemia, hydrops, and even death. Thankfully, the incidence of HDFN has greatly diminished with the prophylactic use of Rh immune globulin. Anti-c can also cause severe HDN; however, anti-C, anti-E, and anti-e do not usually cause HDFN, and when they do, it is usually mild. The most common Rh antigen seen in transfused individuals besides anti-D is anti-E, followed by anti-c, anti-e, and anti-C. Patients with warm autoimmune hemolytic anemia may have autoantibodies that appear to have Rh specificity, often toward e; however, the true epitopes they may be binding to have yet to be determined. This complicates transfusion in these patients, especially since transfusion with antigen-negative RBCs rarely results in better red cell survival.

Anti-G (also known as "anti-CE") is an alloantibody produced to an epitope common to the RhD and RhC antigens and is therefore only formed in individuals who lack both these antigens, most commonly D-negative, G-negative patients with the genotype *rr* (dce). It presents in a D-negative patient who has never received D-positive blood, but has an antibody that looks like a combination of anti-D and anti-C. This may happen because of pregnancy, or transfusion with donor cells that are D-negative, but did carry the G antigen. Anti-G is capable of causing HDN.[37] The distinction between anti-D, anti-C, and anti-G is most important in prenatal workups, as mothers with anti-G only should receive RhIg prophylaxis to prevent anti-D formation. This distinction may be carried out by a double absorption and elution procedure.[38]

EVOLUTION

The *RH* gene duplicated resulting in *RHD* and *RHCE* in some common ancestor of gorillas, chimpanzees, and humans. Chimpanzees and some gorillas also have a third *RH* gene, indicating a third duplication event. *RH* and *RHAG* genes have also been investigated in other species, including other primates and rodents.

SUMMARY

The ABO and Rh systems remain the most important blood group systems in modern transfusion medicine. Many of the complex serologic reactions seen in the past have been solved in today's era using an array of different biochemical, genetic, and genomic techniques. These methodologies will continue to influence transfusion medicine and no doubt contribute to the evolution of the future of the field.

REFERENCES

1. Moore S, Chirnside A, Micklem L. A mouse monoclonal antibody with anti-A,(B) specificity which agglutinates Ax cells. *Vox Sang*. 1984;47(6):427–434.
2. Race RR, Sanger R. *Blood Groups in Man*. 6th ed. Oxford: Blackwell Scientific Publications; 1975.
3. Maitta RW, Choate J, Emre SH. Emergency ABO-incompatible liver transplant secondary to fulminant hepatic failure: outcome, role of TPE and review of the literature. *J Clin Apher*. 2012;27(6):320–329.
4. Yamamoto F, Marken J, Tsuji T, White T, Clausen H, Hakomori S. Cloning and characterization of DNA complementary to human UDP-GalNAc: fuc alpha 1-2Gal alpha 1-3GalNAc transferase (histo-blood group A transferase) mRNA. *J Biol Chem*. 1990;265:1146–1151.

5. Ferguson-Smith MA, Aitken DA, Turleau C, de Grouchy J. Localisation of the human ABO: Np-1: AK-1 linkage group by regional assignment of AK-1 to 9q34. *Hum Genet.* 1976;34(1):35–43.

6. Yamamoto F, McNeill PD, Hakomori S. Genomic organization of human histo-blood group ABO genes. *Glycobiology.* 1995;5(1):51–58.

7. Yamamoto FI. Review: recent progress in the molecular genetic study of the histo-blood group ABO system. *Immunohematology.* 1994;10(1):1–7.

8. Yamamoto F, McNeill PD, Hakomori S. Human histo-blood group A2 transferase coded by A2 allele, one of the A subtypes, is characterized by a single base deletion in the coding sequence, which results in an additional domain at the carboxyl terminal. *Biochem Biophys Res Commun.* 1992;187(1):366–374.

9. Yamamoto F-I, Clausen H, White T, Marken J, Hakomori S. Molecular genetic basis of the histo-blood group ABO system. *Nature.* 1990;345:229–233.

10. Flegel WA. ABO genotyping: the quest for clinical applications. *Blood Transfus.* 2013;11(1):6–9.

11. Bownan JM. RhD hemolytic disease of the newborn. *N Engl J Med.* 1998;339:1775–1777.

12. Levine P, Stetson R. An unusual case of intra-group agglutination. *JAMA.* 1939;113(2):126–127.

13. Daniels G. *Human Blood Groups.* Oxford: Blackwell; 2002.

14. Tippett P. A speculative model for the Rh blood groups. *Ann Hum Genet.* 1986;50(Pt 3):241–247.

15. Wagner FF, Flegel WA. RHD gene deletion occurred in the Rhesus box. *Blood.* 2000;95(12):3662–3668.

16. Daniels G. The molecular genetics of blood group polymorphism. *Transpl Immunol.* 2005;14(3–4):143–153.

17. Sandler SG, Flegel WA, Westhoff CM, et al. It's time to phase-in RHD genotyping for patients with a serological weak D phenotype. *Transfusion.* 2015;55(3):680–689.

18. Wagner FF, Gassner C, Müller TH, Schönitzer D, Schunter F, Flegel WA. Molecular basis of weak D phenotypes. *Blood.* 1999;93(1):385–393.

19. Wagner T, Körmöczi GF, Buchta C, et al. Anti-D immunization by DEL red blood cells. *Transfusion.* 2005;45(4):520–526.

20. Westhoff CM. The structure and function of the Rh antigen complex. *Semin Hematol.* 2007;44(1):42–50.

21. Beck ML, Harding J. Incidence of D category VI among Du donors in the USA. *Transfusion.* 1991;31(suppl):25.

22. Wagner FF, Gassner C, Muller TH, Schonitzer D, Schunter F, Flegel WA. Three molecular structures cause rhesus D category VI phenotypes with distinct immunohematologic features. *Blood.* 1998;91:215768.

23. Mouro I, Colin Y, Chérif-Zahar B, Cartron JP, Le Van Kim C. Molecular genetic basis of the human Rhesus blood group system. *Nat Genet.* 1993;5(1):62–65.

24. Westhoff CM, Siegel DL. Rh and LW blood group antigens. In: Simon TL, Snyder EL, Solheim BG, et al., eds. *Rossi's Principles in Transfusion Medicine.* 4th ed. Wiley-Blackwell; 2009.

25. Faas BHW, Beckers EAM, Simsek S, et al. Involvement of Ser103 of the Rh polypeptides in G epitope formation. *Transfusion.* 1996;36:506–511.

26. Faas BHW, Beckers EAM, Wildoer P, et al. Molecular background of VS and weak C expression in blacks. *Transfusion.* 1997;37:38–44.

27. Westhoff CM. The Rh blood group system in review: a new face for the next decade. *Transfusion.* 2004;44:1663–1673.

28. Noizat-Pirenne F, Lee K, Pennec PY, et al. Rare RHCE phenotypes in black individuals of Afro-Caribbean origin: identification and transfusion safety. *Blood.* 2002;100:4223–4231.

29. Ballas SK, Clark MR, Mohandas N, et al. Red cell membrane and cation deficiency in Rh null syndrome. *Blood.* 1984;63(5):1046–1055.

30. Huang CH, Chen Y, Reid ME, Seidl C. Rhnull disease: the amorph type results from a novel double mutation in RhCe gene on D-negative background. *Blood.* 1998;92(2):664–671.

31. Chérif-Zahar B, Mattéi MG, Le Van Kim C. Localization of the human Rh blood group gene structure to chromosome region 1p34.3-1p36.1 by in situ hybridization. *Hum Genet.* 1991;86(4):398–400.

32. Chérif-Zahar B, Bloy C, Le Van Kim C. Molecular cloning and protein structure of a human blood group Rh polypeptide. *Proc Natl Acad Sci USA.* 1990;87(16):6243–6247.

33. Cartron JP, Agre P. Rh blood group antigens: protein and gene structure. *Semin Hematol.* 1993;30(3):193–208.

34. Avent ND, Reid ME. The Rh blood group system: a review. *Blood.* 2000;95:375–387.

35. Ridgwell K, Spurr NK, Laguda B. Isolation of cDNA clones for a 50 kDa glycoprotein of the human erythrocyte membrane associated with Rh (rhesus) blood-group antigen expression. *Biochem J.* 1992;287(Pt 1):223–228.

36. Ridgwell K, Eyers SA, Mawby WJ, Anstee DJ, Tanner MJ. Studies on the glycoprotein associated with Rh (rhesus) blood group antigen expression in the human red blood cell membrane. *J Biol Chem.* 1994;269(9):6410–6416.

37. Makroo RN, Kaul A, Bhatia A. Anti-G antibody in an alloimmunized pregnant women: report of two cases. *Asian J Transfus Sci.* 2015;9(2):210–212.

38. Vos GH. The evaluation of specific anti-G (CD) eluate obtained by a double absorption and elution procedure. *Vox Sang.* 1960;5:472–478.

CHAPTER 4

Common Significant Non-ABO Antibodies and Blood Group Antigen Alloimmunization

IAN L. BAINE, MD, PHD • JEANNE E. HENDRICKSON, MD • CHRISTOPHER A. TORMEY, MD

RED BLOOD CELL TRANSFUSION AS AN ORGAN TRANSPLANT

Although not traditionally thought of as such, red blood cell (RBC) transfusions are, fundamentally, the most commonly performed organ transplant in all of medicine. Therefore when thinking about the concept of RBC alloimmunization, it makes sense to approach RBC transfusion from the perspective of organ "tolerance" or "rejection."[1,2] A basic concept in transplantation is that if there is immunologic, or antigenic, mismatch between the donor and recipient (host), the recipient is capable of mounting an immune response against the transplanted organ, ultimately leading to its destruction. For the purposes of examining RBC alloimmunization, humoral immune responsiveness is by far the predominant mechanism.[3] Although cellular graft-versus-host disease mechanisms do exist in transfusion medicine in the form of passenger lymphocyte syndrome and are behind the pathogenesis of certain transfusion reactions, they will not be discussed in this chapter. Therefore in general terms, RBC alloimmunization can be thought of as recognition of donor tissue (RBCs) by recipient-generated antibodies.

The basic immunologic mechanism behind RBC alloimmunization is the exact same one that drives our immune system to create antibodies to pathogens that we encounter in the environment, or that are presented to us in the form of vaccines. That is, our immune system recognizes antigens that are not visibly present in our body as foreign. Foreign antigen is recognized by the binding of a specific B-cell clone to its antigen-specific surface-bound immunoglobulin, also known as a B-cell receptor (BCR). Antigen binding to the BCR initiates a signal transduction cascade in the B cell causing it to activate, clonally proliferate, and differentiate into both memory B cells and antibody-producing plasma cells.[4] Throughout this process, the antigenic

specificity of the B-cell clone remains intact. In the case of RBC transfusion, the recipient's B cells recognize an antigen on the surface of the donor RBCs that is not present in the recipient, causing the recipient to generate an antibody response to the red cells bearing the foreign antigen (Fig. 4.1). This can potentially result in the rapid production and binding of the said antibodies to future transfused red cells (termed a secondary immunologic or "antibody recall" response), and their subsequent destruction by either complement fixation and intravascular hemolysis or opsonization and extravascular destruction via the reticuloendothelial system in the spleen. This manifests clinically as either an acute hemolytic transfusion reaction or a delayed serologic transfusion reaction, respectively,[5] processes discussed in detail elsewhere in this text.

One of the earliest classic examples of this process is alloimmunization to the RhD antigen, the most prominent member of the Rh antigen system. In the 1940s, it was observed by Levin and Wiener that mothers of stillborn fetuses who were born with fetal hydrops (intrauterine hemolysis) also had adverse hemolytic reactions to blood transfusions from the father of the stillborn.[6-8] Other studies[9] demonstrated the presence of the RhD antigen, a component of an RBC structural protein, on the RBCs of both the fetus and the father. This dominant trait of RhD expression had, in this case, been inherited by the fetus from the father. The mother, who did not express the RhD antigen, had become exposed to it either from prior pregnancy or via small amounts of maternal-fetal hemorrhage while pregnant. True to our model as we have just explained, her immune system recognized the RhD antigen as foreign and mounted an IgG antibody response to it. These anti-RhD antibodies, once circulating in her blood, crossed the placenta and caused destruction of the fetal red cells, resulting in stillbirth. Likewise, when the

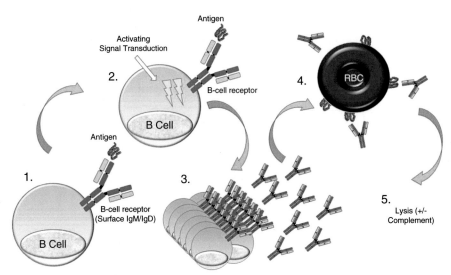

FIG. 4.1 Simplified overview of Steps in RBC antibody production. (1) The B cell recognizes RBC-specific antigen either as free-floating antigen or when bound to RBC membrane (not shown), via its B-cell receptor, which is surface-bound IgM or IgD. (2) After receiving activating signaling to cross an activation threshold via either sufficient binding avidity to antigen or T-cell help, the B cells activate. (3) Upon activation, B cells proliferate clonally and begin to differentiate into antibody-secreting plasma cells or long-lived memory B cells. Usually, B cells undergo class-switch recombination, causing secretion of IgG, and less commonly, IgA and IgE antibodies. Plasma cells generated from a single immune response secrete a specific clone of antibody that is unique to the antigen originally encountered by the B cell in Step 1. (4) These antibodies bind their specific "cognate" antigen on RBCs, causing either endocytosis by cells of the reticuloendothelial system in the spleen (not shown) or (5) fixation of complement and intravascular RBC lysis. *RBC*, red blood cell.

father's RBCs, which bore the RhD antigen, were transfused into the mother, her circulating anti-RhD antibodies recognized and attacked the father's transfused RBCs, causing intravascular hemolysis and an adverse reaction. In the ensuing years, dozens of different protein and carbohydrate antigens have been discovered, although only a small proportion of the alloantibodies to them are typically associated with clinically significant reactions.

HUMORAL IMMUNE RESPONSES–AN OVERVIEW OF THE BASIC MECHANISMS
T-Independent Antibody Responses
As mentioned previously, the fundamental process that drives RBC alloimmunization is the humoral immune response to a foreign antigen. This requires the presence of both the antigen itself and a B cell that recognizes it. Through the complex and intricate process of germline DNA recombination, B cells generate clonal surface-bound immunoglobulins that function as B-cell antigen receptors that are capable of recognizing a specific antigen, be it from a pathogen or an RBC.[10]

Direct binding of the BCR to its cognate antigen results in activation of the B cell and rapid secretion of clonal IgM class antibodies that bear the *exact same specificity* as the BCR. These IgM antibodies are secreted as pentamers and have a relatively weak binding affinity for their cognate antigen (Fig. 4.2, left panel). Because this process involves only the interaction of the B cell and free-floating antigen and does not involve T cells, it is termed a thymus-independent reaction or T-independent reaction. The antigen to which the B cell has responded is therefore termed a T-independent antigen (reviewed in Ref. [4], pp. 379–420). Broadly speaking, antibody responses to T-independent antigens generally are restricted to the IgM class, are traditionally associated with carbohydrate antigens, and are generally clinically *insignificant* from the transfusion compatibility standpoint. Some IgM antibodies are theoretically capable, however, of reacting over a broad thermal amplitude, or range of temperatures, and can therefore cause clinically significant hemolytic transfusion reactions in patients.[6,11] If such an IgM antibody is suspected, thermal amplitude testing is recommended. IgM class antibodies readily bind and activate, or "fix,"

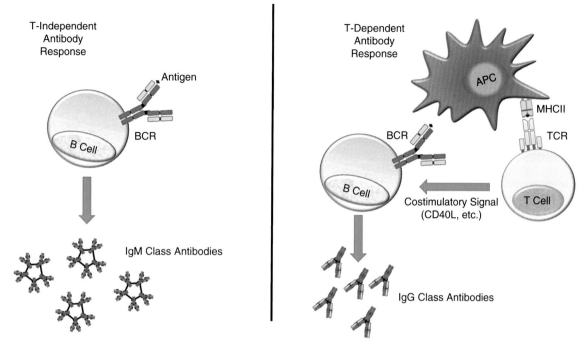

FIG. 4.2 Simplified overview of T-independent and T-dependent antibody responses. (Left) When B cells activate to soluble antigen in the absence of surrounding APCs and T cells, they proliferative and produce primarily IgM pentameric antibodies. These typically bind only at subphysiologic temperatures, although several notable exceptions (ABO and others) will bind at physiologic body temperature. Because IgM readily fixes and activates complement, it can cause intravascular hemolysis. (Right) When B cells activate in the presence of APCs and T cells, they are provided with costimulatory signals that cause them to undergo isotype class switching, allowing them to secrete IgG antibodies. These typically bind antigen at physiologic body temperature and more often will not activate complement [although notable exceptions (Kidd and others) do exist]. Instead they mark the RBCs for clearance from the circulation in the spleen and cause extravascular RBC destruction. *APC*, antigen-presenting cell; *BCR*, B-cell receptor; *MHC*, major histocompatibility complex; *RBC*, red blood cell.

upstream components of the complement cascade, allowing certain IgM antibodies to cause intravascular complement-mediated lysis of RBCs. However, because of their large size (pentamers), IgM antibodies cannot cross the placenta in pregnant women and therefore do not cause hemolytic disease of the fetus/newborn (HDFN).

T-Dependent Antibody Responses
Another way in which B cells recognize antigen and generate an antibody response to it involves "help" from a nearby T cell. Like B cells, T cells also possess surface-bound antigen receptors, called T-cell receptors (TCRs). Similar to formation of the BCR, these TCRs are also clonal and antigen specific and are formed via an analogous process of germline DNA recombination. However, whereas the BCR is able to bind free-floating antigen, the TCR is only able to recognize and bind antigen that is presented by the specialized antigen presentation molecules of the major histocompatibility complex (MHC). Broadly speaking there are two major classes of MHC molecules, termed Class I and Class II. Class I MHC molecules are present on all nucleated cells in humans and traditionally present intracellular peptides to CD8+ T cells. Class II MHC molecules are present on specialized antigen-presenting cells, such as macrophages, dendritic cells, and B cells; class II MHC presents peptides derived from extracellular antigens that have been endocytosed to CD4+ T cells (reviewed in Ref. [4]). Because transfused RBCs are essentially foreign extracellular antigens, we will focus only on Class II MHC in this process.

To generate a T-dependent immune response, the process begins similar to a T-independent response but involves additional cell populations as well. First, the B cell recognizes free-floating antigen via its BCR, which causes B-cell activation. Simultaneously, B cells or other antigen-presenting cells endocytose and process the antigen (or the cell bearing that antigen—like an RBC) and present that antigen to T cells via class II MHC molecules. Upon recognition of the antigen by its TCR, the T cell expresses the costimulatory molecule CD154 (CD40L), which binds to CD40 on B cells. Once the B cell has received this additional costimulatory signal, two processes begin. First, it induces a process called somatic hypermutation, which allows the B cell to further modify the specificity of its secreted antibodies. Second, and most important for transfusion medicine purposes, it undergoes a process termed class-switch recombination, in which it ceases to secrete IgM antibodies and begins to secrete other antibody isotypes, like IgG (Fig. 4.2, Right Panel). Most IgG class anti-RBC antibodies do not efficiently fix complement (with anti-Jk^a being a notable exception) to destroy their targets.[12] Rather, these antibodies opsonize target cells, allowing for their phagocytosis by macrophages, or in the case of RBCs, their removal from circulation by the reticuloendothelial system of the spleen. Clinically, this manifests as a delayed serologic transfusion with a drop in the hematocrit following transfusion, but without acute intravascular hemolysis.

The process of T-dependent antibody responses described earlier constitutes what is known as the primary antibody response, that is, the antibody response formed by the host when the antigen (or transfused RBCs) is seen for the *first time* by its immune system. In addition to antibody production, the formation of populations of long-lived memory B cells and plasma cells also occurs, allowing the host to respond with a much more rapid-onset production of antibody when the antigen is then seen the *second time* by the host. This is known as the secondary response or "memory" antibody response. It is this rapid and strong secondary response that is responsible for the clinical manifestations of antibody-associated transfusion reactions.

From a transfusion medicine perspective, IgG class antibodies are generally directed against protein antigens and react at physiologic body temperatures (approximately 37°C). Therefore they are considered clinically significant when identified in a screen or antibody panel. In contrast to IgM antibodies, IgG class antibodies can fix complement to varying degrees, depending on subtype. IgG1 and IgG3 are notable for complement fixation, whereas IgG2 and IgG4 fix complement poorly.[12] The major consideration regarding IgG alloantibodies in transfusion medicine is their ability to opsonize transfused RBCs and cause their removal from circulation by the recipient's spleen. Additionally, because of their monomeric state and relatively small size, they are able to readily cross the placenta in pregnant women and bind antigens on fetal RBCs, causing their destruction. This is the mechanism underlying immune-mediated hydrops fetalis.

To summarize our understanding of alloimmunization to RBC antigens, the host is exposed to transfused RBCs bearing a protein or carbohydrate antigen that is not present in the host. Recognizing this antigen as foreign, B cells are activated to form a primary antibody response, of either the IgM (T-independent) or IgG (T-dependent) type. As a component of this immune response, long-lived memory B cells are formed, which remain in the secondary lymphoid tissues or the bone marrow, poised to encounter the antigen a second time, at which point they will rapidly secrete antibodies in a secondary immune response. The initial primary antibody response to RBCs is slow, forming over weeks to months. Given the approximate 120 day life span of a circulating RBC, an alloantibody response may not be detected on a screen until long after the inciting transfusion event.[13,14]

ANTIBODY RESPONSVES TO RED BLOOD CELL ANTIGENS

Antibodies formed against red cell antigens can be broadly divided into two major categories, naturally occurring and induced by RBC exposure. Natural antibodies are present either from birth or very early in life and are defined as antibodies formed in the absence of an exposure to the antigen source against which the antibodies are directed.[15] If there is no exposure to antigen, how then are these antibodies made? Although it is still fundamentally true that antibodies cannot be formed by a host unless there is exposure to an immunogenic event, pioneering animal studies by Landsteiner and Weiner in the 1940s and the 1950s showed that exposure to pathogens such as certain strains of *Escherichia coli*, which contain antigens similar to the group B RBC antigens, resulted in anti-B alloimmunization in mice that were never exposed to the B antigen directly.[16] This is likely due to cross-reactivity of these anti-*E. coli* antibodies with the B antigen, and further human studies support this as well.[17–20] Generally speaking, natural antibodies form against carbohydrate antigens and are predominantly IgM in class.[21] By contrast, induced alloantibodies against polypeptide antigen antigens are only produced by the host once exposed to antigen-positive RBCs via either transfusion or pregnancy.

As mentioned previously, alloimmune responses consist of a gradually forming and weaker primary and rapid and strong secondary immune responses. Studies using RhD alloimmunization as the model demonstrated that alloantibodies are detected by standard serologic methods beginning at about 4 weeks postexposure and reach maximum concentration between 6 and 10 weeks.[22] A similar timeframe for primary antibody induction was later demonstrated to be confirmed for a variety of other antigen specificities by Redman and colleagues.[1] Consistent with our understanding of immunogenicity of antigens, there appears to be a minimum threshold model of exposure for RBC antigens, above which an alloantibody response is induced and below which it is not.[23,24] The degree to which a host will respond to allogeneic RBC exposure will vary based on numerous factors intrinsic to both the RBC and the patient.[25] Some patients alloimmunize rapidly and robustly to the initial exposure, whereas others respond poorly. Thus it is proposed that patients who do readily alloimmunize can be classified as "responders" to allogeneic RBC antigens.

Factors That Affect Alloimmunization

There are numerous factors that affect whether or not a patient will become alloimmunized, which can be divided into two major categories. The first are[26] factors intrinsic to the patient, including the underlying disease state, the number of previous transfusions, the patient's intrinsic "immune responder" status, the geographic/ethnic makeup, prior pregnancies, and the human leukocyte antigen (HLA) haplotype. The second group of factors are those extrinsic to the patient. These include the age of the RBC unit, the presence or absence of leukoreduction, the absence of a complete transfusion history, and the method of unit preparation, i.e., washing/volume reduction/irradiation.

In the general transfused population, up to 7% of healthy adults will form an alloantibody.[27] This reflects the overall relatively low frequency of transfusion. By contrast, patient populations who receive numerous transfusions chronically are more likely to form alloantibodies. This includes patients with hemoglobinopathies such as sickle cell disease and β-thalassemia major. Studies show alloimmunization rates ranging from 5% to 36% in β-thalassemia major, with the majority of antibodies being directed against Rh or K antigens. One study showed approximately 21% of patients alloimmunizing after 6 years of transfusion (average 18 units/year), with drastically lower rates present in the group receiving D/C/E/K-matched units (3.7%) when compared with RhD-only-matched units (15.7%).[28–30]

Patients with sickle cell disease (SCD) show higher alloimmunization rates, ranging from 18% to 36%, depending on the study, with patients receiving 100 or more transfusions having a 50% likelihood of alloimmunizing.[26,31] Regarding SCD specifically, the high alloimmunization rates are thought to be due not only to the frequency of transfusions but also to population-level discrepancies in the frequency of the Rh system and K antigens (0.178 allelic frequency in blacks, 0.597 in whites). Therefore many institutions will now procure RhD/C/E-matched and K-antigen-matched units when transfusing patients with SCD. Another related factor is the finding that patients with SCD have been shown to express unique variants of Rh system antigens at a higher frequency than the general population, further complicating the identification of truly matched units. This may account for a study in 2013 showing persistent alloimmunization in patients with SCD, even when receiving D/C/E/K-matched units.[32] This might be addressed in the coming years with increasing use of molecular-based methods of RBC antigen typing. In the case of SCD specifically, it is important to point out that alloimmunization rates in children are lower than those in adults, and studies have shown that alloimmunization rates are lower with RBC exposure via erythrocytapheresis when compared with simple transfusion.[33,34]

The degree of chronic inflammatory state in patients with SCD and other diseases may play a role as well, as patients presenting with acute chest syndrome or vaso-occlusive crises were more likely to alloimmunize than patients with nonacute SCD.[35,36] Further supporting this is the finding that chronic autoimmune conditions in general, such as inflammatory bowel disease, psoriasis, and rheumatoid arthritis, present a higher risk for alloimmunization than patients without inflammation. Studies showing that patients with most types of hematologic malignancies have a greater likelihood to alloimmunize are mixed, with some groups finding higher rates of alloimmunization[37] and advocating for C/D/E/K antigen matching for these patients as well, whereas other groups find lower rates. Conversely, it is also known that patients who are severely immunosuppressed either due to chronic conditions such as human immunodeficiency virus (HIV)/acquired immunodeficiency syndrome or due to medications taken after organ transplantation are less likely to alloimmunize.[38] The role of leukoreduction and the type of leukoreduction (bedside vs. universal) remains unclear, with some studies showing clinical benefit and reduced rates of alloimmunization, whereas others showing no benefit.[39] Additional well-controlled studies are needed to clarify this further. The role of pathogen reduction in preventing alloimmunization is still being defined, with initial studies showing reduced HLA alloimmunization.[14,40-46]

Because many alloantibodies evanesce (or disappear from detection) over time, obtaining a complete transfusion history for a patient is of paramount importance, as it may reveal an undetectable clinically significant alloantibody. It is common for patients to receive transfusions at more than one institution, and to date there is no national centralized database for transfusion or alloantibody identification records, leaving only the patient's recollection as our best option for determining undetectable alloantibodies. One study of just 100 patients revealed a 64% prevalence of discrepancy in alloantibody records when comparing detection at the authors' institution and records obtained from other local and distant hospitals.[47]

Studies on the effect of the age of the RBC unit on the potential for alloimmunization in general show no effect of aged RBC units on alloimmunization,[48-50] whereas other studies showed a correlation with units just 7 days old (hazard ratio [HR] 3.5), which increased with the age of the unit (HR 9.8 at 35 days).[51] However, it should be pointed out that the latter study focused on patients with SCD, and because these patients are known to have a higher baseline risk for alloantibody formation, the results of this study may reflect that fact. Additional studies will be needed to further clarify this topic, ideally factoring in patient disease and immune status.

BLOOD GROUP ANTIGEN SYSTEMS AND ASSOCIATED ALLOANTIBODIES
The Rh System
Aside from the ABO blood groups (which are beyond the scope of this chapter dedicated to non-ABO antigens and alloimmunization), the Rh system (particularly the RhD antigen) represents the most antigenic of all RBC antigens. Initially suspected by Levine in 1941,[52] subsequently inadvertently discovered by Landsteiner and Wiener, and then confirmed by others,[9,53] the Rh system presents up to an 80% risk of alloantibody formation when patients are exposed to antigen-positive blood and is responsible for the most severe forms of HDFN.[54,55] Alloantibodies to Rh antigens represent some of the most common alloantibodies identified and are generally considered clinically significant. To understand the different Rh antibodies, it is best to first have a brief overview of the Rh antigens' genetics and antigenic structure on the RBC membrane.

By the late 1940s, a total of five major Rh antigens were identified. They are RhD, C/c, and E/e, with C/c

and E/e being alternative alleles. By contrast, there is no alternative allele to the D antigen; it is either expressed or not expressed on the RBC. An extensive debate existed as to whether or not these antigens were coded for by a single gene (RhDCE), or by three separate genes (RhD, RhC, and RhE). However, it was later discovered in the 1980s that all the Rh antigens are coded for by two genes, *D* and *CcEe*, both located on chromosome 1.[56-58] They code for the transmembrane proteins RhD and RhCE, respectively. Both are 417 amino acid residues in length and are nearly identical. Predictive modeling shows that they both make 12 passes each through the RBC membrane, resulting in six extracellular domains that are exposed to the immune system. Point mutations in the transmembrane and extracellular domains of the RhCE protein result in amino acid substitutions C16T, I60L, S68N, S103P, and P226A, comprising the major primary sequence differences between the C/c and E/e alleles.[59] It should also be noted that the differences in allelic frequency for the given ABO or Rh phenotypes, as well as Rh genetic haplotypes, vary by ethnicity (Tables 4.1–4.3). These considerations become relevant when determining the statistical likelihood of expression of a given antigen in

TABLE 4.1
ABO Phenotype Frequencies in the United States by Ethnicity

ABO Type	White (%)	Black (%)	Hispanic (%)	Asian (%)
O	45	50	56	40
A	40	26	31	28
B	11	20	10	25
AB	4	4	3	7

TABLE 4.2
Overview of the Percentage of People by Ethnicity Expressing a Specific Rh Allele

Rh Allele Expression	White (%)	Black (%)	Hispanic (%)	Asian (%)
D	85	92	93	99
C	68	27	71[111]	93
E	29	22	41[111]	39
c	80	96	64[111]	47
e	98	98	84[111]	96

a patient or RBC unit in situations in which transfusion is emergent and there is insufficient time to fully phenotype either the patient or the unit.

As mentioned previously, only the *D* gene product (denoted by a capital D) can be expressed and the *d* allele does not exist; in RhD-negative individuals, the *D* gene either is deleted or contains a silencing mutation. This is denoted as a lowercase d when considering the genotype, *even though there is no such thing as the d protein.* As such, a patient's genotype can have heterozygous RhD expression (D/d), homozygous expression (D/D), or no expressed copies (d/d). Phenotypically, both the D/D and D/d patients will express the D antigen, and are termed RhD+ (colloquially called just "Rh+," even though it refers specifically to the D antigen). By contrast the d/d patient will not express any D antigen on the RBC surface and phenotypically will be RhD– (or just "Rh–," again referring to the D antigen specifically). The C/c and E/e alleles are more easily understood, with inheritance and behavior like normal Mendelian allelic variants of many other genes. That is, they can be inherited on a single allele as CE, cE, Ce, or ce. Keep in mind that unlike the D gene, *both alleles of the CE gene are expressed.* This means that each of the aforementioned combinations of C/c and E/e variants are present on each chromosome copy (Table 4.3). It should also be noted that advances in molecular sequencing of the Rh genes have identified Rh-like

pseudogenes and at least 58 different Rh phenotypic variants, some of which are clinically significant in certain select scenarios. Also, genetic recombination events can create novel hybrid genes between RhD and RhCE; a discussion of these concepts is beyond the scope of this text.[60,61]

Alloimmunization to the D antigen can occur to any of the extracellular loops or combination of loops that may function as linear or conformational epitopes (Fig. 4.3). There are at least 30 epitopes that have been defined to date.[62,63] Using the foundation we have built at the beginning of this chapter, we can expect that an RhD– patient who is transfused with RhD+ RBCs will form alloantibodies to the RhD antigen. The antigenicity of the D antigen depends on its density on the transfused RBC. Patients may express the D antigen at a much lower level; this is termed the "weak D" antigen.[64] Although the extracellular portions of the weak D antigen are the same as those in normal RhD+ patients, the weak D antigen results from numerous documented amino acid changes that result in decreased stability of the RhD protein in the RBC membrane. These patients may test as RhD-negative by serologic methods. However, if weak D RBCs are transfused into a truly RhD– patient, the patient may alloimmunize or experience a hemolytic transfusion reaction. Conversely, weak-D-expressing patients who are pregnant with an RhD– fetus will not need RhIg prophylaxis, despite negative results of serologic testing. Alternatively, another mechanism by which patients may express lower levels of D is known as the C-*in trans*/Cepellini effect, in which patients with the C allele present in trans to the D gene (i.e., on the other copy of chromosome 1), express lower levels of D protein on the RBC surface.[61] These patients may also test serologically as RhD– but can have alloimmunization or hemolytic reactions if their RBCs are transfused into true RhD– patients. Other forms of weak D expression such as D_{el} exist as well, but their discussion is beyond the scope of this text. In all these aforementioned cases, molecular sequencing of the patient's RhD gene will reveal the true nature of the patient's RhD status and zygosity.

In addition to the weak D antigen, there is another variant known as the "partial D" antigen. This antigen is formed by the aforementioned hybrid gene rearrangement between the RhD and RhCE genes, resulting in a novel RhD-like protein that is missing certain residues in the extracellular portions of the protein, normally present in the typical RhD. As a result, the host is able to form antibodies against these missing residues and can develop an anti-RhD alloantibody if transfused with RhD+ cells. Partial D can be identified

TABLE 4.3
Overview of the Percentage of People by Ethnicity Expressing a Specific Rh Allelic Haplotype

Rh Haplotype	White	Black	Asian
DCe (R_1)	42%	17%	70%
DcE (R_2)	14%	11%	21%
Dce (R_0)	4%	44%	3%
DCE (R_z)	Very rare	Very rare	1%
ce (r)	37%	26%	3%
Ce (r')	2%	2%	2%
cE (r″)	1%	Very rare	Very rare
CE (rʸ)	Very rare	Very rare	Very rare

Both Fisher-Race and Wiener (in parentheses) terminologies are shown. Alleles that are "very rare" are present at a frequency of less than 1%. Numbers highlighted in red represent significant differences in haplotype prevalence that must be considered to reduce the chances of alloimmunization to Rh-group antigens.

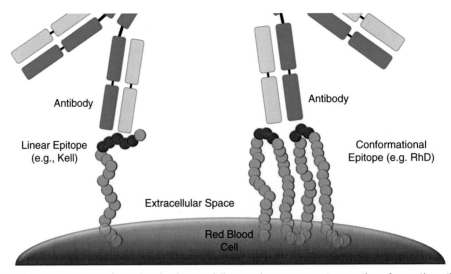

FIG. 4.3 Linear versus conformational epitopes. A linear epitope represents a portion of an antigen that is contiguous in terms of primary sequence. By contrast, a conformational epitope may be composed of multiple regions of an antigen that are distant from each other in terms of the primary sequence, but reside in close proximity when viewed in terms of the three-dimensional conformation of the protein antigen on the cell surface.

via extended anti-D serologic testing with a panel of anti-D reagents, while molecular sequencing continues to reveal the exact nature of these and newly discovered mutations.[65-67]

The anti-C/c and anti-E/e antibodies are produced in response to different epitopes on the RhCE protein. Like RhD, the RhCE protein resides in the RBC membrane and makes 12 passes through it, resulting in six extracellular domains. As mentioned earlier, point mutations throughout the extracellular and transmembrane domains of the protein account for differences between the C and c antigens and the E and e antigens. Also as mentioned earlier, there are two alleles of RhCE, both of which are expressed. Hence, C/c/E/e antigen expression follows typical Mendelian rules of inheritance, but the antigens are codominantly expressed. Like RhD, there are several variants of RhCE, with a variant E antigen being the most common (but still quite rare); these are discussed more extensively in other resources.[65,68,69]

As mentioned before, the D antigen is by far the most immunogenic of the Rh system, with studies showing up an 85% alloimmunization rate when 200 mL or more of RhD+ RBCs are transfused into a RhD− patient,[54] but studies also demonstrate alloantibody formation as little as 0.1 mL of whole cord blood. Therefore transfusion of even a portion of 1 unit of Rh-incompatible cells is more than enough to elicit

an antibody response. Interestingly, the remaining 15% of patients comprise a subset, termed "nonresponders," who do not form detectable anti-D antibodies upon the first exposure. Yet, half of this group will eventually form an anti-D upon subsequent exposure. While these studies were conducted under experimental conditions, retrospective studies of D-negative patients who received numerous intraoperative D+ transfusions showed an alloimmunization rate of 95% when detected with enzyme-treated cells and studies of patients who received fewer or a single unit show lower rates of alloimmunization, but still at very significant rates, especially when "boosted" with a second antigen exposure 6 months later.[22,70,71] Interestingly, patients with either primary or disease-associated immunosuppression make anti-D at relatively low rates, underscoring the role of the recipient's immune status at the time of exposure. Anti-D antibodies may wane over a period of many years, but they have been detected 38 years following exposure.[72] Nonetheless, the patients remain immunized to the D antigen for the rest of their life, even if the antibody is not detectable by serologic methods.

Anti-D is predominantly IgG, although an IgM component can coexist as well; as such it is primarily detected via the IAT, although some antisera can agglutinate RBCs directly. While anti-D IgG1 and IgG3 subclasses have been demonstrated, anti-D generally does not fix complement efficiently, and as such will more often result in a serologic transfusion reaction, with extravascular clearance of antigen-positive RBCs. Additionally, as anti-D is predominantly IgG, it is able to cross the placenta and can cause a severe form of HDFN. Formation of anti-D can be seen as early as 2 months and as late 5 months, and it does not form more rapidly if exposed multiple times.

With the advent of RhIg use in the late 1960s combined with the standardized use of careful RhD typing, including testing for weak D and the most common form of partial D, formation of anti-D antibodies is now increasingly rare. However, women with inadequate prenatal care may not have received prophylaxis during pregnancy and may present with anti-D. Likewise, emergent transfusion of Rh-incompatible units in cases of massive traumatic bleeding can cause the formation of anti-D, although the rates of alloimmunization are lower when compared with healthy recipients.[73] One potentially more commonly encountered scenario is the transfusion of platelets into recipients who are RhD negative. Although platelets do not express the RhD antigen, platelet units necessarily contain a small amount of contaminating RBCs, usually less than 0.5 mL, as part of their preparation. An earlier study of immunosuppressed patients receiving such "Rh-incompatible" platelet units showed that up to 8% develop detectable anti-D, although other studies demonstrate lower rates, or no allommunization at all.[74-76] However, this may be mitigated with the coadministration of RhIg as a prophylactic measure, which binds the RhD+ RBCs and shields them from immune recognition, thereby preventing anti-D formation. Case reports exist of anti-D formation following solid organ transplantation, with one study of 42 patients showing a 5% incidence of anti-D formation after a renal transplant.[77]

Clinically significant antibodies directed against the C, c, E, and e antigens have all been documented and can mediate hemolytic transfusion reactions and HDFN. Of these, the anti-E antibody is the most common with an incidence of 19.4%[78]; however, as described earlier, virtually all cases are naturally occurring anti-E, making the E antigen a very weak one from the perspective of alloimmunization. Anti-C is the next most common antibody, with an incidence of less than 5% in a large study of over 18,700 US military veterans who were transfused. Notably, this study population was largely male and therefore the incidence in the general population is likely higher due to exposure via pregnancy. Anti-c, although rare, is notable because it is solely formed as a result of antigenic exposure; no natural forms of this antibody

are known to exist. Interestingly, patients who are of the R_1/R_1 genotype, and who have already developed an anti-E, have a significant risk (approximately 18% according to one study[79]) of developing a subsequent anti-c if exposed to untyped RBCs. Anti-e has been reported, although studies show the e antigen to be weakly immunogenic; however, the antibody is clinically significant once formed. Studies on the immunogenicity of the e antigen are limited by the relative scarcity of e-antigen-negative patients who are capable of forming anti-e alloantibodies. In the aforementioned large study of veterans, all these anti-Rh alloantibodies were reactive at 37°C, the AHG phase, or both, indicating that they are IgG class antibodies.

The Kell System

After the ABO and Rh systems, the Kell system, which is composed of a total of at least 28 antigens, represents the next most immunogenic system of RBC antigens. For simplicity, we will mention only K, k, Kp[a], Kp[b], Js[a], and Js[b], the most frequently encountered antigens in clinical practice; a comprehensive review of all antigens can be found in numerous texts[61,69,80,81].

The K antigen, and its alternate allele k, is the most commonly encountered clinically within this system, and K is expressed in about 9% of whites and 1.5% of blacks, either in homozygous or in heterozygous (Kk) forms (Table 4.4). Generally speaking, it is about 8- to 10-fold less immunogenic than the RhD antigen. The Kell genetic locus is located at 7q33 and is a part of the CD238 transmembrane protein. Unlike the Rh system, the Kell protein only inserts into the membrane at a single point, with defined extracellular, transmembrane, and intracellular portions. It is also associated with the Xk protein covalently via disulfide bonds with extracellular cysteine residues. Due to multiple extracellular disulfide bonds, the Kell protein is rendered serologically undetectable by treatment with reducing agents, either dithiothreitol or beta-mercaptoethanol. It is not sensitive to trypsin, ficin, or papain.

A single protein encodes both the K and k antigens, with the only difference being a single amino acid substitution, T193M. In contrast to the K antigen, k (also referred to as "Cellano") is present in nearly 100% of patients. Other K alleles, also on 7q33 code for the closely related antigens Kp[a] (2%), Kp[b] (~100%), Js[a] (<1% in whites, ~20% in blacks), and Js[b] (approximately 100% in whites, 80% in blacks, see Table 4.4). The Kp[a] and Kp[b] antigens differ by a single amino acid substitution W281 and R281, respectively. Similarly, Js[a] and Js[b] differ by a single amino acid, P597 and L597, respectively.[59]

TABLE 4.4
Overview of the Percentage of People by Ethnicity Expressing a Specific Kell Allelic Genotype

Kell Phenotype	White	Black
K−k+	91%	98%
K+k+	~9%	2%
K+k−	0.2%	Very rare
Kpª−Kpᵇ+	98%	100%
Kpª+Kpᵇ+	~2%	Very rare
Kpª+Kpᵇ−	Very rare	0%
Jsª−Jsᵇ+	100%	80%
Jsª+Jsᵇ+	Very rare	19%
Jsª+Jsᵇ−		

The K/k, Kpª/Kpᵇ, and Jsª/JSᵇ haplotypes and frequencies are shown individually. Haplotypes that are "very rare" are present at a frequency of less than 1%. Numbers highlighted in red represent significant differences in haplotype frequency that must be considered to reduce the chances of alloimmunization to Rh-group antigens. These are important to note when determining the statistical likelihood of expression of a given antigen in a patient or red blood cell unit. This information, in combination with that found in Tables 4.1 and 4.2, may be of use in situations in which transfusion is emergent and there is insufficient time to fully phenotype either the patient or the unit.

Anti-K is the most common alloantibody aside from the ABO and Rh antibodies; it is predominantly an IgG₁ class antibody, and studies show incidence ranging between 14% and 28%.[82,83] Early studies placed the risk of forming an anti-K at 10% if transfused with at least 1 unit of K-antigen-positive blood,[84,85] making the K antigen one of the more immunogenic ones. Similar to the formation of anti-C antibodies, recipients who form anti-D antibodies are more likely to form anti-K antibodies as well, likely reflecting the general "responder" capability of the individual patient. Although it is able to fix complement, it does so only incompletely and does not cause the formation of the membrane attack complex. Nonetheless, it is capable of causing severe hemolytic transfusion reactions.

In addition to anti-K antibodies causing serologic transfusion reactions, anti-K is also a well-known cause of severe HDFN in K-antigen-positive fetuses, as it not only crosses the placenta and clears fetal red cell from circulation but also is able to bind and destroy fetal erythroid precursors (and possibly myeloid/megakaryocytic precursors as well), which express the K antigen early in lineage development.[86–88] This results

in the suppression of fetal hematopoiesis and severe fetal anemia, requiring intrauterine RBC transfusions. HDFN has also been associated with Jsª and Jsᵇ and Kpª antibodies (k antibodies are rare), but anti-K is by far the most prevalent and severe. The frequency of anti-K in pregnant women is approximately 1/1000,[89,90] and the incidence of HDFN due to anti-K is estimated at 1/20,000. In case series of known maternal-fetal K antigen mismatch in the presence of maternal anti-K antibodies, the rate of hydrops or fetal death ranges from 15% to 38%.[91–95] Due to the severity of HDFN mediated by anti-K, cell-free fetal DNA testing assays have been developed for testing the fetal K genotype in pregnant mothers with a known anti-K. Additionally, unlike other instances of maternal-fetal alloimmunization where the antibody titer generally shows correlation with the severity of fetal anemia, anti-K titers do not correlate well with fetal anemia.

Anti-k is quite rare, due to its status as a high-incidence antigen. Overall, approximately 98% of patients express the k antigen (Table 4.4). Conversely, the incidence of anti-k ranges from 0.005% in blacks to up to 2% in whites in the United States.[69] Anti-Kpª and anti-Kpᵇ are rare, as are anti-Jsª and Jsᵇ, about 0.5% and 0.4%, respectively.[78] Like anti-K they too are capable of mediating hemolytic transfusion reactions.

Another antigen closely related to Kell is the Xk (or XK1) antigen, which is coded for by the XK gene at the locus Xp21.1. This protein has 10 transmembrane domains and is notable here because it is covalently attached to the K protein via a disulfide bond. This link serves to stabilize the K protein in the RBC membrane, and allow for its normal expression. A condition known as McLeod syndrome results from inactivating mutations in the XK gene, resulting in loss of Xk expression. Clinically, it presents with acanthocytosis, and muscular, neurologic, and psychiatric manifestations as well. In RBCs from these patients, there is very weak expression of the K antigen.

The Duffy System

Antigens of the Duffy system are coded for by the DARC protein, located on chromosome 1q21. It functions as a chemokine receptor, binding the inflammatory cytokines interleukin-8, MCP-1, and CXCL1,[96] although its role on the RBC membrane is not fully understood. The most commonly encountered antigens are the Fyª and Fyᵇ, which are expressed codominantly. The Fyª and Fyᵇ antigens differ by a single amino acid substitution, G42 and D42, respectively. Of note, 100% of whites express some combination of Fyª and/or Fyᵇ, whereas about two-thirds of blacks express neither antigen (Table 4.5),

TABLE 4.5
Overview of the Percentage of People by
Ethnicity Expressing a Specific Duffy Haplotype

Duffy Phenotype	White (%)	Black (%)	Asian (%)
Fy^a+Fy^b−	20	10	81
Fy^a+Fy^b+	48%	3%	15
Fy^a−Fy^b+	32%	20%	4%
Fy^a−Fy^b-	0%	67%	0%

Numbers highlighted in red represent potentially clinically significant differences in antigenic frequency between ethnicities. These are important to note for the same reasons previously outlined in Table 4.4.

TABLE 4.6
Overview of the Percentage of People by
Ethnicity Expressing a Specific Kidd Haplotype

Kidd Phenotype	White (%)	Black (%)	Asian (%)
Jk^a+Jk^b−	26	52	23
Jk^a+Jk^b+	50	40	50
Jk^a−Jk^b−	24	8	27

with population studies in Gambia showing 100% of people with a Fy^a/Fy^b phenotype. This is due to a mutation in the promoter of the DARC gene at the binding site of GATA-1, a transcription factor that drives Fy antigen transcription. However, the Fy antigen is still expressed on other tissues, such as the thymus,[97] hence alloantibodies are usually not formed in these cases. However, cases also exist where the Fy^a and Fy^b antigens are missing due to deletions or other inactivating mutations; in these cases, the Fy antigen expression is completely lost in all tissues and these patients can form "pan-anti-Duffy" antibodies, usually either anti-Fy3 or anti-Fy5, which will react with all Fy$^{a/b}$-antigen-positive RBCs. Similarly, Fy^a is more immunogenic in Fy^a-Fy^b+ patients when they are exposed, due to the deletional nature of the lack of Fy^a expression.

Anti-Fy^a is present in about 30% of patients,[78] with anti-Fy^b being much less common. They are predominantly IgG$_1$ class antibodies and are known to cause both acute and delayed hemolytic transfusion reactions, as well as HDFN.[98] Interestingly, there appears to be a strong association between anti-Fy^a formation and the HLA DRB1*04 allele, indicating that the presentation of the Fy^a antigen may depend on a very specific antigen presentation configuration.[99] It was shown in the 1970s that patients with the Fy$^{a/b}$ null phenotype were resistant to RBC infection with *Plasmodium vivax* and *Plasmodium knowlesi* [100,101] and that the Fy antigens serve as a binding site and point of entry for these parasites into the RBCs. This may account for the selective evolutionary pressure toward this phenotype in malaria-endemic regions. Studies have also shown that Fy^{a-b-} RBCs are able to more efficiently bind HIV, raising speculation that these individuals may be more susceptible to HIV infection.[102]

The Kidd System

The Kidd system consists of three antigens, Jk^a, Jk^b, and Jk3, which are coded for by the *Slc14a1* gene located on chromosome 18q12. Like the Rh and Duffy antigens, it too is a multipass transmembrane protein, with 10 transmembrane domains and five extracellular loops.[69] It functions as a urea transporter termed HUT11 and is expressed in numerous tissues throughout the body, most notably in the renal medulla.[105] Similar to other antigens, Jk^a and Jk^b differ by a single amino acid mutation, D280 and N280, respectively.[59] The Jk^a and Jk^b antigens are codominantly expressed, with frequencies depending on the ethnicity (Table 4.6). The Jk3 phenotype, which is present in some ethnicities at an incidence of up to 1.4% in some Pacific Islander populations,[103] represents a null phenotype where the individual has an unexpressed allele at the Jk$^{a/b}$ locus. This is due most commonly to a splice site mutation, or an S291P point mutation.[104]

Most anti-Jk^a and anti-Jk^b antibodies are IgG$_1$ and IgG$_3$, but IgG$_{2/4}$ and IgM components have also been characterized. The anti-Jk^a antibody was present at a frequency of 21% in a large study of transfused US veterans[78]; anti-Jk^b was present at a much lower frequency (~1%). Two important features of anti-Jk^a and anti-Jk^b antibodies are their abilities to completely fix complement and activate the cascade to completion, and their associations with delayed acute and serologic hemolytic transfusion reactions. The latter feature is due to their ability to fall to undetectable levels (via evanescence) by conventional serologic methods, just several months following alloimmunization. This underscores the importance of a complete transfusion history in patients, as it may prevent a potentially serious delayed hemolytic reaction, or potential HDFN, although Kidd-associated HDFN is rare. Another point of consideration is its role as a minor histocompatibility antigen in renal allografts. Due to the high concentration of the Jk antigens on the renal medullary tissue, it is thought that Jk-antigen-mismatched renal transplants are associated with a higher rate of chronic rejection. Studies show that mismatched allografts demonstrate higher degrees of cellular infiltration in early rejection.[106]

The MNSs System

The MNSs system is composed of over 46 different alleles but is divided into two major allelic loci of most frequent clinical significance, the MN and the Ss loci. Both of these alleles are inherited in a Mendelian manner and can be expressed codominantly, meaning that all possible permutations of M/N/S/s can be expressed. The MM, MN, and NN genotypes are found at differing rates across ethnicities (Table 4.7).

The M and N antigens are expressed on the glycoprotein glycophorin A, whereas the S and s (and U) antigens are expressed on glycophorin B; the differences between M and N, and S and s involve alterations in the terminal amino acid sequence of their respective proteins.[59] These are single-pass proteins that contain distinct intracellular, transmembrane, and extracellular domains and may serve as entry receptors for *Plasmodium falciparum*.[107,108] Glycophorin B also serves as a binding site for the C3b component of the complement cascade. The S⁻s⁻ phenotype is rare and found in approximately 1.5% of black people; these individuals

also lack the high incidence U antigen (100% whites, 99% blacks) and are capable of developing an alloantibody to the U antigen,[109] making it exceedingly difficult to obtain compatible units. Serologic immunoreactivity to these antigens is reduced after treatment with ficin or papain.

Anti-M and anti-N alloantibodies are fairly common, and many are naturally occurring, cold-reactive antibodies, all of which are at least partly IgM class; auto-anti-M may be IgG alone. However, up to 4% of infants and adults are found to have anti-M that is reactive at 37°C, making it a clinically significant antibody.[78,110] Anti-M alloantibody been demonstrated to form up to 12% of the time in the context of alloimmunization to other major alloantigens, such as RhD. This indicates that the M antigen itself is not highly immunogenic. These antibodies do not bind complement and do not mediate intravascular hemolysis. There are scattered case reports of delayed hemolytic reactions due to anti-M and anti-N, therefore these antigens are still honored when providing compatible red cell units to patients. Because these antibodies are generally IgM, they are not implicated in HDFN.[61,69]

By contrast, anti-S and anti-s are typically IgG class antibodies that are reactive at 37°C and are known to mediate both hemolytic transfusion reactions and HDFN. As alluded to previously, the high-incidence U antigen is a common component of the S and s antigens; patients who are S-s- are therefore capable of alloimmunizing to U and also forming a clinically significant anti-U, which can cause hemolytic reactions and HDFN as well. Due to its extremely high prevalence in white and black donor populations, it is extremely difficult to find compatible units.[61,69]

SUMMARY

Blood group antigens and their corresponding antibodies are an extremely important aspect of clinical blood banking and form the basis for compatibility testing in transfusion. These antigens/antibodies also play important roles in HDFN. We hope that this chapter has not only enhanced your understanding of the complex facts/figures of blood group antibodies but also has improved your understanding of how and why the human body mounts immunological responses to these antigens. Clearly, much more work remains to be dome to unravel the causes of alloimmunization. With this knowledge and understanding, the blood bank community can continue to improve the safety and compatibility of transfusion therapy.

TABLE 4.7
Overview of the Percentage of People by Ethnicity Expressing a Specific MNS Haplotype

MNS Phenotype	White (%)	Black (%)
M+N-	30	25
M+N+	49	49
M-N+	21	26
S+s-	10	6
S+s+	42	24
S-s+	48	68
S-s-	0%	2% (also U-)

Numbers highlighted in red represent potentially clinically significant differences in antigenic frequency between ethnicities. Note that by definition patients who are negative for both S and s antigen expression cannot express the U antigen, a conformational epitope composed of both the S and s antigens. These S-s-U- patients may form a clinically significant anti-U antibody. It then becomes extremely difficult to find compatible red blood cell units for these patients, as approximately 99% of all red blood cell units will express the high-incidence U antigen. These are important to note for the same reasons previously outlined in the legend for Table 4.4.

REFERENCES

1. Redman M, Regan F, Contreras M. A prospective study of the incidence of red cell allo-immunisation following transfusion. *Vox Sang.* 1996;71(4):216–220.
2. Kissmeyer-Nielsen F, et al. Hyperacute rejection of kidney allografts, associated with pre-existing humoral antibodies against donor cells. *Lancet.* 1966;2(7465): 662–665.
3. Walker RH, Lin DT, Hartrick MB. Alloimmunization following blood transfusion. *Arch Pathol Lab Med.* 1989;113(3):254–261.
4. Murphy K, et al. *Janeway's Immunobiology.* 7th ed. vol. xxi. New York: Garland Science; 2008. 887 pp.
5. Savage WJ. Transfusion reactions. *Hematol Oncol Clin North Am.* 2016;30(3):619–634.
6. Levine P. The pathogenesis of erythroblastosis fetalis - a review. *J Pediatr.* 1943;23:656–675.
7. Levine P, Katzin EM, Burnham L. Isoimmunization in pregnancy - its possible bearing on the etiology of erythroblastosis foetalis. *J Am Med Assoc.* 1941;116: 825–827.
8. Levine P, et al. Pathogenesis of erythroblastosis fetalis: statistical evidence. *Science.* 1941;94(2442):371–372.
9. Landsteiner K, Wiener AS. Studies on an agglutinogen (Rh) in human blood reacting with anti-rhesus sera and with human isoantibodies. *J Exp Med.* 1941;74(4): 309–320.
10. Lewis SM, Wu GE. The origins of V(D)J recombination. *Cell.* 1997;88(2):159–162.
11. Wiener AS. *Blood Groups and Transfusion.* 3rd ed. Springfield, IL: CC Thomas; 1943.
12. Stowell SR, et al. Initiation and regulation of complement during hemolytic transfusion reactions. *Clin Dev Immunol.* 2012;2012:307093.
13. Stack G, Tormey CA. Detection rate of blood group alloimmunization based on real-world testing practices and kinetics of antibody induction and evanescence. *Transfusion.* 2016;56(11):2662–2667.
14. Schonewille H, et al. Red blood cell alloantibodies after transfusion: factors influencing incidence and specificity. *Transfusion.* 2006;46(2):250–256.
15. Landsteiner K. *The Specificity of Serological Reactions.* Boston, MA: Harvard University Press; 1945.
16. Wiener AS. Origin of naturally occurring hemagglutinins and hemolysins; a review. *J Immunol.* 1951;66(2): 287–295.
17. Drach GW, Reed WP, Williams Jr RC. Antigens common to human and bacterial cells: urinary tract pathogens. *J Lab Clin Med.* 1971;78(5):725–735.
18. Drach GW, Reed WP, Williams Jr RC. Antigens common to human and bacterial cells. II. *E. coli* 014, the common Enterobacteriaceae antigen, blood groups A and B, and *E. coli* 086. *J Lab Clin Med.* 1972;79(1):38–46.
19. Wittels EG, Lichtman HC. Blood group incidence and *Escherichia coli* bacterial sepsis. *Transfusion.* 1986; 26(6):533–535.
20. Springer GF, Horton RE. Blood group isoantibody stimulation in man by feeding blood group-active bacteria. *J Clin Invest.* 1969;48(7):1280–1291.
21. Chattoraj A, Gilbert Jr R, Josephson AM. Immunologic characterization of anti-H isohemagglutinins. *Transfusion.* 1968;8(6):368–371.
22. Samson D, Mollison PL. Effect on primary Rh immunization of delayed administration of anti-Rh. *Immunology.* 1975;28(2):349–357.
23. Zipursky A, et al. The transplacental passage of foetal red blood-cells and the pathogenesis of Rh immunisation during pregnancy. *Lancet.* 1963;2(7306):489–493.
24. Cohen F, et al. Mechanisms of isoimmunization. I. The transplacental passage of fetal erythrocytes in homospecific pregnancies. *Blood.* 1964;23:621–646.
25. Hendrickson JE, Eisenbarth SC, Tormey CA. Red blood cell alloimmunization: new findings at the bench and new recommendations for the bedside. *Curr Opin Hematol.* 2016;23(6):543–549.
26. Aygun B, et al. Clinical significance of RBC alloantibodies and autoantibodies in sickle cell patients who received transfusions. *Transfusion.* 2002;42(1):37–43.
27. Ngoma AM, et al. Red blood cell alloimmunization in transfused patients in sub-Saharan Africa: a systematic review and meta-analysis. *Transfus Apher Sci.* 2016; 54(2):296–302.
28. Dhawan HK, et al. Alloimmunization and autoimmunization in transfusion dependent thalassemia major patients: study on 319 patients. *Asian J Transfus Sci.* 2014; 8(2):84–88.
29. Azarkeivan A, et al. RBC alloimmunization and double alloantibodies in thalassemic patients. *Hematology.* 2015;20(4):223–227.
30. Azarkeivan A, et al. Blood transfusion and alloimmunization in patients with thalassemia: multicenter study. *Pediatr Hematol Oncol.* 2011;28(6):479–485.
31. Josephson CD, et al. Transfusion in the patient with sickle cell disease: a critical review of the literature and transfusion guidelines. *Transfus Med Rev.* 2007;21(2): 118–133.
32. Chou ST, et al. High prevalence of red blood cell alloimmunization in sickle cell disease despite transfusion from Rh-matched minority donors. *Blood.* 2013;122(6): 1062–1071.
33. Wahl SK, et al. Lower alloimmunization rates in pediatric sickle cell patients on chronic erythrocytapheresis compared to chronic simple transfusions. *Transfusion.* 2012;52(12):2671–2676.
34. Michot JM, et al. Immunohematologic tolerance of chronic transfusion exchanges with erythrocytapheresis in sickle cell disease. *Transfusion.* 2015;55(2): 357–363.
35. Fasano RM, et al. Red blood cell alloimmunization is influenced by recipient inflammatory state at time of transfusion in patients with sickle cell disease. *Br J Haematol.* 2015;168(2):291–300.

36. Telen MJ, et al. Alloimmunization in sickle cell disease: changing antibody specificities and association with chronic pain and decreased survival. *Transfusion.* 2015;55(6):1378–1387.

37. Baia F, et al. Phenotyping Rh/Kell and risk of alloimmunization in haematological patients. *Transfus Med.* 2016;26(1):34–38.

38. Evers D, et al. Treatments for hematologic malignancies in contrast to those for solid cancers are associated with reduced red cell alloimmunization. *Haematologica.* 2017;102(1):52–59.

39. Mishima Y, et al. Effects of universal vs bedside leukoreductions on the alloimmunization to platelets and the platelet transfusion refractoriness. *Transfus Apher Sci.* 2015;52(1):112–121.

40. Jackman RP, et al. Reduced MHC alloimmunization and partial tolerance protection with pathogen reduction of whole blood. *Transfusion.* 2017;57(2):337–348.

41. Seftel MD, et al. Universal prestorage leukoreduction in Canada decreases platelet alloimmunization and refractoriness. *Blood.* 2004;103(1):333–339.

42. Blumberg N, Heal JM, Gettings KE. WBC reduction of RBC transfusions is associated with a decreased incidence of RBC alloimmunization. *Transfusion.* 2003;43(7):945–952.

43. Fast LD. Recipient elimination of allogeneic lymphoid cells: donor CD4(+) cells are effective alloantigen-presenting cells. *Blood.* 2000;96(3):1144–1149.

44. Schonewille H, Brand A. Alloimmunization to red blood cell antigens after universal leucodepletion. A regional multicentre retrospective study. *Br J Haematol.* 2005;129(1):151–156.

45. Strauss RG, et al. Comparing alloimmunization in preterm infants after transfusion of fresh unmodified versus stored leukocyte-reduced red blood cells. *J Pediatr Hematol Oncol.* 1999;21(3):224–230.

46. van de Watering L, et al. HLA and RBC immunization after filtered and buffy coat-depleted blood transfusion in cardiac surgery: a randomized controlled trial. *Transfusion.* 2003;43(6):765–771.

47. Unni N, et al. Record fragmentation due to transfusion at multiple health care facilities: a risk factor for delayed hemolytic transfusion reactions. *Transfusion.* 2014;54(1):98–103.

48. Yazer MH, Triulzi DJ. Receipt of older RBCs does not predispose d-negative recipients to anti-d alloimmunization. *Am J Clin Pathol.* 2010;134(3):443–447.

49. Dinardo CL, et al. Transfusion of older red blood cell units, cytokine burst and alloimmunization: a case-control study. *Rev Bras Hematol Hemoter.* 2015;37(5):320–323.

50. Lacroix J, et al. Age of transfused blood in critically ill adults. *N Engl J Med.* 2015;372(15):1410–1418.

51. Desai PC, et al. Alloimmunization is associated with older age of transfused red blood cells in sickle cell disease. *Am J Hematol.* 2015;90(8):691–695.

52. Levine P, Burnham L, Katzin EM, et al. The Role of Isoimmunization in the pathogenesis of erythroblastosis fetalis. *Am J Obstet Gynecol.* 1941;42(925).

53. Rosenfield RE. Who discovered Rh? A personal glimpse of the Levine-Wiener argument. *Transfusion.* 1989;29(4):355–357.

54. Pollack W, et al. Studies on Rh prophylaxis. II. Rh immune prophylaxis after transfusion with Rh-positive blood. *Transfusion.* 1971;11(6):340–344.

55. Urbaniak SJ, Robertson AE. A successful program of immunizing Rh-Negative male-volunteers for anti-d production using frozen-thawed blood. *Transfusion.* 1981;21(1):64–69.

56. Colin Y, et al. Genetic-basis of the Rhd-positive and Rhd-negative blood-group polymorphism as determined by southern analysis. *Blood.* 1991;78(10):2747–2752.

57. Colin Y, Bailly P, Cartron JP. Molecular-genetic basis of Rh and Lw blood-groups. *Vox Sang.* 1994;67:67–72.

58. Mouro I, et al. Molecular-genetic basis of the human rhesus blood-group system. *Nat Genet.* 1993;5(1):62–65.

59. Reid M, et al. *The Blood Group Antigens Factbook.* 3rd ed. Cambridge, MA: Academic Press; 2012.

60. Nardozza LM, et al. The molecular basis of RH system and its applications in obstetrics and transfusion medicine. *Rev Assoc Med Bras (1992).* 2010;56(6):724–728.

61. Fung MK, Grossman B, Hillyer CD, Westhoff CM. *Technical Manual of the American Association of Blood Banks.* 18th ed. Bethesda, MD: American Association of Blood Banks (AABB); 2014.

62. Scott ML, et al. Epitopes on Rh proteins. *Vox Sang.* 2000;78(suppl 2):117–120.

63. Avent ND, et al. Site directed mutagenesis of the human Rh D antigen: molecular basis of D epitopes. *Vox Sang.* 2000;78(suppl 2):83–89.

64. Agre PC, et al. A proposal to standardize terminology for weak D antigen. *Transfusion.* 1992;32(1):86–87.

65. Flegel WA. Molecular genetics of RH and its clinical application. *Transfus Clin Biol.* 2006;13(1–2):4–12.

66. McGowan EC, et al. Diverse and novel RHD variants in Australian blood donors with a weak D phenotype: implication for transfusion management. *Vox Sang.* 2017;112(3):279–287.

67. Srivastava K, et al. The DAU cluster: a comparative analysis of 18 RHD alleles, some forming partial D antigens. *Transfusion.* 2016;56(10):2520–2531.

68. Prisco Arnoni C, et al. RHCE variants inherited with altered RHD alleles in Brazilian blood donors. *Transfus Med.* 2016;26(4):285–290.

69. Klein HG, Anstee DJ. *Mollison's Blood Transfusion in Clinical Medicine.* 12th ed. West Sussex, United Kingdom: John Wiley & Sons; 2014.

70. Mollison PL, et al. Suppression of primary RH immunization by passively-administered antibody. Experiments in volunteers. *Vox Sang.* 1969;16(4):421–439.

71. Woodrow JC, et al. Mechanism of Rh prophylaxis: an experimental study on specificity of immunosuppression. *Br Med J.* 1975;2(5962):57–59.

72. Stratton F. Rapid Rh-typing: a sandwich technique. *Br Med J.* 1955;1(4907):201–203.

73. Meyer E, Uhl L. A case for stocking O D+ red blood cells in emergency room trauma bays. *Transfusion.* 2015;55(4):791–795.

74. Goldfinger D, McGinniss MH. Rh-incompatible platelet transfusions–risks and consequences of sensitizing immunosuppressed patients. *N Engl J Med.* 1971; 284(17):942–944.

75. Weinstein R, et al. Prospective surveillance of D- recipients of D+ apheresis platelets: alloimmunization against D is not detected. *Transfusion.* 2015;55(6):1327–1330.

76. Cid J, et al. Low frequency of anti-D alloimmunization following D+ platelet transfusion: the Anti-D Alloimmunization after D-incompatible Platelet Transfusions (ADAPT) study. *Br J Haematol.* 2015;168(4):598–603.

77. Quan VA, et al. Rhesus immunization after renal transplantation. *Transplantation.* 1996;61(1):149–150.

78. Tormey CA, Fisk J, Stack G. Red blood cell alloantibody frequency, specificity, and properties in a population of male military veterans. *Transfusion.* 2008;48(10): 2069–2076.

79. Shirey RS, Edwards RE, Ness PM. The risk of alloimmunization to c (Rh4) in R1R1 patients who present with anti-E. *Transfusion.* 1994;34(9):756–758.

80. Daniels GL, et al. Terminology for red cell surface antigens. ISBT working party oslo report. International society of blood transfusion. *Vox Sang.* 1999;77(1):52–57.

81. Daniels G, et al. International Society of Blood Transfusion Committee on terminology for red cell surface antigens: Macao report. *Vox Sang.* 2009;96(2):153–156.

82. Grove-Rasmussen M. Routine compatibility testing: standards of the aabb as applied to compatibility tests. *Transfusion.* 1964;4:200–205.

83. Tovey GH. Preventing the incompatible blood transfusion. *Haematol (Budap).* 1974;8(1–4):389–391.

84. Wiener AS, et al. Studies on immunization in man. III. Immunization experiments with pooled human blood cells. *Exp Med Surg.* 1955;13(4):347–352.

85. Maurer C, Buttner J. The frequency of irregular erythrocyte antibodies (author's transl). *Dtsch Med Wochenschr.* 1975;100(30):1567–1570, 1573.

86. Daniels G, Green C. Expression of red cell surface antigens during erythropoiesis. *Vox Sang.* 2000;78(suppl 2):149–153.

87. Vaughan JI, et al. Inhibition of erythroid progenitor cells by anti-Kell antibodies in fetal alloimmune anemia. *N Engl J Med.* 1998;338(12):798–803.

88. Vaughan JI, et al. Erythropoietic suppression in fetal anemia because of Kell alloimmunization. *Am J Obstet Gynecol.* 1994;171(1):247–252.

89. Caine ME, Mueller-Heubach E. Kell sensitization in pregnancy. *Am J Obstet Gynecol.* 1986;154(1):85–90.

90. Mayne KM, Bowell PJ, Pratt GA. The significance of anti-Kell sensitization in pregnancy. *Clin Lab Haematol.* 1990;12(4):379–385.

91. Goh JT, et al. Anti-Kell in pregnancy and hydrops fetalis. *Aust N Z J Obstet Gynaecol.* 1993;33(2):210–211.

92. Bowman JM, et al. Maternal Kell blood group alloimmunization. *Obstet Gynecol.* 1992;79(2):239–244.

93. Frigoletto Jr FD. Anti-Kell and hydrops. *Am J Obstet Gynecol.* 1978;130(3):376.

94. Frigoletto FD, Davies IJ. Erythroblastosis fetalis with hydrops resulting from anti-Kell isoimmune disease. *Am J Obstet Gynecol.* 1977;127(8):887.

95. Scanlon JW, Muirhead DM. Hydrops fetalis due to anti-Kell isoimmune disease: survival with optimal long-term outcome. *J Pediatr.* 1976;88(3):484–485.

96. Hadley TJ, Peiper SC. From malaria to chemokine receptor: the emerging physiologic role of the Duffy blood group antigen. *Blood.* 1997;89(9):3077–3091.

97. Rojewski MT, Schrezenmeier H, Flegel WA. Tissue distribution of blood group membrane proteins beyond red cells: evidence from cDNA libraries. *Transfus Apher Sci.* 2006;35(1):71–82.

98. Goodrick MJ, Hadley AG, Poole G. Haemolytic disease of the fetus and newborn due to anti-Fy(a) and the potential clinical value of Duffy genotyping in pregnancies at risk. *Transfus Med.* 1997;7(4):301–304.

99. Noizat-Pirenne F, et al. Relative immunogenicity of Fya and K antigens in a Caucasian population, based on HLA class II restriction analysis. *Transfusion.* 2006;46(8): 1328–1333.

100. Miller LH, et al. The resistance factor to *Plasmodium vivax* in blacks. The Duffy-blood-group genotype, FyFy. *N Engl J Med.* 1976;295(6):302–304.

101. Horuk R, et al. A receptor for the malarial parasite *Plasmodium vivax*: the erythrocyte chemokine receptor. *Science.* 1993;261(5125):1182–1184.

102. He W, et al. Duffy antigen receptor for chemokines mediates trans-infection of HIV-1 from red blood cells to target cells and affects HIV-AIDS susceptibility. *Cell Host Microbe.* 2008;4(1):52–62.

103. Woodfield DG, et al. The Jk(a-b-) phenotype in New Zealand polynesians. *Transfusion.* 1982;22(4):276–278.

104. Lawicki S, Covin RB, Powers AA. The Kidd (JK) blood group system. *Transfus Med Rev.* 2016;31(3).

105. Hamilton JR. Kidd blood group system: a review. *Immunohematology.* 2015;31(1):29–35.

106. Rourk A, Squires JE. Implications of the Kidd blood group system in renal transplantation. *Immunohematology.* 2012;28(3):90–94.

107. Li X, et al. Identification of a specific region of *Plasmodium falciparum* EBL-1 that binds to host receptor glycophorin B and inhibits merozoite invasion in human red blood cells. *Mol Biochem Parasitol.* 2012;183(1): 23–31.

108. Wang HY, et al. Rapidly evolving genes in human. I. The glycophorins and their possible role in evading malaria parasites. *Mol Biol Evol.* 2003;20(11):1795–1804.

109. Issitt PD. Heterogeneity of anti-U. *Vox Sang.* 1990; 58(1):70–71.

110. Murakami J. MNSs blood group system and antibodies (anti-M, -N, -S and -S antibodies). *Nihon Rinsho.* 2010; 68(suppl 6):743–747.

111. Badjie KS, Tauscher CD, van Buskirk CM, et al. Red blood cell phenotype matching for various ethnic groups. *Immunohematology.* 2011;27(1):12–19.

CHAPTER 5

Pretransfusion Testing

LANCE A. WILLIAMS III, MD • SIERRA C. SIMMONS, MD, MPH •
HUY P. PHAM, MD, MPH

MEMBERS OF THE TRANSFUSION MEDICINE (OR BLOOD BANK) TEAM

A discussion of pretransfusion testing should begin with an introduction to the members of the transfusion medicine/blood bank team who perform, interpret, and/or oversight blood bank testing to ensure the quality and safety of blood products that are provided to patients. First, transfusion medicine physicians are typically pathologists subspecialized in transfusion medicine via a fellowship. Transfusion medicine fellowships provide an in-depth knowledge of all aspects of blood banking and typically educate the fellow on hemostasis/thrombosis as well. These physicians are usually ultimately responsible for the service with regard to regulatory perspective. They also interpret test results and are available for consultation to other clinical services.

Next, we have medical technologists (MTs) or medical laboratory technicians (MLTs). These individuals are trained to perform all the testing that both blood products and patient samples must undergo to be safely transfused. They are also trained in quality management and proficiency testing.

Last, a part of some transfusion medicine programs in the United States is the Transfusion Safety Officer (TSO). The TSO is responsible for being a bridge between the blood bank and the clinical services to ensure that the quality and safety of the blood product from the blood bank to the patient's bedside and beyond is as safe as possible. Furthermore, they help establish proper blood utilization and assist the hospital administration in minimizing blood product wastage. Oftentimes, the TSO is a registered nurse or a senior MT who can easily interact with multiple disciplines to enhance transfusion safety.[1,2]

PREPARATION OF BLOOD COMPONENTS

Briefly, blood bank products consist of mainly red blood cells (RBCs), plasma, platelets, and cryoprecipitate. Fig. 5.1 is a representation of how a unit of donated whole blood (WB) is processed to produce the aforementioned components. First, WB is lightly spun to produce platelet-rich plasma (PRP) and RBCs. The PRP is then placed in a hard spin to produce a platelet concentrate and plasma. Typically, the plasma is frozen, the platelets are kept at room temperature, and the RBCs are refrigerated. If the cryoprecipitate is desired, the fresh frozen plasma can be slowly thawed and spun to produce cryoprecipitate and cryopoor plasma.[2,3]

BASICS OF BLOOD BANK TESTING

Proper sample identification is one of the key aspects of pretransfusion safety that has evolved over many years. As you may know, both sample and blood product misidentifications are the leading causes of ABO-incompatible blood transfusions, which can lead to potentially fatal acute hemolytic transfusion reactions (AHTRs). AHTRs are sometimes a deadly consequence of ABO-incompatible transfusions.[4] To that end, regulatory and accrediting agencies [e.g., the American Association of Blood Banks (AABB)] require that samples be labeled with identifying information such as the patient's name, patient's medical record number, date and time of sample collection, and the phlebotomist identification or initials (Fig. 5.2).

Any blood sample that is mislabeled or not labeled with *all* the required information is rejected by the

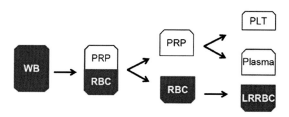

FIG. 5.1 Production of blood components from a unit of whole blood. *LRRBC*, leukoreduced RBCs; *PRP*, platelet-rich plasma; *RBC*, red blood cell; *WB*, whole blood. (From Williams LA, Fritsma MG, Marques MB. *Quick Guide to Transfusion Medicine*. 2nd ed. Washington, DC: AACC Press; 2014; with permission.)

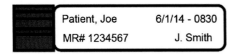

| Patient, Joe | 6/1/14 - 0830 |
| MR# 1234567 | J. Smith |

FIG. 5.2 Proper sample labeling. (From Williams LA, Fritsma MG, Marques MB. *Quick Guide to Transfusion Medicine*. 2nd ed. Washington, DC: AACC Press; 2014; with permission.)

blood bank staff, and the nurse/clinician is asked to recollect the sample.[5] All this is done to prevent what is termed 'Wrong Blood in Tube' (WBIT). A WBIT is where it is suspected that the wrong patient's blood is in a mislabeled tube. A WBIT has obvious negative consequences in that the wrong blood type may be assigned to the patient, thereby resulting in the wrong blood type being transfused to that patient.[2]

The next basic blood bank responsibility includes determination of the patient's blood type, performance of the antibody screen, and crossmatching. These will all be discussed in more detail later in this chapter. Determination of the patient's blood type involves determining the ABO and Rh type of the patient to ensure that ABO-compatible products are transfused. Antibody screening tries to detect any antibodies that are present with subsequent antibody identification, if necessary, via antibody panels. Finally, the crossmatch methods discussed later serve as a final safety check to verify compatibility between the recipient and donor.[6]

PRINCIPLES AND METHODOLOGIES OF BLOOD BANK TESTING

The most basic reactions that we observe in blood bank testing involve the idea of positive versus negative. In order for the blood bank technologist to identify whether an antibody and antigen reaction is occurring, the reaction is visualized in a tube, a gel column, or within a solid-phase well. A 'positive' reaction is the appearance of agglutination, graded 1+ to 4+, or the appearance of hemolysis within the sample. If there is no evidence of agglutination or hemolysis, then the reaction is considered 'negative.'

There are three general methodologies used to detect antigen-antibody reactions in the blood bank. The first and most basic form of testing is called "tube testing." This involves mixing the patient's plasma with either reagent red cells or donor red cells to test for antigen-antibody interactions. Tube testing may also utilize enhancement reagents such as polyethylene glycol (PEG) or low-ionic strength solution (LISS). After

incubation of the patient's plasma and reagent/donor's RBCs, the mixture is washed to remove any unbound IgG, and anti-human globulin (AHG) is added to facilitate IgG binding. The sample is then centrifuged and checked for agglutination or hemolytic reaction (i.e., a 'positive' reaction).[7]

The next type of testing that has evolved over the last 20 years is gel methodology. This involves mixing the patient's plasma with reagent or donor red cells on top of a gel column, followed by centrifugation to see if the mixture is able to pass through an AHG/IgG-coated well. The theory is that if the mixture of patient plasma and reagent or donor red cells is unable to pass cleanly through the IgG-coated gel then antigen-antibody binding has occurred, thus this is a positive test result. If the cells are able to pass all the way through the gel without getting 'stuck,' thus producing a pellet at the end of the column, then this is considered a negative test result.[8]

The last methodology commonly used in blood banks is termed solid-phase testing. It involves the use of wells coated with RBC antigens. The wells are incubated with the patient's plasma followed by addition of indicator cells coated with AHG. Next, the solid-phase well is centrifuged to see if an antigen-antibody interaction has occurred. If the antigen-antibody interaction has taken place, the well will show a diffuse pattern as the antigens and antibodies have attached to the AHG and IgG on the surface of the well. A negative reaction is represented by the formation of a small solid pellet at the center of the reaction well.[9]

ABO/Rh TYPING

ABO/Rh typing involves both a forward and a reverse reaction. During ABO forward type testing, the patient's RBCs are tested against commercial anti-A, anti-B, and anti-D reagents. The resulting reaction will determine what A, B, and Rh antigens are on the patient's RBC surface, if any. For example, a patient who is A+ will have both A and D antigens on their red cell surface. Therefore the anti-A tube will have agglutination, or be positive; the B tube will be negative; and the D or Rh tube will also have a positive reaction (see Table 5.1). Conversely, a patient with O negative (O–) blood type will have negative reactions, in the A, B, and D or Rh tubes.[4,6]

Next, the blood bank technologist will perform what is called a 'reverse type' reaction, where the patient's plasma is mixed with reagent A1 or B RBCs. This serves as verification of the accuracy of the forward blood type results. For example, the patient

TABLE 5.1
Examples of Forward and Reverse Typing Results for ABO/Rh

FORWARD TYPING			REVERSE TYPING		
Anti-A	**Anti-B**	**Anti-D**	**A1 RBCs**	**B RBCs**	**Interpretation**
Positive	Negative	Positive	Negative	Positive	*A positive*
Negative	Positive	Negative	Positive	Negative	*B negative*
Positive	Positive	Positive	Negative	Negative	*AB positive*
Negative	Negative	Negative	Positive	Positive	*O negative*

RBC, red blood cell.

TABLE 5.2
ABO Types: Antigens, Antibodies, and Frequencies

			PREVALENCE IN THE UNITED STATES	
ABO Type	**Antigens on RBC**	**Antibodies in Plasma/Plasma**	**Caucasian (%)**	**African American (%)**
O	None	Anti-A and anti-B	45	49
A	A	Anti-B	40	27
B	B	Anti-A	11	20
AB	A and B	none	4	4

RBC, red blood cell.
From Williams LA, Fritsma MG, Marques MB. *Quick Guide to Transfusion Medicine*. 2nd ed. Washington, DC: AACC Press; 2014; with permission.

mentioned earlier with blood type A would have anti-B in his or her plasma. Therefore in the reverse type of that particular patient the A1 antigen tube would be negative and the B antigen tube would show a positive reaction because he or she has anti-B that reacts against the reagent B-antigen RBCs. Conversely, the patient with O blood type will have results that are positive on the reverse type for both anti-A and anti-B. This is because patients with blood type O do not have any A or B antigens on their RBCs, therefore they will have anti-A and anti-B in their bloodstream to prevent them from being exposed to any blood that has those antigens (see Table 5.1). Of note, since anti-D is not a "naturally occurring" antibody, it is not part of reverse typing.[3]

ABO/Rh type determination is performed on patient blood as a way to prevent the patient from being transfused with the wrong ABO blood type. Typing is also performed on donor blood that is received into any blood bank before transfusion of that blood takes place. Regulatory agencies require that the ABO blood type be confirmed by the blood bank personnel before the blood is placed into the

inventory.[5] The various blood types and their representative percentages in the general population are shown in Table 5.2.[2]

Due to the concern over the transfusion of ABO-incompatible blood types to patients, regulatory and accrediting agencies have begun to ask blood banks to confirm the ABO type of the patient twice before transfusing any blood to that particular patient, unless the blood is needed emergently.[5] In the past, this was often accomplished by having two blood bank technologists test a single sample of blood from the patient. However, this policy has recently come under scrutiny, because of the thought that even though two blood bank technologists were testing the sample, the sample could have been initially drawn from the wrong patient. Thus new policies are aimed at having two different samples drawn at two different time periods. Hopefully, this will ensure that the correct patient's blood is being drawn. Any discrepancy between these two different samples would require investigation and possibly involve a third tube of blood being drawn from the patient. Of course, there are always human work-arounds to such a policy,

TABLE 5.3
ABO Discrepancy Examples

FORWARD TYPING		REVERSE TYPING		Screening Cells	Autocontrol	Possible Cause	Possible Resolution
Anti-A	Anti-B	A1 RBCs	B RBCs	Reagent RBCs	Patient RBCs		
0	0	0	0	0	0	Newborn or elderly patient with low immunoglobulin levels	Check medical record; incubate test at 4°C
4+	2+	0	4+	0	0	Acquired B phenotype	Check patient history for colon cancer diagnosis; test with anti-B lectin
0	0	4+	4+	4+	0	Bombay (O_h)	Test with anti-H lectin
4+	0	1+	4+	0	0	A subgroup with anti-A1	Test with anti-A1 lectin/*Dolichis biflorus*

RBC, red blood cell.
From Williams LA, Fritsma MG, Marques MB. *Quick Guide to Transfusion Medicine*. 2nd ed. Washington, DC: AACC Press; 2014; with permission.

and therefore, the challenge is to ensure that the two samples are not being drawn at the same time. This remains a logistical challenge for the blood bank leadership and for the TSO to accomplish/solve.[1]

Some complications that arise during ABO typing of the patient involve ABO discrepancies. An ABO discrepancy is considered to take place when the forward and reverse types are not in agreement. For example, a patient who types as A+ in the forward type but has both anti-A and anti-B in the reverse type would be considered have a discrepancy that requires investigation. There are many different reasons for ABO discrepancies, as described in Table 5.3[2] When there is a discrepancy in the patient's blood type, it is imperative that not only the blood bank technologist but also the transfusion medicine physician investigate it to solve the discrepancy, so that the patient may be safely transfused the correct blood type.[3]

Another complication during ABO/Rh testing is the concept of variant D (formerly known as weak D and/or partial D). Weak D, as described by most textbooks, is the presence of a decreased amount of D antigen on a patient's RBCs, leading to a weaker agglutination reaction when the patients RBCs are mixed with the anti-D reagent. In contrast, a patient with a mutated D antigen (i.e., partial D) is considered to have an altered form of the Rh/D antigen but will also typically have weaker than expected reactions when mixed with anti-D reagent.[4]

The controversy that has evolved over the past 5–10 years is how to differentiate between patients with weak-D and partial D RBCs. The clinical implication is that patients with most types of weak-D are not at risk of forming an anti-D after transfusion with D+ RBCs, whereas patients with partial D would be at risk of forming anti-D. The other clinical implication of such testing is whether mothers with the aforementioned D variants will require Rh immunoglobulin during or after delivery of their babies and/or at times when there is significant fetomaternal hemorrhage.

To date there has not been a truly reliable way of making this distinction serologically. However, recent guidelines from the College of American Pathologist and AABB direct blood banks to send out samples for genomic testing to clarify the patient's D antigen type, be it weak D or D variant. This is the only reliable method to correctly categorize these patients.[10,11]

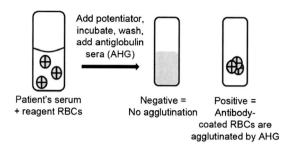

FIG. 5.3 Tube testing illustration. *AHG*, anti-human globulin; *RBC*, red blood cell. (From Williams LA, Fritsma MG, Marques MB. *Quick Guide to Transfusion Medicine*. 2nd ed. Washington, DC: AACC Press; 2014; with permission.)

TABLE 5.4										
Sample Antibody Screening Panel										
Screen Cell	**D**	**C**	**E**	**c**	**e**	**K**	**k**	**Fy^a**	**Fy^b**	**AHG**
I	+	+	0	0	+	0	+	0	+	4+
II	+	0	+	+	0	0	+	0	+	4+
III	0	0	0	+	+	+	+	+	+	0√

√, check cells were added and the negative reaction is valid; *AHG*, anti-human globulin phase (also called IAT or indirect anti-globulin test phase);

ANTIBODY SCREENING

Antibody screening is performed to identify previously undetected antibodies or to reconfirm antibodies that have been identified in the past. Antibody screening is often performed as part of a preoperative testing panel for patients who may require blood during surgery and is also performed during a hospital admission if blood transfusion is required.

If a patient has a previous history of antibodies or a recent history of transfusion, the antibody screen must be performed every 3 days to ensure that an antibody that would require special antigen requirements has not formed. Practically speaking, this is every 4 days, since the first day is counted as day 0. For example, if the patient had a screen performed on July 1, practically speaking, this screen will be good until midnight of July 4th.[5]

As stated in the introduction to this chapter, an antibody screen is performed by mixing the patient's plasma with reagent RBCs (see Fig. 5.3). These reagent RBCs are chosen for the variety of common clinically significant RBC antigens expressed on their surface. Typically, an antibody screen consists of three different reagent RBC mixtures, which contain a particular variety/mixture of common clinically significant RBC antigens (see Table 5.4). If the patient has an antibody to one of these reagent RBC antigens, then a positive reaction (i.e., agglutination or hemolysis) should occur. If the patient does not have an antibody to the reagent RBC antigen, then you would expect a negative reaction (i.e., no agglutination/no hemolysis).[12]

An antibody screen can be positive in only one or two of the test cells, or it can be positive in all the cells tested (i.e., panreactive). A negative reaction implies that there is no antibody present or that the antibody is not currently at a detectable level. The latter situation is the reason that once patients have a documented antibody, they must receive blood negative for that antigen for the rest of their life.[4] For example a patient

may have a negative antibody screen but has an undetectable Kidd antibody (termed evanescence). Once the patient is exposed to Kidd antigen–positive blood, antibody production will rapidly increase leading to the destruction of the antigen-positive transfused RBCs.

In essence, a positive antibody screen means that there is an antigen-antibody reaction that needs to be investigated further to determine its clinical significance. This is investigated within the blood bank by doing a full antibody panel, which is discussed in the next section.

As seen in Table 5.5, antibody testing performed in tubes is interpreted during three main phases: immediate spin (IS) phase, 37°C phase, and AHG phase. IS phase is performed by spinning the sample immediately after mixing the patient's plasma with the reagent or donor RBCs. A reaction at this phase is typical for cold antibodies or ABO antibodies (i.e., IgM antibodies that do not require enhancement to react). Antibodies detected in IS phase are typically not clinically significant, with the exception of anti-A and anti-B antibodies.

After interpreting the IS phase, enhancement media such as LISS or PEG are added (to allow the cells to come closer together) and the sample is incubated at 37°C. This phase is used to detect strong IgM or IgG antibodies that react at warmer temperatures. The sample can be centrifuged and checked for a positive reaction (typically hemolysis) after incubation. In the AHG phase, after washing, AHG is added to the sample to enhance IgG antibody agglutination. Since IgG is a monomer, it is necessary to add AHG to bind enough red cells together to cause agglutination visible to the naked eye. Antibodies discovered in this phase are typically considered to be clinically significant.[12]

ANTIBODY PANELS (ALSO CALLED ANTIBODY WORKUPS)

The purpose of an antibody panel is to more fully investigate the positive antibody screen because it contains only three reagent RBCs. Antibody panels are

TABLE 5.5
Example of an Antibody Panel

	RH						MNS				LU		P	LEWIS		KELL		DUFFY		KIDD		PEG		
	D	C	E	c	e	f	M	N	S	s	Lu^a	Lu^b	P1	Le^a	Le^b	K	k	Fy^a	Fy^b	Jk^a	Jk^b	IS	37	IAT
1	+	+	0	0	+	0	+	+	+	+	0	+	+	+	0	0	+	0	+	0	+	0	NHS	2+
2	0	0	0	+	+	+	+	0	+	0	0	+	0	0	+	+	0	+	+	+	0	0	NHS	0√
3	0	0	+	+	0	0	0	+	0	+	0	+	+	0	+	+	+	+	0	0	+	0	NHS	2+
4	+	0	+	+	0	0	+	+	+	+	0	+	+	0	+	0	+	0	+	+	+	0	NHS	0√
5	+	0	0	+	+	+	+	+	0	+	0	+	+	0	0	0	0	+	0	0	+	0	NHS	0√
6	0	0	0	+	+	+	+	0	+	+	0	+	+	+	0	0	+	+	+	0	+	0	NHS	0√

√, check cells were added and the negative reaction is valid; *IAT*, indirect anti-globulin test phase; *NHS*, no hemolysis seen; *PEG*, polyethylene glycol.

much more extensive than the antibody screen in that they mix the patients plasma with anywhere from 10 to 20 reagent RBCs that have various mixes of RBCs with defined antigenic profiles on their surface (see Table 5.5 for an example of an antibody panel). It is important to point out that reagent red cells will always be of blood type O. Therefore any anti-A or anti-B (e.g., a type A patient will have naturally occurring anti-B, and vice versa) that is present in the patient's plasma will not interfere with the interpretation of the panel. Essentially, the purpose of an antibody panel is to detect antibodies that are present in the patient's plasma that are not ABO antibodies.[3]

Additionally, at the end of any antibody panel the blood bank technologist will often run what is called an 'autocontrol'. An autocontrol is performed by mixing the patient's plasma with their own RBCs. A positive autocontrol implies that the patient has antibodies to self-antigens in their plasma. Typically, an autoantibody will cause all the panel cells to be positive or 'panreactive.' An autoantibody is an antibody against a very common RBC antigen, sometimes with Rh-like specificity. In this setting, patients have almost the same reaction against their own red cells as they would have against transfused red cells.[13]

The interpretation of antibody panels can run from simple to very complex. A very simple example would include an antibody to anti-E. Anti-E is very easily identified by using the process for ruling in and ruling out antibodies (see later discussion for further explanation). However, most antibody panels are not that simple.

For example, if a patient has multiple antibodies, the blood bank technologists will often have to run multiple panel cells or run multiple panels to confirm

the multiple antibodies that are present and rule out those that are not.

Process for ruling in or ruling out antibodies:
1. Review the overall pattern of reactivity and the phases in which the reactivity occurs.
2. Review the results of the autocontrol.
3. Use negative cells to rule out antigens that are present on the panel cell.
4. After you have ruled out as many cells as possible, see if any of the remaining antibodies fit the pattern of positive reactions that remain.
5. If necessary, choose another panel to complete the rule out process and positively identify the antibody present.

Another complicated antibody panel result is when the patient has an antibody against a high-frequency antigen. This pattern of antibody reactivity often involves somewhat panreactivity of the antibody panel but has a negative autocontrol. The negative autocontrol lets the blood bank technologist know that the patient does not have an autoantibody but rather an antibody against a very common antigen. This also differs from an autoantibody in that it is an alloantibody, meaning it was formed after exposure to the foreign antigen. In these instances, often special panels will be performed to confirm the presence of antibody against the high-frequency antigen or the patient sample will have to be sent out to a reference laboratory to confirm its presence.[3]

Last, there is the antibody pattern that results in an interpretation of nonspecific antibodies. These are antibodies that do not fit a particular pattern within the antibody panel, but reactivity is still present, therefore the presence of a yet unknown antibody is still possible. This also could be the result of a nonspecific

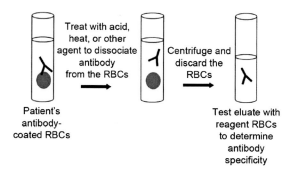

FIG. 5.4 Elution procedure. *RBC*, red blood cell. (From Williams LA, Fritsma MG, Marques MB. *Quick Guide to Transfusion Medicine*. 2nd ed. Washington, DC: AACC Press; 2014; with permission.)

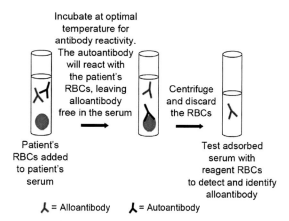

FIG. 5.5 Autoadsorption procedure. *RBC*, red blood cell. (From Williams LA, Fritsma MG, Marques MB. *Quick Guide to Transfusion Medicine*. 2nd ed. Washington, DC: AACC Press; 2014; with permission.)

antigen-antibody reaction that is not likely to be of clinical significance.[7]

As mentioned earlier, warm autoantibodies represent another common antibody pattern to interpret (panreactive screen, panreactive panel, and positive autocontrol). The screen and the panel are typically only reactive in the AHG phase but not in the IS or the 37°C phase. Another clue to a patient having a warm autoantibody is a positive direct agglutination test (DAT). This test can detect the presence of IgG and C3 on the surface of the patient's RBCs. In patients with a warm autoantibody the polyspecific (IgG and C3) DAT is positive, the monospecific IgG is positive, and the monospecific C3 is positive about 50% of the time. In contrast, the DAT for patients with a cold autoantibody will be positive for C3 but negative for IgG. As mentioned earlier, the presence of warm autoantibodies imply that patients have a similar risk of hemolyzing their own cells as they hemolyze any donor cells that are transfused. However, the true danger of warm autoantibodies is that they may mask or "cover up" clinically significant alloantibodies, such as anti-C and anti-E; thus special techniques are required to uncover these underlying alloantibodies.[14]

The first such technique is called elution (see Fig. 5.4). This is performed with using acid or heat to remove antibodies from the patient's RBCs. The antibodies that are attached will be washed off and transferred into another tube, called the "eluate," which is essentially a concentrate of the detached antibodies. This eluate will then be mixed with an antibody panel to determine the type of antibodies that are causing the positive DAT. If reactivity is present on scattered panel cells, this could indicate that an alloantibody is present with no autoantibody. However, if the panel is panreactive, this could indicate either a lone autoantibody or an autoantibody with underlying/concealed alloantibodies.[7]

If the latter is true, additional special techniques will be necessary to separate the autoantibodies from the alloantibodies. Therefore the next step in the workup of a warm autoantibody is to perform an autoadsorption (see Fig. 5.5). An autoadsorption attempts to remove the autoantibody from the eluate while leaving any underlying alloantibodies behind for possible detection.[12]

As long as the patient has not been transfused within the past 90 days, an autoadsorption can be performed. An autoadsorption is performed by mixing the patient's plasma with the patient's own RBCs. The theory behind this is that the patient's own blood cells will adsorb the autoantibody that is present in the plasma. If the reactivity is removed after the autoadsorption is performed, the presence of alone autoantibody is confirmed. Therefore the blood bank will confirm that no clinically significant antibodies to common RBC antigens are present. If, however, reactivity remains after the autoadsorption has taken place, then additional panels must be performed to identify the potentially clinically significant alloantibodies. As mentioned earlier, the blood bank usually performs an autoadsorption only if a patient has not been exposed to foreign RBCs via transfusion during the last 90 days. If they have been exposed during the last 90 days, then a special technique called alloadsorption will need to take place, typically at a reference laboratory.[13] The details of alloadsorption are beyond the scope of this chapter.

Cold autoantibodies are the last complicated antibody panel that we will discuss. Cold autoantibodies demonstrate panreactivity to the IS and 37°C phase of testing, but unlike warm autoantibodies they are typically negative at the AHG phase of testing.

Like warm autoantibodies, cold autoantibodies can conceal other antibodies, although this is less common because most clinically significant antibodies are reactive only at the AHG phase.

One of the techniques that will resolve cold autoantibody reactivity is prewarming, which involves warming the patient's plasma/donor or reagent RBC mixture during antibody identification. Once the sample is warmed the reaction is typically negative, since the antibody in these cases is not reactive at warmer temperatures and thus cannot create an antigen-antibody interaction.[7,12] After confirming the presence of the cold autoantibody, the clinical strategy involves infusion of any transfused blood via a blood warmer. A blood warmer is a device in which the blood infusion tubing is wrapped around a warm cylinder, thus warming the blood right before it reaches the patient's vascular access site.

In some instances, the blood bank technologist will be asked to confirm the exact temperature at which a cold antibody is reacting, termed thermal amplitude testing.[12] This is particularly important for patients who might undergo surgery during which the temperature of the room is decreased, such as coronary artery bypass grafting (CABG) surgeries. During CABG surgeries, the temperature is often decreased during a portion of the surgery. During this period of lower temperature, a patient's cold autoantibody could become reactive and start hemolyzing either his or her own red cells or any transfused red cells. Thus thermal amplitude testing maybe performed to find the exact temperature at which the antibody is reactive (i.e., causing agglutination or hemolysis). Results of thermal amplitude testing will let the surgeon know how cool the room can be made without having any adverse effect on the patient.

Any of these additional manipulations of patient samples take additional time to finalize the workup, and clinicians need to know that these steps cannot be shortened because of the inherent complexities of testing. In case of emergent transfusion, although the workup is not completed, RBC units can be released but the patient's physician needs to sign an "emergency release" form accepting the risk of hemolysis and that the benefit of transfusion outweighs these risks.

PHENOTYPING

The final step on identification of an antibody is called phenotyping. Theoretically, in order for a patient to form an antibody the corresponding antigen must be lacking. If the patient is exposed to the antigen then he or she may form an antibody. For example, for a patient to form an anti-E, the E antigen must be lacking, therefore at the end of an antibody identification panel the blood bank technologist will often test the patient's RBCs for the absence of that particular antigen unless the patient was recently transfused.[12]

CROSSMATCHING

Crossmatching can be thought of as the final step in ensuring the safety of transfusion between a donor and a patient. Typically, crossmatching is performed on RBC products that will be transfused to a given recipient. The only time that platelets require crossmatching is when they contain 2 mL RBCs or more per the AABB Standards. Plasma and cryoprecipitate do not require any crossmatching because they are devoid of RBCs.[5]

Crossmatching (see Table 5.6) is performed by mixing patient plasma with donor RBCs. If a patient has a negative antibody screen, there are two options for crossmatching the patient. Because the patient does not have any apparent antibodies present and there is no history of antibodies or any recent history of pregnancy/transfusion, the patient is potentially eligible for two types of crossmatching. The first type is termed IS crossmatching. In this type of crossmatching, the patient's plasma is mixed with a few drops of donor blood; the mixture is centrifuged, washed, and centrifuged again; and then the reaction is read as positive or negative. The second type is termed electronic crossmatch. This is simply done by a computer using the patient's existing information. The unit of blood is scanned into the system, and the patient's known blood type is compared with the blood type of this particular unit. If the two types are compatible, then the unit is released to the patient. Patients are eligible for electronic crossmatching if their blood type has been confirmed twice, they have no history of transfusion or pregnancy within the past 90 days, and they have no known history of antibodies.[2,5,6]

For patients with a known antibody history or a current antibody history, a third type of crossmatching is required, known as extended crossmatching. In this type of crossmatching, a sample of the patient's plasma and the donor RBCs are mixed together with an enhancement agent, such as LISS or PEG. The mixture is allowed to incubate for a period of 30–45 min to allow for the antigen-antibody interaction to occur. After incubation and washing, AHG is added to further enhance any agglutination, the specimen is washed and spun, and the sample is read for reactivity. If

TABLE 5.6
Comparison of Crossmatch Methods

Type of Crossmatch	Procedure	Detects	Indication/Requirements
Immediate spin	Patient plasma and donor red cells are mixed, centrifuged, and examined for agglutination or hemolysis	ABO incompatibility	No clinically significant antibodies shown by antibody detection test or history review
Antiglobulin	Patient plasma and donor red cells are incubated at 37°C and an antiglobulin test is performed	Incompatibility due to ABO or other clinically significant antibodies (including autoantibodies)	Must be performed if clinically significant antibodies are shown in antibody detection test or history review
Electronic	Validated computer system is used to verify ABO compatibility between donor and recipient	ABO incompatibility	No clinically significant antibodies shown by antibody detection test or history review. Requires two separate determinations of ABO type and extensive computer system validation

antigen-negative units have been chosen because of the patient's antibodies, then you would expect the extended crossmatch to be negative.[12] One caveat to this situation is if a patient has a warm autoantibody, in this setting, the crossmatch can still be incompatible, especially if the adsorptions were unsuccessful, or if "neat" (i.e., unabsorbed) patient plasma is used for the crossmatch.

In the end, a unit of blood will be either compatible or incompatible with its intended recipient. Compatible blood will result in a negative (i.e., no agglutination or visible hemolysis) reaction. Incompatible results will demonstrate agglutination or hemolysis, thus another unit should be chosen or further investigation should take place for an antibody that was missed during the initial testing.

It is important to note that "compatibility" at the time of crossmatch does not always guarantee that the blood will be compatible in vivo. As an example, due to their evanescence, Kidd antibodies (mentioned earlier) are notorious for causing in vivo hemolysis in patients with recently negative antibody screens (i.e., their presence is below the level of detection by the test). Kidd antibodies often disappear initially but come back briskly once the patient is exposed to the Kidd antigen again via transfusion. Thus a patient with a Kidd antibody will often have a negative antibody screen but will hemolyze units transfused rather briskly once antigen reexposure has taken place.[3,15]

The process of selecting compatible units for patients is determined by whether or not the patient

TABLE 5.7
Compatible ABO Types for Transfusion of RBCs and Plasma

Recipient Type	RBCs No Foreign Antigen Infused	Plasma No Antibody against Recipient RBC Infused
A	A or O	A or AB
B	B or O	B or AB
AB	AB, A, B, or O	AB
O	O	O, A, B, or AB

RBC, red blood cell.

has any antibodies. If a patient has no history of previous antibodies and has a negative antibody screen, the blood bank technologist will select blood that is ABO compatible with the patient (see Table 5.7 for compatible types). Once this blood is selected, the crossmatch will take place, and if compatible, the blood will be released to the patient.

In patients who have a current or previous history of antibodies, the so-called antigen-negative units will be selected for crossmatching and transfusion. For example, if a patient has an Fy^a antibody, Fy^a-antigen-negative units will be selected for crossmatching and transfusion. In patients with only one or two antibodies, this typically is not a difficult process; however, some patients have multiple antibodies or they

TABLE 5.8
Blood Group Systems and Antigen Frequencies

Blood Group System	Antigen	Antigen Frequency %	% Donor Blood Compatible (Antigen Negative)
Rh	D	85	15
	C	70	30
	E	30	70
	c	80	20
	e	98	2
Kell	K	9	91
	Kp^a	2	98
	Js^a	0.1 Caucasians 19.5 African Americans	99.9 Caucasians 80 African Americans
	k, Kp^b, Js^b	99.9	0.1
Duffy	Fy^a	*66	34
	Fy^b	*85	15 *Note: 68% of African Americans are Fy(a–b–)
Kidd	Jk^a	77	23
	Jk^b	72	28
MNS	M	78	22
	N	72	28
	S	55	45
	s	89	11
P	P$_1$	80	20
Lewis	Le^a	22	78
	Le^b	72	28 *Note: 22% of African Americans are Le(a–b–)
Lutheran	Lu^a	8	92
	Lu^b	99.9	0.1

have antibodies to high-frequency antigens, which may require obtaining blood from outside sources, sometimes even including a national search among rare units. For example, it would be difficult to obtain blood for a patient with anti-E, anti-Jk^b, anti-Fy^a, and anti-s, as it would be for a patient with anti-e.

The difficulty of finding compatible units can be determined by utilizing antigen frequency charts (see Table 5.8) and/or by calculating the percentage of antigen-negative units likely found in the donor population. For instance, if a patient has anti-E, finding units will be relatively easy because 70% of donors will lack this antigen. However, if a patient has anti-E and Fy^b, the likelihood of finding antigen-negative units drops to only 11%. This is determined by multiplying the antigen-negative frequencies together as follows: antigen negative for E = 70% or 0.70, antigen negative for Fy^b = 15% or 0.15, thus $0.70 \times 0.15 = 0.11$ or 11%. For cases where blood will be difficult to find, the transfusion medicine physician will often notify the clinical team in case a surgery may need to be postponed until compatible units are found.[2]

CONCLUSION
This chapter has provided an overview of the testing that takes place within the blood bank/transfusion service to ensure the highest quality and safest possible blood products transfused to patients in need. This chapter has also provided an overview of the basic interpretation that takes place by the transfusion medicine specialist(s), while outlining the role of the TSO in the blood bank/hospital system. Put together, these elements are an essential component toward ensuring that patients receive the safest blood products available.

REFERENCES
1. Brown M, Fritsma M, Marques M. Transfusion safety: what has been done; what is still needed? *MLO Med Lab Obs.* 2005;37(11). 20, 22–23, 26.
2. Williams LA, Fritsma MGF, Marques MB. *Quick Guide to Transfusion Medicine.* 2nd ed. Washington, DC: AACC Press; 2014.
3. Pham HP, Williams LA, eds. *Transfusion Medicine, Apheresis, and Hemostasis: Review Questions and Case Studies.* London, UK: Elsevier; 2017.
4. Fung MK, Grossman BJ, Hillyer CD, Westhoff CM, eds. *Technical Manual.* 18th ed. Bethesda, MD: AABB Press; 2014.
5. Ooley PW, ed. *AABB Standards.* 30th ed. Bethesda, MD: AABB Press; 2016.
6. PR H. *Basic and Applied Concepts of Blood Banking and Transfusion Practices.* 3rd ed. St. Louis, MO: Mosby; 2013.
7. Blaney KD, Howard PR. *Basic and Applied Concepts of Immunohematology.* 2nd ed. St. Louis, MO: Elsevier-Mosby; 2008.
8. Nathalang O. The gel test: twelve-year's experience in Thailand. *J Med Assoc Thai.* 2005;88(suppl 3):S325–S329.

9. Dwyre DM, Erickson Y, Heintz M, Elbert C, Strauss RG. Comparative sensitivity of solid phase versus PEG enhancement assays for detection and identification of RBC antibodies. *Transfus Apher Sci.* 2006;35(1):19–23.

10. Sandler SG, Flegel WA, Westhoff CM, et al. It's time to phase in RHD genotyping for patients with a serologic weak D phenotype. College of American Pathologists transfusion medicine resource committee work group. *Transfusion.* 2015;55(3):680–689.

11. Flegel WA, Westhoff CA, Denomme GA, Delaney M, Keller MA. *Joint Statement on Phasing-in RHD Genotyping for Pregnant Women and Other Females of Childbearing Potential with a Serologic Weak Phenotype.* http://www.aabb.org/advocacy/statements/Pages/statement150722.aspx. Accessed Dec 12, 2017.

12. Harmening DM. *Modern Blood Banking and Transfusion Practices.* 6th ed. Chicago, IL: F.A. David; 2012.

13. Reardon JE, Marques MB. Laboratory evaluation and transfusion support of patients with autoimmune hemolytic anemia. *Am J Clin Pathol.* 2006;125(suppl 1):S71–S77.

14. Wheeler CA, Calhoun L, Blackall DP. Warm reactive autoantibodies; clinical and serologic correlations. *Am J Clin Pathol.* 2004;122(1):680–685.

15. Reid ME, Lomas-Francis C, Olsson ML. *The Blood Group Antigens FactsBook.* 3rd ed. London, UK: Elsevier; 2012.

CHAPTER 6

Indications for Transfusion and Dosing of Blood Components

MICHELLE L. ERICKSON, MD, MBA

MODIFICATION OF BLOOD PRODUCTS

Understanding the modifications that can be made to blood products is essential for improving patient safety and tolerability. Many blood banks are capable of modifying products on site, or they can order specific product modifications. All blood product modifications are costly and time consuming. Clinician understanding of available and appropriate modifications preserves valuable blood bank time and resources while leading to better outcomes for patients. All blood modification requires precise labeling and oversight by the Food and Drug Administration (FDA).[1]

Leukoreduction

Leukocyte reduction is the process of filtering blood to remove the donor white blood cells (WBCs) from the product, ideally at the time of donation but sometimes at the bedside of the patient. Bedside leukoreduction is associated with hypotensive transfusion reactions[2] and does not mitigate the effects of the stored leukocytes releasing cytokines and pyrogens into the transfusion media.[3] Prestorage removal of leukocytes is preferred because it reduces the risk of cytomegalovirus (CMV) transmission, febrile nonhemolytic transfusion reaction, transfusion-related immunomodulation (TRIM), postoperative infection, alloimmunization, and platelet refractoriness.[4] Leukoreduced units are CMV safe and can be used for immunosuppressed patients.[5–7] Although the need for universal leukoreduction has been controversial, most patients meeting strict guidelines for transfusion also meet the indications for leukopoor blood products. Prestorage leukodepleted blood products are now the standard of care in many institutions.

Standards for leukoreduction in the United States are defined and required by the FDA and the American Association of Blood Banks (AABB).[8] Leukocyte-reduced products are filtered soon after donation during their initial preparation, depleting the numbers of red blood cells (RBCs) or platelets. After a brief cooling period, the RBC products are passed through a filter that removes significant numbers of WBCs, reducing the number of WBCs from $1–3 \times 10^9$[9,10] to less than 5×10^6, with a residual product of at least 85% of the original RBC content, as required by the FDA.[11] For platelets isolated from a whole blood donation, standards require WBCs to be reduced to less than 8.3×10^5 per unit, for 95% of products tested, with at least 75% of the products containing a minimum of 5.5×10^{10} platelets.[12]

Leukoreduction is not an alternative for irradiation or washing and does not prevent graft-versus-host disease (GvHD) or allergic transfusion reactions.

Washed Blood Products

Washing is a pretransfusion process in which a unit of RBCs or platelets is rinsed, centrifuged, and resuspended in saline before transfusion, to remove cellular debris, potassium, and plasma protein component. Plasma (fresh frozen plasma [FFP]) and cryoprecipitate, of course, cannot be washed. Washing compromises the blood product, shortens the shelf life, and tends to reduce the volume of the product by about 20% for RBCs and 33% for platelets.[13] Additionally, it requires significant technologist time. Because of the damage to the product and the cost and time involved in preparation, washed blood products should be ordered only when absolutely required for patient benefit. The classic clinical indications for washing include known patient hypersensitivity to specific plasma components, for example, anti-IgA antibody in IgA-deficient patients.[14] Patients with multiple severe or escalating allergic transfusion reactions to blood products containing plasma also may require washed RBCs and platelet products to remove the offending plasma protein. Neonatal exchange transfusions and pediatric patients may require washed products to remove plasma components, potassium, and anticoagulant preservative solutions. Washing of a blood product does not reduce the risk of transfusion reactions other than allergic reactions and is not a substitute for irradiation or leukoreduction. Placing a washed product restriction on a patient increases the turnaround time for product preparation and may cause significant delay in procuring plasma products if the patient needs them.

Irradiated Blood Products

Blood irradiation is accomplished by exposing blood to a minimum of 25 Gy (2500 cGy) of radiation at the center of the container, thus preventing the replication and engraftment of immunologically competent donor T leukocytes to the recipient. Because GvHD caused by donor engraftment is fatal in most cases,[15] irradiated blood products should be provided to patients at risk whenever time and resources allow. Patients at high risk for GvHD include those with severe immunosuppression, bone marrow or stem cell transplant, cytotoxic chemotherapy (especially purine analogs), congenital immune deficiency, neonatal or intrauterine transfusion, genetically similar recipient-donor pairs, human leukocyte antigen (HLA)–matched platelet infusion, and Hodgkin disease. Other clinical indications for irradiation of blood components include acute leukemia, lymphoma, solid tumors with intensive chemotherapy or radiotherapy, exchange transfusions, solid organ transplant recipients, and premature infants. Patients with human immunodeficiency virus/acquired immunodeficiency syndrome have not been reported to be susceptible to transfusion-related GvHD and thus do not require irradiation of their blood products.[16] Irradiation damages the RBC membrane, causing potassium leakage and a shortened shelf-life for the unit.[17]

Cytomegalovirus-Negative Blood Products

CMV dwells in the leukocytes of blood components and thus can be transmitted via transfusion to susceptible, CMV-negative and immunosuppressed patients. Donors can be tested for CMV, and those found negative provide CMV-negative blood units. However, studies show that leukoreduced blood is as efficacious as CMV-negative blood at preventing CMV transmission. The benefit of a CMV-negative unit over a CMV-safe leukoreduced unit is theoretical, thus CMV-negative and leukoreduced units are recommended only in cases in which the patient is known to be CMV negative and the CMV infection would be occult and untreatable, for example, for intrauterine transfusions.[5,6]

Volume-Reduced Red Blood Cells and Platelets

In cases of severe cardiac compromise and high risk for transfusion-associated circulatory overload (TACO), a product may be centrifuged and the supernatant storage media removed. This is mostly used for infants and intrauterine transfusions, where minute volumes are being transfused and patients are at high risk. Reducing the volume of a product causes loss of RBCs and platelets and may affect platelet function. The procedure requires extra time for processing and results in a shortened shelf life of 24 h at 1–6 °C, or 4 h at 20–24 °C.[18]

USE OF RED BLOOD CELLS

RBC transfusion is indicated to improve oxygen carrying capacity during periods of profound anemia when there is evidence of severe symptomology or end organ damage. This may be via simple transfusion or RBC exchange transfusion, for example, to patients with sickle cell anemia. Because of the potential for serious transfusion reactions, lack of evidence for improved patient outcomes, and growing concern for worse outcomes, liberal transfusion strategies are no longer recommended for the majority of patients. For many physicians, this is a dramatic change in practice from prior years. Numerous publications have advocated restrictive transfusion guidelines, with abundant supporting evidence. Transfusion should be viewed as a simple risk-benefit evaluation, with the acuity of need for oxygen delivery balanced against the evidence of risk associated with each unit delivered. Unless a patient is acutely hemorrhaging, units can be given slowly with reassessment between each unit to prevent overtransfusion. Best practice utilizes the minimum dose required to correct the deficiency.

Assessment and Communication of the Patient's Clinical Status

It is essential that an evaluation of the patient's clinical status be completed and communicated to the blood bank along with complete patient information when ordering or retrieving products. Many hospital systems now use electronic ordering. However, orders often do not distinguish acutely bleeding patients from those who are stable. The individual tasked with communicating with the blood bank should be prepared with all relevant patient information and a basic history to help the blood bank prioritize and plan for the patient's course of care. For the massively bleeding patient, personnel and extensive resources will need to be devoted, inventory assessed, and products prepared. For a stable, chronically anemic patient, care can be planned around the timeline of transfusion. The usual response given to blood bank technologists requesting more information is "the patient is bleeding" or "the patient is anemic," but of course all transfused patients meet these descriptions. Also unhelpful is the courier who appears at the blood bank window demanding blood products for "the bleeding guy." More useful information to the blood bank are brief descriptions such as "massive trauma due to a motor vehicle accident," "splenic rupture," "maternal hemorrhage after delivery with 2 L lost," or "stable elderly patient with severe iron deficiency." Computerized ordering is accurate and reliable, but a brief phone call confirms the situation and urgency.

Indications for Red Blood Cell Transfusion
Severe hemorrhage or massive transfusion
Massive transfusion is defined as the rapid replacement of a significant portion of the patient's blood volume due to a hemorrhage that compromises not only the oxygen carrying capacity but also coagulation and platelet function. Clinical signs and symptoms should guide the assessment for massive hemorrhage. Patients with acute hemorrhage of 40% or more or with 30% hemorrhage and signs of instability should be transfused. Laboratory testing should be done immediately and repeated frequently until hemostasis is attained. Testing should include hemoglobin and/or hematocrit, platelet count, prothrombin time, international normalized ratio (INR), and fibrinogen level to evaluate the needs for transfusion support. Some facilities use viscoelastic testing such as thromboelastography (TEG) or rotational thromboelastometry, whereas others may offer more traditional laboratory panels. If a massive transfusion program or protocol is available, it should be initiated for best outcomes. Once the trigger for massive transfusion has been recognized, it is essential to begin a 1:1:1 transfusion regimen with a focus on infusion of the "yellow" products (FFP and platelets) as soon as possible to prevent development of coagulopathy. Transfusion of appropriate ratios of products continues until hemostasis is achieved.[19]

Acute hemorrhage in the unstable patient
Patients with ongoing bleeding and a hematocrit less than 30% or hemoglobin less than 10.0 g/dL qualify for transfusion. These patients are prone to rapid decompensation and may not show an adequate response to crystalloids alone. Signs and symptoms indicating the need for transfusion include systolic blood pressure less than 90, acute decrease of systolic or diastolic blood pressure, tachycardia, tachypnea greater than 30–40 bpm, oliguria or anuria, delayed capillary refill, diaphoresis, cold and pale skin, or acute mental status changes with anxiety, confusion,

and lethargy. Other immediate indications for transfusion in the acutely bleeding patient include pretransfusion hemoglobin less than 8.0 g/dL or hematocrit less than 24%. Patients with trauma with hemoglobin less than 10 g/dL or hematocrit less than 30% during the acute resuscitation phase may require transfusion even when the massive transfusion protocol is not initiated. Transfusion should be considered for the patient with traumatic brain injury and hemoglobin less than 10 g/dL or hematocrit less than 30%. Patients with ongoing bleeding and hematocrit less than 30% or hemoglobin less than 10.0 g/dL usually qualify for transfusion. Possible exceptions are patients with acute upper gastrointestinal tract bleeding, for whom evidence shows better outcomes with restrictive transfusion (less than 7.0 g/dL).[20]

Patients in the intensive care unit who are critically ill
Multiple studies have examined the hemodynamically stable but critically ill patient in the intensive care unit. In this cohort, a restrictive transfusion policy is recommended, with avoidance of transfusion unless hemoglobin is less than 7.0 g/dL or hematocrit is less than 21%.[21-27] A review examining evidence for this guideline summarized that 12,587 patients in 31 studies were evaluated and lower mortality rates were observed in the restrictive transfusion group.[28] Overall, patients on a restrictive transfusion protocol have outcomes as good or better than those on a liberal protocol.[29]

Stable patients with chronic anemia
Patients with stable or chronic anemia adapt remarkably well to their lower hemoglobin and hematocrit baseline and should not be transfused until they meet the guidelines. Whenever possible, the reason for anemia must be elucidated and corrected. For example, iron deficiency anemia should be treated with iron replacement and blood transfusion should be avoided. For otherwise "healthy" patients, a transfusion can be deferred until the hematocrit and hemoglobin levels are less than 21% and 7.0 g/dL, respectively. Some chronically anemic patients tolerate levels lower than this and still perform their daily activities without adverse effect. A patient who has been functioning in the community or who is asymptomatic does not necessarily warrant a transfusion. For other patients with comorbidities putting them at risk of end organ damage, a guideline of 8.0% and 24% is appropriate. Comorbidities to consider include congestive heart failure, renal dysfunction, chronic obstructive pulmonary disease, and coronary artery disease.

Anemia in the elderly

The elderly patient poses a challenge to the treating physician because they have higher rates of anemia and are more likely to have underlying comorbidities, slower recovery times, and less capability to tolerate a physiologic insult. Rates of anemia in those older than 65 years are estimated at 10%, increasing to over 20% in the population older than 85 years.[30] About a third of these cases are due to renal failure and another third are due to iron, folate, or B12 deficiencies. For the stable elderly patient, a thorough assessment of the clinical status is first recommended to assess evidence of end organ damage, comorbidities, risk for fall, functional status, and the cause of the anemia. Laboratory workup and correction of iron and vitamin deficiencies are indicated. A subset of elderly patients will require transfusion support, and for those with symptoms or comorbidities, hemoglobin of 8 g/dL and hematocrit of 24%–25% are appropriate minimum triggers. For the elderly patient who remains symptomatic and at risk for syncopal events, or shows evidence of end organ compromise, higher goals of hemoglobin above 9 are appropriate.[31] Studies have not shown benefit to transfusion above a hemoglobin of 10 g/dL and hematocrit of 30%.[32] Furthermore, these patients are at high risk for transfusion reactions, including an increased risk for TACO.[33] When needed, slow transfusion of a single unit with posttransfusion reassessment is recommended.

Anemia in the patient with cancer

Studies have begun to evaluate transfusion for patients with cancer, some raising concern that the immunomodulatory effect of RBC transfusion potentiates more rapid growth of the tumor with shorter time until recurrence.[34] Some studies have shown increased adverse events and cancer recurrence associated with intraoperative transfusion for cancer,[35,36] whereas others warn about increased major postoperative complications in patients who are undertransfused.[37] For gynecologic, colon, esophageal, gastric, colorectal liver metastatic, hepatobiliary, bladder, and ovarian cancers, studies are beginning to indicate poor outcomes associated with perioperative transfusion.[38–45] TRIM remains poorly understood, but for the patients with cancer, this potential for early tumor recurrence is concerning. Although no generalized guidelines for patients with cancer are yet available, careful consideration is warranted before transfusion.

Patients with cancer are at high risk for severe anemia due to marrow suppressive chemotherapy, anemia of chronic disease, and tumor invasion of bone marrow.[46] A risk-benefit analysis is recommended for each

patient with cancer with consideration of the goals of treatment. As with other transfusion indications, the minimum transfusion required to alleviate symptomatology and provide adequate oxygenation is endorsed because each unit transfused carries risk and side effects.

Anemia in the perioperative patient

The American Society of Anesthesiologists as well as other groups have published guidelines for blood management of the perioperative patient.[47] These are largely in agreement in recommending a comprehensive approach involving preoperative, perioperative, and postoperative interventions to mitigate and reduce transfusion levels. Before surgery, medical history, laboratory testing, and physical examination are used to identify and treat anemia, and to identify patients at increased risk of bleeding. During this time, patients may require iron therapy, erythropoietin, cessation of anticoagulant or antiplatelet drugs, and crossmatching of blood products for anticipated hemorrhage. During surgical procedures, urgent reversal of anticoagulants, antifibrinolytics, hemodilution, and patient monitoring can be used to limit transfusion. If anemia develops, clinical assessment and laboratory studies together should drive the decision to transfuse. Transfuse single units, with clinical reassessment after each product. Transfusion in the surgical patient is warranted for hemoglobin below 10 g/dL and hematocrit below 30%, with ongoing or uncontrolled bleeding, evidence or high risk for end organ damage, poor cardiopulmonary reserve, or intravascular collapse. When available, cell salvage and reinfusion are recommended. Maximum surgical blood order schedules, massive transfusion protocols, laboratory testing protocols, or viscoelasticity measurement may help guide transfusion support. Because several studies have now demonstrated increased risks for infection and poor outcomes due to intraoperative transfusion,[48–50] transfusion should be avoided for the stable surgical patient with adequate hemostasis.

Anemia in the cardiac patient

Studies in the cardiac patient population are divided into those undergoing cardiovascular surgery and those who are being followed as medical patients.[51] For the cardiovascular surgical population, some evidence-based literature has failed to show a benefit with a liberal transfusion policy, in terms of morbidity or cost,[52,53] and has recommended further studies. Horvath et al., however, found a 29% increase in postoperative infection with every unit transfused perioperatively.[54] An evaluation of Jehovah's Witness patients who refused transfusion with cardiac surgery, versus a control population, found that the Witnesses had fewer acute complications, shorter length of stay, and better survival at 1 year.[55] These findings suggest that while a benefit of liberal transfusion above a hemoglobin of 9 g/dL has not been identified, restrictive transfusion may lead to improved outcomes.

Research has shown that patients undergoing percutaneous coronary intervention are transfused at a rate of about 2% and that transfusion was associated with adverse events including myocardial infarction, stroke, and death.[56] Another study revealed a strong association between transfusion and acute kidney injury in this population.[57] One analysis found that transfusion of RBCs was independently associated with new-onset conduction abnormalities and cardiac arrhythmias after myocardial infarction.[58] For the non-surgical cardiac population, the anemic (hematocrit less than 30%) patient having active chest pain, angina, or evidence of infarction may require transfusion to mitigate end organ damage and improve cardiac oxygenation.[59] The stable cardiac population seems to be at risk for acute coronary syndrome when maintained on restrictive strategy (<7.0 g/dL). Hemoglobin of 8.0 g/dL or higher is recommended to preserve cardiac function; however, overtransfusion should also be avoided because some studies suggest that even in patients having myocardial infarction, transfusion may be associated with increased all-cause mortality and increased risk of repeat infarction.[60] It is reasonable to adopt a strategy of maintaining hemoglobin at or above 8.0 g/dL for stable cardiac patients, with transfusion of the minimal dose RBCs necessary for active angina or evidence of infarction.

Anemia in the patient on palliation

For the patient on palliation or in hospice, transfusion may be used to maintain the quality of life with the goal of comfort and deescalation of care. The transfusion guideline should be the minimum dosage necessary to maintain function, in the lowest appropriate level care setting. Avoiding and mitigating transfusion reactions is paramount. Given the option, many patients in hospice prefer a shorter infusion appointment; however, it does not follow that rapid blood administration is warranted. For example, for an anemic hospice outpatient at risk for TACO it may be appropriate to opt for a slow infusion of only a partial unit over 3 h. Patients on palliation may be maintained with transfusion to keep their hematocrit between 7 and 10 for symptomatic relief, or they may choose to refuse transfusion altogether. Double unit transfusions are discouraged

because of the length of time required to safely transfuse these and the unacceptably high risk of transfusion reaction.

Dosing Guidelines for Red Blood Cells

Because of the risks and side effects associated with transfusion, as well as extensive evidence that restrictive transfusion strategy is often as good or better than liberal transfusion strategy, units of RBCs should be ordered in the lowest dose required to treat the patient. Due to the risks associated with transfusion, it is never advisable to transfuse 2 units of RBCs at once. In most patients, 1 unit is sufficient. For nonemergent severe anemia, a trial of 1 unit followed by reassessment is ideal.

For an adult patient weighing 70 kg, 1 unit of RBCs is expected to increase the hematocrit by 3% and the hemoglobin by 1 g/dL.[61] For pediatric patients, 8–10 mL/kg raises the hematocrit by about 6% and the hemoglobin by 2 g/dL. Calculations for expected increase in hemoglobin and hematocrit are as follows:

Estimated blood volume (EBV) (Box 6.1) = (weight kg) × (70 mL/kg)

1 unit of RBCs = 160–275 mL RBCs[15] (average of 200 mL)

Hematocrit increment = ~200 mL/EBV.

Frequent confusion about dosing includes:
1. adhering to older protocols advising 2 units be given routinely
2. not accounting for patient blood volume in anticipating an expected increase in hematocrit.

For patients who are obese, a less-than-average increase should be expected in hemoglobin/hematocrit because the patient's blood volume is larger. For very small or underweight patients, dosage should be

---

BOX 6.1
Standard Estimated Blood Volumes

	mL/kg
Premature Infants	95
Neonates	85
Infants	80
Children	80
Women	75
Pregnant women	80
Men	65
Average adult	70

carefully considered because transfusion overload is a serious potential risk. Aliquots or split (divided) units can be given slowly, if necessary. It is always preferable to transfuse the *minimum* required blood units to provide symptomatic relief to a patient.

Contraindications and Precautions for Red Blood Cell Administration

RBC transfusion is indicated only to improve the oxygen carrying capacity for patients with a critical deficit. RBC transfusion is not indicated for increasing colloid osmotic pressure or volume expansion. In patients in whom anemia can be corrected by other means, those alternatives are preferable over RBC transfusion. For example, known iron, B12, or folate deficiencies should be treated with supplements or intravenous infusion. Erythropoietin deficiency should be treated medically if appropriate. Transfusion of RBCs neither improves wound healing or performance in physical therapy nor should it be used to improve subjective well-being. Artificial guidelines imposed by outpatient care facilities or a desire to "transfuse up" before a discharge are inappropriate.

At most risk from RBC transfusion may be patients with a history or high risk of hyperhemolysis. These patients often have a hemolytic syndrome, such as sickle cell disease, warm autoimmune hemolysis, or β-thalassemia, and may present with profound anemia. However, when transfused, they may hemolyze the unit given as well as more of their own blood. Transfusion should be reserved for life-threatening circumstances.[62]

USE OF PLATELETS

Platelets are essential for hemostasis because they are the primary component of the thrombotic plug. Platelets, also called thrombocytes, are nonnucleated cell fragments derived from megakaryocytes in the bone marrow. These circulate as small 2- to 3-μm disks until they encounter a defect in the vascular wall, where various combinations of exposed collagen, fibronectin, phospholipids, von Willebrand factor (vWF), and thrombin trigger a process of platelet adhesion, activation, and aggregation.[63] At the disrupted endothelial surface, collagen binds to platelet glycoprotein (GP) VI receptor and integrin $\alpha_2\beta_1$, whereas vWF binds to integrin $\alpha_{IIb}\beta_3$ and GP1b/V/IX receptor, adhering platelets to the site of injury.[64] The tyrosine kinase cascade is triggered by collagen binding, causing calcium release and phospholipase C gamma 2 (PLC-γ2) activation. Simultaneously, tissue factor exposed by injury binds factor VII initiating the extrinsic coagulation cascade and subsequent thrombin formation. Platelets are further activated by thrombin. Physically, the platelets change from discoid to stellate and become sticky, releasing their factor V and fibrinogen to further potentiate coagulation. Aggregation occurs as the GPIIb/IIIa receptor activates and binds with fibrinogen or vWF.[65] Activation of just a few of these receptors causes an intraplatelet signaling cascade leading to morphologic change of the tens of thousands of GPIIb/IIIa receptors on the platelet surface from curly to straight, making them capable of binding fibrinogen for aggregation.[66] Additionally, the platelet surface secretes adenosine diphosphate (ADP) and presents active integrins $\alpha_{IIb}\beta_3$, causing intercellular calcium signaling through the aggregated platelet population. At this point, the platelets have morphed from stellate figures to wide, flat fried-egg-shaped structures, layering themselves into a clot. Depending on the shear forces, various receptors and integrins control calcium flux adapting the clot to the stress, velocity, and rheology of the local environment.

In considering platelets, the transfusing physician needs only to remember that platelets are highly adaptable to their surroundings, can be activated via multiple mechanisms, and serve to potentiate and facilitate activation in one another. A "normal" platelet count (150,000–350,000/μL of blood) is more than sufficient for hemostasis. For most procedures, a platelet count of 50,000/μL is adequate, and for stable patients with hypoproliferative thrombocytopenia, studies have shown that a platelet count of 10,000/μL prevents spontaneous bleeding.[67,68]

Platelets are collected either from whole blood donation ("random" pooled platelets) or via the apheresis procedure. Pooled platelets usually consist of four to six pooled random whole blood donor platelets, with at least 5.5×10^{10} platelets each, in 40–70 mL plasma. Apheresis platelets contain at least 3.0×10^{11} platelet and can be considered an equivalent dose to pooled platelets.[69] These doses can be expected to raise the platelet count of a stable 70-kg patient by 50–60,000/μL.

Platelets are stored at room temperature (20–24°C) for up to 5 days with constant gentle agitation. Current regulations allow extension of the outdate to 7 days with negative rapid pangenera bacterial testing.[70] Whole blood platelets may be prepooled and tested for bacterial contamination, but random donor pools usually are prepared at the time of dispensing. Apheresis and prepooled platelets are cultured for bacteria at the time of collection, are rapidly available for transfusion and thus are appropriate for emergent bleeding.

Indications for Platelet Transfusion

Platelets are indicated for treatment of bleeding in patients with marked or symptomatic thrombocytopenia and nonimmune platelet dysfunction, for planned procedures in patients with thrombocytopenia, and for prophylactic dosing of marked thrombocytopenia. Guidelines for platelet transfusion are fairly consistent and have been published by various groups, including the AABB and the British Committee for Standards in Haematology.[71,72]

Prophylactic platelet transfusions

Hypoproliferative thrombocytopenia (bone marrow failure). Stable patients with a platelet count less than 10,000/μL should be transfused to maintain levels at 10,000 or greater. Platelet counts less than 5000 have been associated with spontaneous hemorrhage. Even a partial platelet product, such as half of an apheresis platelet, or a random platelet pool of 3–4 units is sufficient to prevent hemorrhage, although giving an entire unit of apheresis platelets is not unreasonable. Higher doses or multiple transfusions confer no added benefit.[73] Some guidelines have specified these goals for adults without making a recommendation for children. The Analysis of the Effects of Prophylactic Platelet Dose on Transfusion Outcomes (PLADO) trial shows that although children do have higher rates of bleeding, these seem to be unrelated to platelets because children showed more hemorrhage events over a wide range of platelet counts.[74] Because of the chronic nature of bone marrow insufficiency, some patients benefit from a routine transfusion schedule. In cases in which patients with thrombocytopenic are transfusion dependent, leukoreduction is recommended to reduce the risk for alloimmunization.[75]

Patients with severe thrombocytopenia less than 20,000/μL and an additional risk factor, such as hypersplenism, fever, sepsis, coincident coagulopathy, or an anatomic lesion predisposing them to bleeding, may be transfused to maintain their platelet count at or above 20,000/μL.

Preprocedural thrombocytopenia: minor procedures. The AABB recommends platelet transfusion for minor procedures, such as central venous catheter placement, when the platelet count is less than 20,000/μL. These procedures have low risk for bleeding, and when bleeding does occur it tends to not be platelet related.

For minor procedures involving the central nervous system, such as lumbar puncture, a higher threshold of platelet count above 50,000/μL is recommended because of the unacceptable consequences of a neurologic accident.

Preprocedural thrombocytopenia: major (nonneuraxial) surgical procedures. Patients undergoing major surgical procedures, not including neurosurgery, spinal surgery or eye surgery, may be maintained at a platelet count above 50,000/μL. There is no evidence of increased bleeding risk for major elective procedures with platelet counts above 50,000/μL in the absence of platelet dysfunction, and for these platelet transfusion is not recommended.

For patients undergoing cardiopulmonary bypass (CPB), platelet transfusion is not recommended if the platelet count is over 50,000/μL without evidence of bleeding or coagulopathy. CPB inhibits platelet activity, and patients who have hemorrhage due to platelet dysfunction after cardiac surgery may require platelet transfusion. It is reasonable to delay the consideration of platelet transfusion until the patient is off CPB and then assess for bleeding while platelet counts are measured. Many patients will stabilize without platelet transfusion, and in these cases, transfusion is not indicated.[76]

Preprocedural thrombocytopenia: major neurosurgical or ophthalmic procedures. Surgical intervention involving the brain, spinal column, or posterior part of the eye involves significant risk for hemorrhage and unacceptably devastating sequelae of hemorrhage. For these reasons, these procedures demand the highest level of preoperative platelet counts, at greater than 100,000/μL. There is no evidence that maintaining higher levels of platelet counts confers additional benefit.

Therapeutic platelet transfusions

Massive transfusion or multiple trauma. In cases of massive transfusion or multiple trauma, platelets should be transfused in a "1:1:1" ratio with RBCs and FFP to maintain platelet count at least above 50,000 and ideally above 100,000/μL. Early studies demonstrated, and more recent studies have confirmed, that for healthy adults with massive trauma, platelet counts drop rapidly during resuscitation from normal to less than 100,000/μL with transfusion of 10 units of RBC.[77] Thus early implementation of platelet administration is encouraged. For calculating the product ratio, an apheresis platelet is at least equivalent to six RBCs.

For hemorrhagic cerebrovascular accident, intracranial hemorrhage, or other neuro-ocular hemorrhage, maintain platelet counts greater than 100,000/μL. For severe nonneuraxial hemorrhage, maintain levels of platelets above 50,000/μL.

Congenital or acquired platelet dysfunction

If possible, congenital platelet dysfunction is treated with appropriate pharmacologic therapy, for example, recombinant activated factor VIIa for Glanzmann thrombasthenia or desmopressin (DDAVP) with tranexamic acid for other platelet dysfunction disorders. When these are unavailable, consider transfusion of a single apheresis platelet or platelet pool.

More commonly encountered is acquired platelet dysfunction due to platelet-inhibiting drugs or CPB. Platelet transfusion should be initiated after removal of the cause of the acquired dysfunction (discontinuation of platelet-toxic drugs or CPB) and is indicated for bleeding events or for emergent procedures. In cases in which risk precludes cessation of platelet-inhibiting medication, the procedure can be attempted with platelets on reserve in case of hemorrhage.

As discussed previously, platelets are remarkably resilient and have multiple activation pathways. Therefore it is not necessary to replace the entire platelet population to achieve functionality. Instead, 10%–20% replacement is sufficient. Usually one dose of apheresis or pooled platelets will suffice to recruit adequate platelet activity.

Dosing Guidelines

For most patients, one pool or one apheresis platelet is sufficient for thrombocytopenia or platelet dysfunction. In many cases, a small pool or half apheresis platelet is enough. The recommended dosing is the equivalent of 1 random unit per 10–15 kg body weight to increase the platelet count by 5,000–10,000/μL per unit. Thus one pool or one apheresis platelet can be expected to raise the platelet count of a stable 70-kg patient by 40,000–60,000/μL.

For massive, emergent transfusion, attempt to maintain a "1:1:1" ratio of RBC, FFP, and platelets. As an example, a protocol may consist of six RBCs, six FFP, and one pool or one apheresis platelet. It is prudent to monitor platelet counts to ensure levels above at least 50,000/μL until hemostasis is controlled.

For acquired or congenital platelet inhibition, replace 10%–20% of circulating platelets with transfusion. For most patients, one apheresis platelet or one pool is sufficient.

Alloimmunization should be considered when patients are transfused but show no appreciable improvement in platelet count. Before ordering costly HLA-matched or HLA-crossmatched platelets,

a corrected platelet count increment should be calculated to determine if the patient has become platelet refractory due to immune-mediated platelet removal. It is necessary to measure the platelet count immediately before and within 1 h after the completion of a platelet transfusion. The following equation may be utilized to determine corrected count increment (CCI):

$$CCI = ([Postcount-Precount] \times BSA)/platelets$$ transfused,

where BSA is the body surface area in m^2 and platelets transfused = number of administered platelets × 10^{11}

CCI calculated at 7500 or above usually indicates nonimmune clearance of platelets, whereas CCI of 5000 or less indicates immune-mediated clearance, or alloimmunization. CCI may be repeated twice and the scores utilized with consideration of patient clinical history and status.[69]

Rate of administration of platelets can be as tolerated by the patient, with consideration for volume status and susceptibility to TACO, but it must be completed within 4 h of initiation. Some clinicians will request slow infusion of a "platelet drip," with half a unit of platelets administered over 4 h, and then repeat administration, to ensure a constant source of platelets. Although this is controversial, some clinicians advocate this as an administration technique for the patient who has rapid nonimmune clearance of platelets.

Contraindications and Precautions for Platelet Transfusion

Platelets should not be transfused when bleeding is unrelated to thrombocytopenia or platelet dysfunction. Platelets are not indicated for patients having a platelet count above 100,000/μL unless there is a known or suspected platelet abnormality of function. Transfusion of platelets is not helpful to the patient who is not bleeding on antiplatelet medication, with hyperglobulinemia, or with some types of von Willebrand disease. Extraneous platelet transfusion increases the risk of platelet alloimmunization.

Except in life-threatening emergencies, platelet transfusions have historically been contraindicated for thrombotic thrombocytopenic purpura (TTP) and heparin-induced thrombocytopenia. Some recent studies have demonstrated that platelets can be given safely in these conditions and should not be withheld when clinically indicated.[78–80] Other studies, including a review in 2009, indicate that at least for TTP, the risk for harm is uncertain.[81] Nevertheless, official published guidelines continue to list thrombotic microangiopathies as a contraindication to platelet transfusion.[72] In these situations, a discussion with the clinical team, blood bank, and patient as to the risks and benefits of platelet transfusion is recommended. Platelet transfusion may not benefit patients with idiopathic immune thrombocytopenic purpura, untreated disseminated intravascular coagulation (DIC) without active bleeding, septicemia, or hypersplenism.

Platelet transfusion is not indicated for uremic platelet dysfunction or renal failure. In cases of renal dysfunction, any platelets transfused are also rapidly inhibited by the uremic plasma. Alternative treatment may include dialysis, DDAVP (vasopressin), estrogen, or cryoprecipitate to improve platelet activation. Platelet transfusion in these cases does not improve functionality and only serves to increase the risk for platelet alloimmunization.

Routine prophylactic transfusion before CPB is not indicated because the transfused platelets will be impaired during the procedure. Alternatives include hemodilution, with postoperative reinfusion of autologous blood and delay of platelet transfusion until postprocedure.

USE OF FRESH FROZEN PLASMA

Of all the blood components dispensed, plasma seems to create the most clinical confusion with misperception regarding the indications, dosing, and timing of administration. These can be remedied by recalling that FFP is simply plasma, containing all the coagulant and anticoagulant factors found in normal blood. For the hemorrhaging patient losing whole blood, or for the patient with a yet unknown coagulation deficiency, plasma provides every component available.[82] Laboratory studies have demonstrated that single factor deficiencies are well compensated, unless the deficiency reaches very low levels, usually less than 5%. However, combined or multiple factor deficiencies lead to coagulopathy at levels beginning as high as 60%.[83–85] By understanding the components of FFP, as well as the patient's coagulopathy, weight, estimated blood volume and goal for transfusion, we can calculate proper dosing for transfusion. Although this sounds complex, it is actually simpler and more accurate in daily patient care than placing an order for plasma by units.

FFP is collected, separated, and frozen within 8 h of phlebotomy from the donor, preserving the labile coagulation factors V and VIII. Plasma frozen within 24 h (FP24) may also be available. Frozen plasma can be stored at −18°C or less for up to 1 year. Once thawed, FFP and plasma may be stored at 1–6°C. The levels of factor VIII, FV and protein C decline in vitro

while plasma is in the liquid state; however, factor V levels remain above the 35% required for adequate hemostasis. FP24 and/or thawed plasma is adequate for most plasma transfusions, but for patients with consumptive coagulopathy, FFP is the preferred treatment. In an emergency situation or with massive hemorrhage, rapidly available prethawed plasma may be lifesaving and should be used while additional plasma is thawed. Although the typical volume of a unit of plasma is 200–250 mL, units are variable. Ordering FFP in milliliters is an option for more accurate dosing.

Plasma transfusion cannot be expected to "normalize" the INR to 1.0. A 2006 study in which FFP was transfused to patients with an INR of 1.1–1.9 showed that less than 1% of patients had complete INR correction and only 15% corrected by 50%.[86] Additionally, the measurement of prothrombin time (PT) and INR largely depend on factor VII levels. Factor VII in vivo has the shortest half-life of all the coagulation factors, at about only 4 h. Therefore laboratory values for PT and INR can change over the course of hours and also have implications for timing of FFP administration, especially for preprocedural reversal of warfarin.[87] Without vitamin K repletion, FFP provides only a short-lived reversal of INR. Although this is helpful when a temporary or incomplete reversal is planned, it means that timely coordination with nursing is required to ensure that FFP is administered immediately before a procedure for correction of INR during the period of highest risk.

Indications for Fresh Frozen Plasma

Plasma transfusion is indicated for patients with multiple coagulation deficiencies who are hemorrhaging or undergoing invasive procedures. These situations often are due to warfarin (Coumadin) therapy, but may also be found with vitamin K deficiency due to malnourishment. When available, the use of four-factor prothrombin complex concentrate (PCC) is recommended as first-line therapy over FFP.[88] PCC has the benefits of faster INR reversal without the risk of volume overload and transfusion reaction. Additional causes of coagulation deficiency include liver failure, massive blood loss, aggressive volume resuscitation, and disseminated intravascular coagulopathy. FFP may be used for treatment of specific coagulation/anticoagulant factor deficiencies for which factor concentrates are not available. FFP may be used for rare plasma protein deficiencies when specific recombinant products are unavailable. For patients with TTP, FFP is indicated as part of plasma exchange.

Patients identified as having an elevated, nontherapeutic PT and INR who are not bleeding nor urgently needing an invasive procedure may be treated more conservatively with vitamin K supplementation and/or with warfarin dose reduction.

Dosing Guidelines

For massive transfusion, the goal is to maintain a "1:1" ratio of RBCs and FFP. It is also important also that FFP is started promptly and continues to be administered frequently throughout the protocol.[89,90]

For acute bleeding or a planned invasive procedure in a patient who is coagulation factor deficient, the appropriate dosing is 10–15 mL/kg (when PCC is not available). For prophylactic preprocedural dosing, consider the following guideline:

1. INR 1.6–2.0: Transfuse 2 units of FFP, if clinically indicated.
2. INR 2.1–4.0: Transfuse 10 mL/kg, maximum of 4 units (round to nearest unit).
3. INR 4.0–8.0: Transfuse 15 mL/kg, maximum of 6 units (round to nearest unit).
4. INR above 8.0: Begin FFP administration; give vitamin K; monitor PT, partial thromboplastin time (PTT), and INR frequently; contact hematology or blood bank for consultation if needed.

Administration

Plasma infusion should be timed to finish *within 1 h* of the planned procedure. Give premedications as appropriate for the individual patient. Administer each unit FFP over 15–20 min, with a maximum of 15 min between units if the patient can tolerate volume load. Send laboratory studies for PT, INR, and PTT within 20 min of completion of infusion.

Guidelines for performing procedure after fresh frozen plasma administration for initial international normalized ratio

1. INR 1.6–2.0: Can go directly to procedure without repeat INR result
2. INR 2.1–4.0: Can go directly to procedure without repeat INR result
3. INR 4.1–8.0: Wait for repeat INR result (draw 15 min after transfusion and run statim (STAT))
   - Repeated INR < 1.6: proceed directly with procedure.
   - Repeated INR 1.6–2.0: administer 2 units of FFP and proceed directly to procedure.
   - Repeated INR 2.1–4.0: administer 3 units of FFP and recheck INR.

Contraindications and Precautions for Plasma Administration

Due to the risks of transfusion transmitted diseases and transfusion reactions, plasma should never be transfused for volume expansion, for specific factor replacement when factor concentrate is available, or for protein replacement for nutritionally deficient patients. Plasma transfusion will not reverse the effects of coagulation factor inhibitors. It does not enhance wound healing or subjective well-being.

FFP/plasma is not indicated for reversal of minimally elevated PT, PTT, or INR in stable, nonbleeding patients. Minor coagulation deficiencies as shown by minimally elevated PT, INR, and PTT have not been shown to correlate with adverse bleeding risk or surgical bleeding and cannot be completely corrected by plasma transfusion in the majority of cases.

FFP/plasma is not indicated for nonemergent warfarin (or vitamin K deficiency) reversal. Vitamin K deficiency (and warfarin therapy) leads to the deficiency of factors II, VII, IX, and X and proteins C and S. Nonurgent reversal of warfarin should be treated with vitamin K. Vitamin K should be administered in addition to plasma if reversal is needed for bleeding or an urgent procedure.

Isolated elevation of PTT is usually due to heparin administration or lipid anticoagulant, in which case FFP/plasma administration will not correct the PTT (and may cause exacerbation of bleeding in cases of heparin dosing). Contact factor deficiencies are not associated with bleeding and do not require replacement. Isolated factor XI deficiency may require plasma replacement.[91]

Because of the short in vitro half-life of factor VII (2–6 h), dosing of plasma before the procedure should be timed to complete transfusion within 1 h of initiating the procedure, with the option of continued transfusion during the procedure. Plasma administered several hours or the day before a procedure will have little effect and constitutes an unnecessary transfusion.

USE OF CRYOPRECIPITATE

Cryoprecipitate, which is produced by allowing FFP to thaw slowly at 1–6 °C, contains five protein precipitates that are extremely useful in specific clinical settings. It is important to understand the components of the cryoprecipitate and their impact on coagulation and hemostasis to utilize this resource correctly and to avoid the misimpression that cryoprecipitate is "concentrated" plasma. Properly used, cryoprecipitate plays an essential role in transfusion medicine.

When plasma is frozen and then slowly thawed at near-freezing temperatures between 1 and 6 °C, the high-molecular-weight proteins naturally present in fresh plasma solidify and precipitate to the bottom of the bag, forming a whitish, pasty, or powdery substance. The remaining cryodepleted plasma called cryosupernatant is then decanted off and the protein solids are dissolved into the residual plasma and refrozen. This is whole blood–derived cryoprecipitate. Usually, cryoprecipitate is pooled into batches of four to six before being refrozen. The concentrate primarily contains:

- Factor VIII–activates intrinsic coagulation cascade
- vWF–activates platelets
- Fibrinogen–precursor to fibrin, essential for clot structure
- Factor XIII–strengthens and cross-links fibrin
- Fibronectin–attaches integrins to collagen, essential to wound repair

The key in thinking about cryoprecipitate and its core components is to consider these, especially fibrinogen, as the "mortar" required to build the clot "wall." Fibrinogen is a soluble GP hexamer, which is broken down by thrombin (factor IIa) to form fibrin, an *essential* component of clot formation. Also known as factor I, it is synthesized in the liver and then circulates in the plasma in the soluble form until converted into insoluble fibrin strands by thrombin. These fibrin strands act to physically tie platelets and RBCs together, forming a clot. The process is further aided by FXIII, which cross-links the strands and also recruits and binds fibrinolysis inhibitors (α2-antiplasmin, thrombin activatable fibrinolysis inhibitor). Furthermore, fibrin catalyzes the activation of factor XIII and plasminogen activator.

Cryoprecipitate also potentiates clotting through FVIII and vWF, which ordinarily circulate together in the plasma until activated by tissue injury. At this point they separate, and the activated FVIII triggers the coagulation cascade, whereas the vWF enhances binding of platelets to exposed collagen. The close proximity of platelet GP VI to collagen activates tight binding and initiates a signaling cascade of activated platelet integrins. Soluble fibronectin binds integrins, collagen, and fibrin. Activated platelets morph from spherical to stellate, release the contents of their granules further activating other platelets, and increase their affinity for fibrinogen.

Thus cryoprecipitate contains core factors required to activate the coagulation cascade, activate platelets, and build the fibrin strands essential to clotting. It is no surprise that this product is therefore useful for patients with uremic platelet dysfunction, massive bleeding, fibrinogen deficiency, and dysfibrinogenemia. Studies have shown that transfusion of cryoprecipitate to those who are massively bleeding is widely variable.[92] The Fibrinogen Early In Severe Trauma Study (FEISTY)

will determine whether consistent early administration of cryoprecipitate or fibrinogen concentrate improves measures of coagulation and patient outcomes.[93]

Indications for cryoprecipitate

Indications for transfusion of cryoprecipitate include repletion of fibrinogen levels; activation of platelets; emergent replacement of factor VIII, vWF, or factor XIII when recombinant factors are unavailable; and as part of a massive transfusion protocol.[94]

Platelet activation: uremic platelet dysfunction

Although DDAVP (vasopressin) is the preferred first-line treatment, cryoprecipitate also can be used to activate platelets with uremic platelet dysfunction. Vasopressin works by stimulating endothelial cells to release factor VIII and vWF, whereas cryoprecipitate provides these directly. Uremic platelet dysfunction often goes unrecognized during acute bleeding events. It is important to recognize it and avoid transfusing platelets instead of giving DDAVP or cryoprecipitate.

Massive bleeding, cardiovascular surgery, labor, and delivery

During massive hemorrhage situations, a massive transfusion protocol or rapid testing with TEG or viscoelastography may be used to guide dosing. In either case, studies have shown that massive replacement should consist of all lost components of blood. Whether measured by TEG or by traditional laboratory measures, low fibrinogen during massive bleeding or postpartum hemorrhage must be rapidly corrected to preserve coagulation. Fibrinogen levels should be kept above 150 mg/dL for massive bleeding and above 200 mg/dL for pregnancy.[95] If a fibrinogen concentrate is not readily available, cryoprecipitate is appropriate in these instances.

Fibrinogen deficiency (hypofibrinogenemia; <100 mg/dL) or dysfibrinogenemia

Patients with a known deficiency or dysfunctionality of fibrinogen will have impaired or ineffective clotting capability. There are fibrinogen concentrates that should be used as first-line therapy for patients with known hypo- or dysfibrinogenemia before a planned obstetric delivery or surgical procedure. However, in an emergency or during massive hemorrhage, cryoprecipitate can be used to rapidly increase fibrinogen levels.

Factor XIII deficiency

When there is a documented deficiency of factor XIII, cryoprecipitate may be an acceptable treatment option in an emergency. The preferred treatment is a factor XIII concentrate, such as Corifact or Tretten. Factor XIII deficiency is a rare, congenital autosomal recessive trait, leading to poor clot stability. Acquired factor XIII deficiency due to autoantibody formation may be related to certain drugs, such as isoniazid or phenytoin, or to various underlying conditions, such as renal failure, myeloid leukemia, or autoimmune disorders. The disease presents with easy bruising, soft tissue bleeding, poor wound healing, central nervous system bleeding, spontaneous early miscarriage, and delayed or recurrent bleeding following trauma.

Hemophilia and von Willebrand disease. For hemophilia and von Willebrand disease, the standard-of-care treatment is purified factor products to replace the specific known deficiency. However, in an emergency situation, cryoprecipitate containing factor VIII and vWF can be administered making it an effective option for these patients.

Dosing guidelines
Cryoprecipitate contains at least 80 IU of factor VIII and 150 mg of fibrinogen per unit, although most units actually contain about 200 mg of fibrinogen. Other components include vWF, factor XIII, and fibronectin. Many blood banks order prepooled cryoprecipitate, which comes in pools of 5 or 6 units, whereas other banks pool their own product. A typical adult dose is 10–15 units of cryoprecipitate (2–3 pools), which in a 70-kg adult will raise the fibrinogen level by 70–80 mg/dL. A frequent mistake is the ordering of a single 5-unit pool of cryoprecipitate to treat an adult. It is important to understand the product available at your institution for appropriate dosing.

Fibrinogen replacement:
Dose (units) = (Desired fibrinogen increment [mg/dL] × Plasma Volume)/250 mg/unit
Plasma Volume = ([1 − HCT] × 0.7 dL/kg × Weight [kg])

Contraindications
Contraindications to the administration of cryoprecipitate include known hypersensitivity to any component of cryoprecipitate. Because cryoprecipitate contains only the five components listed earlier, it is not appropriate for other types of factor replacement. It is not a substitute for activated factor VIIa, and it will not reverse vitamin K deficiency (warfarin). Cryoprecipitate is not a "stronger" or concentrated form of FFP and should not be used in place of plasma. Cryoprecipitate is not the first-line treatment for hemophilia A, von Willebrand disease, factor XIII deficiency, or known hypo- or

dysfibrinogenemia. These should be treated with factor concentrates or complexes whenever possible.

CONCLUSION
In administering RBCs, transfuse only when clinically indicated and in the smallest dose possible to relieve the symptomatology. For platelet transfusions, usually a single dose is sufficient to correct dysfunction, improve thrombocytopenia, or prepare a patient for a procedure. Plasma should be ordered based on the patient's weight and given timely to correct the coagulopathy. Cryoprecipitate contains only five proteins, but is very useful for fibrinogen replacement and platelet activation.

REFERENCES
1. FDA. Guideline for the uniform labeling of blood and blood components. In: *U.S. Food & Drug Administration Vaccines, Blood & Biologics*. 1985. Available at: https://www.fda.gov/downloads/BiologicsBloodVaccines/GuidanceComplianceRegulatoryInformation/Guidances/Blood/UCM080974.pdf.
2. Zoon KC, Jacobson ED, Woodcock J. Hypotension and bedside leukocyte reduction filters. *Int J Trauma Nurs*. 1999;5:121–122.
3. Federowicz I, Barrett BB, Andersen JW, Urashima M, Popovsky MA, Anderson KC. Characterization of reactions after transfusion of cellular blood components that are white cell reduced before storage. *Transfusion*. 1996;36(1):21–28.
4. Dumont LJ, Papari M, Aronson CA, Dumont DF. Whole-blood collection and component processing. In: Fung MK, Grossman BJ, Hillyer CD, Westhoff CM, eds. *Technical Manual*. 18th ed. Bethesda: AABB Press; 2014:154.
5. Laupacis A, Brown J, Costello B, et al. Prevention of posttransfusion CMV in the era of universal WBC reduction: a consensus statement. *Transfusion*. 2001;41:560–569.
6. Bowden RA, Slichter SJ, Sayers M, et al. A comparison of filtered leukocyte-reduced and cytomegalovirus (CMV) seronegative blood products for the prevention of transfusion-associated CMV infection after marrow transplant. *Blood*. 1995;86:3598–3603.
7. Vamvakas EC. Is white blood cell reduction equivalent to antibody screening in preventing transmission of cytomegalovirus by transfusion? A review of the literature and meta-analysis. *Transfus Med Rev*. 2005;19(3):181–199.
8. Ooley PW, ed. *Standards for Blood Banks and Transfusion Services*. 30th ed. Bethesda, MD: AABB Press; 2016.
9. Meryman HT, Hornblower M. The preparation of red cells depleted of leukocytes. *Transfusion*. 1986;26:101–106.
10. Sirchia G, Rebulla P, Parravicini A, et al. Leukocyte depletion of red cell units at the bedside by transfusion through a new filter. *Transfusion*. 1987;27:402–405.

11. FDA. Guidance for industry: pre-storage leukocyte reduction of whole blood and blood components Intended for transfusion. In: *U.S. Food & Drug Administration Vaccines, Blood & Biologics.* 2012. Available at: https://www.fda.gov/BiologicsBloodVaccines/GuidanceComplianceRegulatoryInformation/Guidances/Blood/ucm320636.htm.

12. FDA. Guidance for industry and FDA review staff: collection of platelets by automated methods. In: *U.S. Food & Drug Administration Vaccines, Blood & Biologics.* 2007. Available at: https://www.fda.gov/biologicsbloodvaccines/guidancecomplianceregulatoryinformation/guidances/blood/ucm073382.htm.

13. Dunbar N. Hospital storage, monitoring, pretransfusion processing, distribution and inventory management of blood components. In: Fung MK, Grossman BJ, Hillyer CD, Westhoff CM, eds. *Technical Manual.* 18th ed. Bethesda: AABB Press; 2014:223.

14. Sandler SG, Mallory D, Malamut D, Eckrich R. IgA anaphylactic transfusion reactions. *Transfus Med Rev.* 1995; 9(1):1–8.

15. Schroeder ML. Transfusion associated graft vs host disease. *Br J Haematol.* 2002;117:275–287.

16. Dwyre DM, Holland PV. Transfusion-associated graft-versus-host-disease. *Vox Sang.* 2008;95:85–93.

17. Weiskopf RB, Schnapp S, Rouine-Rapp K, Bostrom A, Toy P. Extracellular potassium concentrations in red blood cell suspensions after irradiation and washing. *Transfusion.* 2005;45(8):1295–1301.

18. AABB, American Red Cross, America's Blood Centers, Armed Services Blood Program. *Circular of Information for the Use of Human Blood and Blood Components;* 2013:30. Available at: http://www.aabb.org/tm/coi/Documents/coi1113.

19. Callum JL, Nascimento B, Alam A. Massive haemorrhage protocol: what's the best protocol? *ISBT Sci Ser.* 2016;11(suppl 1):297–306.

20. Villanueva C, Colomo A, Bosch A, et al. Transfusion strategies for acute upper gastrointestinal bleeding. *N Engl J Med.* 2013;368(1):11–21.

21. Hebert PC, Tinmouth A, Corwin H. Anemia and red cell transfusion in critically ill patients. *Crit Care Med.* 2003;31(12):S672–S677.

22. Hebert PC, Wells G, Blajchman MA, et al. A multicenter randomized controlled clinical trial of the transfusion requirements in critical care. *New Engl J Med.* 1999;340(6):409–417.

23. Haitsma IK, Maas AI. Advanced monitoring in the intensive care unit: brain tissue oxygen tension. *Curr Opin Crit Care.* 2002;8(2):115–120.

24. Corwin HL, Gettinger A, Pearl RG, et al. The CRIT study: anemia and blood transfusion in the critically ill. Current clinical practice in the United States. *Crit Care Med.* 2004;32(1):39–52.

25. Corwin HL, Surgenor SD, Gettinger A. Transfusion practice in the critically ill. *Crit Care Med.* 2003;31(12): S668–S671.

26. Vincent JL, Baron JF, Reinhart K, et al. Anemia and blood transfusion in critically ill patients. *JAMA.* 2002;288(12): 1499–1507.

27. Fowler RA, Berenson M. Blood conservation in the intensive care unit. *Crit Care Med.* 2003;31(12):S715–S720.

28. Carson JL, Guyatt G, Heddle NM, et al. Clinical practice guidelines from the AABB red blood cell transfusion thresholds and storage. *JAMA.* 2016;316(19):2025–2035.

29. Carson JL, Sieber F, Cook DR, et al. Liberal versus restrictive blood transfusion strategy: 3-year survival and cause of death results from the FOCUS randomised controlled trial. *Lancet.* 2015;385(9974):1183–1189.

30. Patel KV. Epidemiology of anemia in older adults. *Semin Hematol.* 2008;45(4):210–217. http://dx.doi.org/10.1053/j.seminhematol.2008.06.006.

31. Goodnough LT, Schrier SL. Evaluation and management of anemia in the elderly. *Am J Hematol.* 2014;89(1): 88–96.

32. Holst LB, Petersen MW, Haase N, Perner A, Wetterslev J. Restrictive versus liberal transfusion strategy for red blood cell transfusion: systematic review of randomised trials with meta-analysis and trial sequential analysis. *BMJ.* 2015;350:1354.

33. Regan DM, Markowitz MA. *Transfusion-associated Circulatory Overload (TACO). Association Bulletin # 15-02.* AABB; 2015. Available at: http://www.aabb.org/programs/publications/bulletins/Pages/ab17-01.aspx.

34. Goubran HA, Elemary M, Radosevich M, Seghatchian J, El-Ekiaby M, Burnouf T. Impact of transfusion on cancer growth and outcome. *Cancer Growth Metastasis.* 2016;9: 1–8.

35. Al-Refaie WB, Parsons HM, Markin A, Abrams J, Habermann EB. Blood transfusion and cancer surgery outcomes: a continued reason for concern. *Surgery.* 2012;152(3): 344–354.

36. Ørskov M, Iachina M, Guldberg R, Mogensen O, Mertz Nørgård B. Predictors of mortality within 1 year after primary ovarian cancer surgery: a nationwide cohort study. *BMJ Open.* 2016;6(4):1–7.

37. de Almeida JP, et al. Transfusion requirements in surgical oncology patients: a prospective, randomized controlled trial. *Anesthesiology.* 2015;122(1):29–38.

38. Ejaz A, Spolverato G, Kim Y, et al. Impact of blood transfusions and transfusion practices on long-term outcome following hepatopancreaticobiliary surgery. *J Gastrointest Surg.* 2015;19(5):887–896.

39. Komatsu Y, Orita H, Sakurada M, Maekawa H, Hoppo T, Sato K. Intraoperative blood transfusion contributes to decreased long-term survival of patients with esophageal cancer. *World J Surg.* 2012;36:844–850.

40. Sun C, Wang Y, Yao HS, Hu ZQ. Allogeneic blood transfusion and the prognosis of gastric cancer patients: systematic review and meta-analysis. *Int J Surg.* 2015;13: 102–110.

41. Schiergens TS, Rentsch M, Kasparek MS, Frenes K, Jauch KW, Thasler WE. Impact of perioperative allogeneic red blood cell transfusion on recurrence and overall survival after resection of colorectal liver metastases. *Dis Colon Rectum.* 2015;58(1):74–82.

42. De Oliveira GS, Schink JC, Buoy C, Ahmad S, Fitzgerald PC, McCarthy RJ. The association between allogeneic perioperative blood transfusion on tumour recurrence and survival in patients with advanced ovarian cancer. *Transfus Med.* 2012;22(2):97–103.

43. Prescott LS, Aloia TA, Brown AJ, et al. Perioperative blood transfusion in gynecologic oncology surgery: analysis of the National surgical quality improvement program database. *Gynecol Oncol.* 2015;136(1):65–70.

44. Uccella S, Ghezzi F, Cromi A, et al. Perioperative allogenic blood transfusions and the risk of endometrial cancer recurrence. *Arch Gynecol Obstet.* 2013;287(5):1009–1016.

45. Linder, et al. Impact of perioperative blood transfusion on cancer recurrence and survival following radical cystectomy. *Eur Urol.* 2013;63:839–845.

46. Rogers GM, Gela D, Cleeland C, et al. *NCCN Guidelines Version 2. 2014 Cancer- and Chemotherapy-induced Anemia. NCCN Clinical Practice Guidelines in Oncology.* Fort Washington, PA: National Comprehensive Cancer Network; 2013.

47. American Society of Anesthesiologists Task Force on Perioperative Blood Management. Practice guidelines for perioperative blood management: an updated report by the American Society of Anesthesiologists task force on perioperative blood management. *Anesthesiology.* 2015;122(2):241–275.

48. Bernard AC, Davenport DL, Chang PK, Vaughan TB, Zwischenberger JB. Intraoperative transfusion of 1 U to 2 U packed red blood cells is associated with increased 30-day mortality, surgical-site infection, pneumonia, and sepsis in general surgery patients. *J Am Coll Surg.* 2009; 208(5):931–937.

49. Rohde JM, Dimcheff DE, Blumberg N, et al. Health care-associated infection after red blood cell transfusion: a systematic review and meta-analysis. *JAMA.* 2014;311(13): 1317–1326.

50. Clevenger B, Mallett SV, Klein AA, Richards T. Patient blood management to reduce surgical risk. *Br J Surg.* 2015;102(11):1325–1337.

51. Qaseem A, Humphrey LL, Fitterman N, Starkey M, Shekelle P. Clinical guidelines committee of the American College of physicians. Treatment of anemia in patients with heart disease: a clinical practice guideline from the American College of physicians. *Ann Intern Med.* 2013; 159(11):770–779.

52. Murphy GJ, Pike K, Rogers CA, et al. Liberal or restrictive transfusion after cardiac surgery. *NEJM.* 2015;372(11): 997–1008.

53. Curley GF, Shehata N, Mazer CD, Hare GMT, Friedrich JO. Transfusion triggers for guiding RBC transfusion for cardiovascular surgery: a systemic review and meta-analysis. *Crit Care Med.* 2014;42:2611–2624.

54. Horvath KA, Acker MA, Chang H, et al. Blood transfusion and infection after cardiac surgery. *Ann Thorac Surg.* 2013;95:2194–2201.

55. Pattakos G, Koch CG, Brizzio ME, et al. Outcomes of patients who refuse transfusion after cardiac surgery. A natural experiment with severe blood conservation. *Arch Intern Med.* 2012;172(15):1154–1160.

56. Sherwood MW, Wang Y, Curtis JP, Peterson E, Rao SV. Patterns and outcomes of red blood cell transfusion in patients undergoing percutaneous coronary intervention. *JAMA.* 2014;311(8):836–843.

57. Karrowni W, Vora AN, Dai D, Wojdyla D, Dakik H, Rao SV. Blood transfusion and the risk of acute kidney injury among patients with acute coronary syndrome undergoing percutaneous coronary intervention. *Circ Cardiovasc Interv.* 2016;9:e003279. http://dx.doi.org/10.1161/CIRCINTERVENTIONS.115.003279.

58. Athar MK, Bagga Nair N, Punjabi V, Vioto K, Schorr C, Gerber DR. Risk of cardiac arrhythmias and conduction abnormalities in patients with acute myocardial infarction receiving packed red blood cell transfusions. *J Crit Care.* 2011;26:335–341.

59. Docherty AB, O'Donnell R, Brunskill S, et al. Effect of restrictive versus liberal transfusion strategies on outcomes in patients with cardiovascular disease in a non-cardia surgery setting: systemic review and meta-analysis. *BMJ.* 2016;352:i1351.

60. Chatterjee S, Wetterslev J, Sharma A, Lichstein E, Mukherjee D. Association of blood transfusion with increased mortality in myocardial infarction. A meta-analysis and diversity-adjusted study sequential analysis. *JAMA Intern Med.* 2013;173(2):132–139.

61. Petrides M. Indications for transfusion. In: Petrides M, Stack G, Cooling L, Maes LY, eds. *Practical Guide to Transfusion Medicine.* 2nd ed. Bethesda: American Association of Blood Banks Press; 2007:203–207.

62. Win N. Hyperhemolysis syndrome in sickle cell disease. *Expert Rev Hematol.* 2009;2(2):111–115.

63. Movat HZ, Weiser WJ, Glynn MF, Mustard JF. Platelet phagocytosis and aggregation. *J Cell Biol.* 1965;27(3): 531–543.

64. Dubois C, Panicot-Dubois L, Merrill-Skoloff G, Furie B, et al. Glycoprotein VI-dependent and -independent pathways of thrombus formation in vivo. *Blood.* 2006;107 (10):3902–3906.

65. Jackson SP, Nesbitt WS, Kulkarni S. Signaling events underlying thrombus formation. *J Thromb Haemost.* 2003;1(7):1602–1612.

66. O'Halloran AM, Curtin R, O'Connor F. The impact of genetic variation in the region of the GPIIIa gene, on PlA-2expression bias and GPIIb/IIIa receptor density in platelets. *Br J Haematol.* 2006;132(4):494–502.

67. Stanworth SJ, Estcourt LJ, Powter G, et al., TOPPS Investigators. A no-prophylaxis platelet-transfusion strategy for hematologic cancers. *N Engl J Med.* 2013;368(19):1771–1780.

68. Wandt H, Schaefer-Eckart K, Wendelin K, et al. Study Alliance Leukemia. Therapeutic platelet transfusion vs routine prophylactic transfusion in patients with haematological malignancies: an open-label, multicenter, randomized study. *Lancet.* 2012;380:1309–1316.

69. AABB, American Red Cross, America's Blood Centers, Armed Services Blood Program. *Circular of Information for the Use of Human Blood and Blood Components*; 2013:23–27. Available at: http://www.aabb.org/tm/coi/Documents/coi1113.

70. FDA. Draft guidance for industry: bacterial risk control strategies for blood collection establishments and transfusion services to enhance the safety and availability of platelets for transfusion. In: *U.S. Food & Drug Administration Vaccines, Blood & Biologics.* 2016. Available at: https://www.fda.gov/downloads/biologicsbloodvaccines/%20guidancecomplianceregulatoryinformation/guidances/blood/ucm425952.pdf.

71. Kaufman RM, Djulbegovic B, Gernsheimer T, et al. Platelet transfusion: a clinical practice guideline from the AABB. *Ann Intern Med.* 2015;162:205–213.

72. Estcourt LJ, Birchall J, Allard S, et al. The British Committee for standards in Haematology. Guidelines for the use of platelet transfusions. *Br J Haematol.* 2017;176:365–394.

73. Slichter SJ, Kaufman RM, Assmann SF, et al. Dose of prophylactic platelet transfusions and prevention of hemorrhage. *The New Engl J Med.* 2010;362(7):600–613.

74. Josephson CD, Granger S, Assmann SF, et al. Bleeding risks are higher in children versus adults given prophylactic platelet transfusions for treatment-induced hypoproliferative thrombocytopenia. *Blood.* 2012;120(4):748–760.

75. Slichter SJ. The Trial to Reduce Alloimmunization to Platelets Study Group. Leukocyte reduction and ultraviolet B irradiation of platelets to prevent alloimmunization and refractoriness to platelet transfusions. *N Engl J Med.* 1997;337:1861–1869.

76. Kaufman RM, Djulbegovic B, Gernsheimer T, et al. Platelet transfusion: a clinical practice guideline from the AABB. *Ann Intern Med.* 2015;162:205–213.

77. Miller RD. Massive blood transfusions: the impact of Vietnam military data on modern civilian transfusion medicine. *Anesthes.* 2009;110(6):1412–1416.

78. Hopkins CK, Goldfinger D. Platelet transfusions in heparin-induced thrombocytopenia: a report of four cases and review of the literature. *Transfusion.* 2008;48(10):2128–2132.

79. Otrock ZK, Liu C, Grossman BJ. Platelet transfusion in thrombotic thrombocytopenic purpura. *Vox Sang.* 2015; 109(2):168–172.

80. Refaai MA, Chuang C, Menegus M, Blumberg N, Francis CW. Outcomes after platelet transfusion in patients with heparin-induced thrombocytopenia. *J Thrombosis Haemostasis.* 2010;8:1419–1421.

81. Swisher KK, Terrell DR, Vesely SK, Kremer Hovinga JA, Lämmle B, George JN. Clinical outcomes after platelet transfusions in patients with thrombotic thrombocytopenic purpura. *Transfusion.* 2009;49(5):873–887.

82. AABB, American Red Cross, America's Blood Centers, Armed Services Blood Program. *Circular of Information for the Use of Human Blood and Blood Components;* 2013:16–21. Available at: http://www.aabb.org/tm/coi/Documents/coi1113.

83. Holland LL, Brooks JP. Toward rational fresh frozen plasma transfusion: the effect of plasma transfusion on coagulation test results. *Am J Clin Pathol.* 2006; 126:133–139.

84. Hirshberg A, Dugas M, Banez EI, Scott BG, Wall Jr MJ, Mattox KL. Minimizing dilutional coagulopathy in exsanguinating hemorrhage: a computer simulation. *J Trauma.* 2003;54(3):454–463.

85. Dzik WH. *Component Therapy before Bedside Procedures.* 2nd ed. Baltimore, MD: AABB Press; 2005.

86. Abdel-Wahab OI, Healy B, Dzik WH. Effect of fresh-frozen plasma transfusion on prothrombin time and bleeding in patients with mild coagulation abnormalities. *Transfusion.* 2006;46:1279–1285.

87. Yazer MH. The how's and why's of evidence based plasma therapy. *Korean J Hematol.* 2010;45(3):152–157.

88. Holbrook A, Schulman S, Witt DM, et al. Evidence-based management of anticoagulant therapy: antithrombotic therapy and prevention of thrombosis. 9th ed: American College of Chest Physicians Evidence-based Clinical Practice Guidelines. *Chest.* 2012;141(2 suppl):e152S–e184S.

89. Holcomb JB, del Junco DJ, Fox EE, et al. The prospective, observational, multicenter, major trauma transfusion (PROMMTT) study: comparative effectiveness of a time-varying treatment with competing risks. *JAMA Surg.* 2013;148(2):127–136.

90. Holcomb JB, Tilley BC, Baraniuk S, et al. Transfusion of plasma, platelets, and red blood cells in a 1:1:1 vs a 1:1:2 ratio and mortality in patients with severe trauma: the PROPPR randomized clinical trial. *JAMA.* 2015; 313(5):471–482.

91. Holland L, Sarode R. Should plasma be transfused prophylactically before invasive procedures? *Curr Opin Hematol.* 2006;13:447–451.

92. Holcomb JB, Fox EE, Zhang X, et al. Cryoprecipitate use in the prospective observational multicenter major trauma transfusion study (PROMMTT). *J Trauma Acute Care Surg.* 2013;75(1 suppl 1):S31–S39.

93. Winearls J, Wullschleger M, Wake E, et al. Fibrinogen Early in Severe Trauma studY (FEISTY): study protocol for a randomised controlled trial. *Trials.* 2017;18:241.

94. Droubatchevskaia N, Wong MP, Chipperfield KM, Wadsworth LD, Ferguson DJ. Guidelines for cryoprecipitate transfusion. *BCMJ.* 2007;49(8):441–445.

95. Levy JH, Goodnough LT. How I use fibrinogen replacement therapy in acquired bleeding. *Blood.* 2015;125(9): 1387–1393.

CHAPTER 7

Noninfectious Complications of Transfusion: Adverse Events

SARA RUTTER, MD • CHRISTOPHER A. TORMEY, MD • AMIT GOKHALE, MD

A BACKGROUND ON TRANSFUSION-ASSOCIATED ADVERSE EVENTS

Over the past several decades, as medicine has advanced, the practice of transfusion has also advanced in parallel. In particular, there have been dramatic increases in the safety of transfusions, with the administration of blood or blood components being a routine practice in the management of patients. Transfusion, however, still carries risks. Although transfusion-associated fatalities are significantly less common today, adverse events do occur. Studies estimate the rate of adverse reactions at 77.5–239.5 per 100,000 blood components transfused.[1-3] These may be minor and have no significant clinical implications or may be severe and life-threatening.

Until very recently, there were few rigorously developed standards or guidelines for the definition of various transfusion-associated adverse events in the United States. However, as part of an effort to develop a national hemovigilance network, the Centers for Disease Control and Prevention (CDC) created a very useful document to better classify the myriad types of hazards associated with transfusion. At present, the CDC recognizes 12 categories of adverse reactions, which we will refer to as transfusion reactions throughout the rest of this chapter.[4] In writing this chapter, we have organized reactions according to the CDC criteria and present them as those associated with high morbidity/mortality rates followed by those with low morbidity/mortality. Each reaction category is discussed in depth, with sections devoted to incidence, pathophysiology, treatment, and prevention. However, before beginning a detailed discussion of transfusion reactions, it is first important for the reader to appreciate the general concepts of transfusion reactions, including how they are evaluated. As such, we will begin with a basic approach to a patient with a suspected transfusion reaction. Finally, note that although we are discussing "noninfectious" adverse events in this chapter, we have included a brief discussion of septic transfusion reactions (STRs) because they are an important acute-onset adverse event; the specifics of transmission of nonbacterial agents (e.g., viruses, prions) that do not typically manifest as an acute transfusion reaction is beyond the scope of this chapter.

APPROACH TO A REACTION: GENERAL CONSIDERATIONS

The timeline of a transfusion reaction can vary greatly based on the suspected reaction type. Some adverse events may occur almost immediately, whereas others may not be evident for days or even weeks after transfusion. Although the presentation and timing vary, many key concepts in the approach to a transfusion reaction remain the same. The three most fundamental, immediate steps for a clinician caring for a patient with a suspected transfusion reaction are to:

- stop the transfusion,
- stabilize the patient, and
- report the reaction to the blood bank or transfusion medicine service.[2]

Box 7.1 summarizes these and the additional steps to be taken when initially consulted about a possible reaction, or when in the midst of a formal reaction evaluation.

If a patient displays symptoms of even a *possible* reaction during a transfusion, the transfusion must also stop. The initial symptoms may be vague and are often nonspecific (see our discussion of febrile reactions later in this chapter, for example). Because a definite distinction between reactions cannot be made quickly, ending the transfusion is the safest course of action. If necessary, measures should be taken to ensure hemodynamic stability and prevent respiratory compromise.[2]

Once the patient is stable, the clinician should notify the blood bank or transfusion medicine service that a suspected transfusion reaction has occurred. Pathologists or blood bank medical personnel should be prepared to obtain a clinical summary of the patient, the start time (and completion time, if applicable) of the transfusion, and a description of the patient's

---

BOX 7.1
Flowchart Representation of the Approach to a Transfusion Reaction From the Blood Bank/Clinical Pathology Perspective

Reaction Suspected
↓
If not already done, recommend an immediate stop to the infusion!
↓
Advise clinical team to complete the steps of a reaction evaluation:
- Return the product(s) & compatibility paperwork to the blood bank
- Collect a post-reaction blood bank specimen

↓
Gather relevant information from the patient or clinical team including:
- Specific chief complaint & reaction signs / symptoms
- Changes in vital signs above / below baseline values
- Physical exam changes from baseline
- A transfusion reaction review of systems, particularly focused on any new cardiovascular, pulmonary, abdominal / flank issues or pain at the infusion site
- History of prior reactions / products received that day

↓
Evaluate the need for additional testing, which may include in some cases:
- Urinalysis
- Culture of the patient and/or blood product
- Brain-natriuretic peptide
- Hemolysis markers
- Coagulation studies
- Imaging (e.g., chest x-ray)

↓
Review the results of the blood bank-specific evaluation & results of any additional testing ordered
↓
Discuss findings with the clinical team and make treatment or preventative recommendations (as applicable)
↓
Complete a formal consultation note

---

symptoms. Note should be made of any premedication before the transfusion (e.g., diphenhydramine, acetaminophen) and any history of transfusion reactions. The remainder of the blood product (or the empty product bag) should be returned to the blood bank, if possible. The blood bank will perform a review to ensure that the patient's blood type is correct and that the patient received the correct blood product and unit. There may be variation between institutions regarding what laboratory testing is performed in a given situation. Some blood banks may standardly evaluate for hemolysis. Additional testing may be necessary based on the patient's symptoms and the suspected reaction[2]; such testing will be discussed in more detail later.

REACTIONS ASSOCIATED WITH HIGH MORBIDITY AND MORTALITY

Transfusion-Related Acute Lung Injury

Transfusion-related acute lung injury (TRALI) was first recognized in 1926 and was previously known as pulmonary hypersensitivity reaction.[5] Of all the transfusion reactions, TRALI is associated with the highest mortality, ranging from 5% to 35% in some series; according to the Food and Drug Administration (FDA), TRALI accounted for 38% of all transfusion-related deaths from 2011 to 2015.[3,5,6] Per data from the American Red Cross, the risk of fatal TRALI is 1:202,673 for plasma, 1:320,572 for apheresis platelets, and 1:2,527,437 for red blood cell (RBC) units.[5]

Pathophysiology

The current "two-hit" model of TRALI's pathogenesis revolves around the transfusion of antibodies and/or other nonimmunologic mediators to a susceptible patient.[5,7] The most frequently implicated antibodies are human leukocyte antigen (HLA) class I, HLA class II, and human neutrophil antibodies (HNA)[5,7]; these antibodies activate the leukocytes, which bind to the endothelium in the lungs, causing endothelial injury and edema.[5,7] Other nonimmune mediators such as CD40L and various lipids accumulate during blood product storage and can also activate leukocytes, leading to the same end result.[5,7,8]

Plasma-rich products like fresh frozen plasma (FFP) and platelets are the most likely blood components to be involved in TRALI because donor antibodies are present in the plasma; it is important to note, however, that TRALI can also be seen following RBC transfusion.[5] In an effort to prevent TRALI, the International Society for Blood Transfusion has recommended that donors be screened for antileukocyte antibodies.[9] HLA and human neutrophil antibodies (HNA) antibodies are more commonly identified in the plasma of women, specifically those who have been pregnant. For this reason, plasma products may be collected primarily from men.[5,7] These measures have proved to be effective in decreasing the incidence of TRALI.[5,7]

Diagnostic criteria

The CDC defines TRALI as acute lung injury occurring within 6 h of a transfusion, as evidenced by hypoxemia and bilateral pulmonary infiltrates on x-ray. There must not be evidence of cardiac overload or acute lung injury before the transfusion[4]; all criteria must be met to make the diagnosis. Although not specifically listed as criteria by the CDC or the TRALI Consensus Guidelines,[4,10] fever, hypotension, tachypnea, transient neutropenia,

and dyspnea frequently accompany the lung injury.[2] Because management differs, it is imperative that TRALI be distinguished from other respiratory reactions discussed in this chapter. Any patient with suspected TRALI should have a chest radiograph as part of the reaction workup; brain natriuretic peptide (BNP) levels may be helpful in evaluating a patient's cardiovascular status (expected to be elevated in volume overload and normal in TRALI), and such testing can to help exclude other diagnoses. Notably, however, there are no acute care tests currently available to help establish the diagnosis of TRALI–it is a diagnosis made on clinical grounds. Although testing of the donors of a product implicated in TRALI for HLA or HNA antibodies should be performed, this testing is not acute in nature and generally will not be useful in the establishment of a diagnosis of TRALI in "real time."

Treatment

As with all transfusion reactions, immediate cessation of the transfusion and stabilization of the patient are critical. Respiratory support may range from supplemental oxygen to intubation. Steroids have not been proven to be beneficial. TRALI reactions usually resolve over the course of a few days with only supportive measures being needed.[2,5,7] Reporting of suspected TRALI is vital; as a risk reduction strategy, donors of units associated with TRALI are removed from the donor pool based on the testing described earlier.[5,11]

Transfusion-Associated Circulatory Overload/Transfusion-Associated Dyspnea

Transfusion-associated circulatory overload (TACO) is generally the most common high-morbidity transfusion reaction encountered in clinical practice, and it is currently the second leading transfusion-associated cause of death in the United States, accounting for 24% of such deaths between 2011 and 2015.[2,3,6,11] This statistic is made more concerning by the knowledge that cardiopulmonary transfusion reactions, including TACO, are frequently unrecognized and go unreported.[11] Certain patient characteristics are known to increase the risk of TACO, including older age, renal disease, cardiac disease, positive fluid balance, and critically ill status.[2,12] Certain transfusion practices are also known to be associated with TACO, such as transfusion of large volumes of plasma, rapid infusion rates, and transfusion of multiple products.[2,11,12]

The clinical criteria for TRALI and TACO are strict, and a number of reactions with cardiopulmonary symptoms do not necessarily meet the standards necessary for diagnosis. This may be due to the variation in presentation,

TABLE 7.1
Signs, Symptoms, and Diagnostic Testing Findings in Various Pulmonary Transfusion-Associated Adverse Events

	TRALI	TACO	TAD
Time frame	During or within 6 h of transfusion completion	During or within 6 h of transfusion completion	During or within 24 h of transfusion completion
Pathophysiology	Immunologic; often antibody mediated	Circulatory overload	Unclear mechanism
Radiologic findings	New, diffuse, bilateral pulmonary infiltrates	Pulmonary edema or effusions; may or may not be bilateral	Highly variable; no definitive need for pulmonary edema or effusions
Fever?	Yes, often	Not typical	Not typical
Neutropenia?	Yes, occasional	Not typical	Not typical
BNP elevation?	Not typical	Yes, frequent	Not typical
Blood pressure?	Normo- or hypotension	Hypertension	Variable
Central venous pressure elevation?	Not typical	Yes, frequent	Not typical
Treatment	Aggressive pulmonary support; no clear role for immunosuppression	Diuresis; aggressive pulmonary support if nonresponsive to diuresis	Aggressive pulmonary support; no clear role for immunosuppression

BNP, brain natriuretic peptide; *TACO*, transfusion-associated circulatory overload; *TAD*, transfusion-associated dyspnea; *TRALI*, transfusion-related acute lung injury.

the temporal relationship between the transfusion and symptom onset, or an incomplete reaction workup. If not meeting strict consensus criteria, but in cases in which there is high likelihood that a pulmonary reaction is attributable to transfusion, such adverse events may be classified as transfusion-associated dyspnea (TAD), which acts as a "catch-all" category for pulmonary reactions wherein there is strong implication of a recent transfusion, but the reaction cannot be otherwise definitively classified.[4]

Pathophysiology
Unlike the majority of transfusion reactions, which are immunologically mediated, TACO's pathophysiology invokes simple physics—too much fluid is added to the system too quickly (or in volumes that cannot be tolerated) for the transfusion recipient. Because the circulatory system cannot cope with the additional volume of the transfused products, pulmonary edema and respiratory distress result as fluid "backs up" into the lungs.[2]

Diagnostic criteria
To diagnose TACO, the CDC requires that at least three of the following six criteria be met within 6 h of the transfusion: acute respiratory distress, elevated BNP, increased central venous pressure, signs of left-sided heart failure, positive fluid balance, and pulmonary

edema on radiology.[4] Acute respiratory distress may include cough, dyspnea, orthopnea, or tachypnea.[2,4]

TACO and TRALI may be difficult to differentiate at the initial presentation, and although the clinical diagnostic criteria are similar, there are certain features that may be useful in acutely differentiating between these entities. As discussed in Table 7.1 and later in the chapter, TACO is not an inflammatory condition, therefore fever is not typically seen, and when present, should be more indicative of TRALI.[2] Patients with TACO also frequently show improvement within 24 h of their symptoms; lack of improvement or worsening of respiratory status should prompt reconsideration of TRALI.[13] The usefulness of BNP in distinguishing TACO and TRALI is debatable[12]; however, in light of the CDC criteria, we recommend that BNP levels be measured for the evaluation of any transfusion reaction involving pulmonary edema to better evaluate for TACO.[13]

As mentioned previously, many reactions that present with TRALI or TACO-like symptoms do not meet the criteria for a diagnosis of TACO. In such situations, the diagnosis of TAD may be used.[4] As also outlined in Table 7.2, TAD may be diagnosed if the patient experiences acute respiratory distress within 24 h of the transfusion and the reaction cannot otherwise be classified as TACO, TRALI, or an allergic/anaphylactic reaction.[4]

TABLE 7.2
Signs, Symptoms, and Laboratory Findings in Acute and Delayed Hemolytic Transfusion Reactions

	Acute Hemolytic Transfusion Reactions	Delayed Hemolytic Transfusion Reactions
Site of hemolysis	Intravascular	Extravascular
Degree of anemia	Moderate to severe	Mild to moderate
LDH	Marked increase (↑↑↑)	Mild increase (↑)
Total and indirect bilirubin	Marked increase (↑↑↑)	Mild increase (↑)
Haptoglobin	Marked decrease (↓↓↓)	No or mild decrease (↓)
Hemoglobinemia	Present	Absent
Hemoglobinuria	Present	Absent
Pain at flank or infusion site	Present	Absent
Direct antiglobulin test	Positive (C3 +/− IgG)	Positive (IgG +/− C3)
Peripheral smear findings	Schistocytes + microspherocytes	Microspherocytes

LDH, lactate dehydrogenase.

Treatment

If the transfusion is still running, it should be stopped immediately. In some cases, the patient will improve with simply stopping the infusion. More commonly, patients will require some form of respiratory support, at least temporarily; a mild reaction may only necessitate supplemental oxygen, whereas intubation and ventilator support may be needed in more severe cases.[2] In contrast with TRALI, diuretics are useful in the treatment of TACO; the decrease in circulatory volume relieves cardiovascular stress, improving the pulmonary edema.

Discussion of the treatment of TACO must also include an acknowledgment that in many cases, it can be prevented altogether. The cause of the reaction is understood; patients at risk of fluid overload are likely to be at increased risk of TACO and should be transfused at a slow rate.[2] In addition, transfusion of multiple products within a short time should be avoided in these patients, if clinically possible. Unfortunately, multiple studies have shown that TACO is underreported. Proper reporting of cardiopulmonary reactions, specifically TACO, may help identify patients who may be at increased risk for subsequent occurrences and lead to better transfusion strategies to avoid these reactions in such patients.[11]

Hemolytic Reactions

Transfusions leading to RBC hemolysis can be among the most devastating and feared complications of blood product administration. According to data accrued by the US FDA, hemolytic reactions are a leading cause of transfusion-associated fatalities in the United States, often cited as the second or third most common cause of death due to transfusion over the past 10 years.[6] Data from other large hemovigilance networks around the globe (such as the UK Serious Hazards of Transfusion database) also implicate hemolytic reactions as having high rates of morbidity and mortality.[14] As such, recognizing and preventing the occurrence of hemolysis is a major goal of the international blood bank community.

When considering hemolytic reactions from a general standpoint, it is important to recognize that these adverse events do not come in a "one size fits all" categorization, but rather represent a spectrum of signs and symptoms and, depending on the clinical scenario, may be acute or delayed, intra- or extravascular, attributable to ABO or non-ABO antibodies, and in some circumstances, may even be caused by mechanical forms of hemolysis due to improper infusion techniques![2] For the purposes of this chapter, our discussion of hemolytic reactions will focus on those that are immune mediated (i.e., driven by antibodies and/or the complement cascade). The remainder of the distinctions will be further detailed in the next section on reaction pathophysiology.

Pathophysiology

As discussed previously, there are many different ways the immune system can react to, and lyse, transfused red cells. For our characterization of hemolytic reactions, we will delve first into where the clearance of

RBCs is taking place, namely, the intra- or extravascular space. Dividing reactions up into sites of clearance will reveal that the clinical presentations, as well as the antibodies driving these reactions, typically demonstrate unique characteristics and distinct pathophysiology.

Intravascular hemolysis. In the setting of intravascular hemolysis, RBCs are most often cleared after an antibody binds to the incompatible cells, resulting in fixation of complement.[15] Once the complement cascade has been fixed and activated on the incompatible cells, the resulting membrane attack complex punches holes in the red cell, resulting in its lysis and destruction. Most often it is the IgM class antibodies that are most efficient at fixing complement and, therefore, acute intravascular hemolysis is strongly associated with incompatibilities within ABO antibodies (which are most likely to be IgM in nature among all blood group antigen/antibody families).[15]

Acute intravascular hemolysis can be devastating to a transfusion recipient. In addition to acute, significant anemia due to rapid hemolysis of incompatible RBCs, the systematic activation of complement can have substantial physiologic consequences.[15] For instance, destruction of RBCs and generation of free RBC membranes in the intravascular space can cause concomitant activation of the coagulation system, resulting in the development of disseminated intravascular coagulation (DIC). Moreover, complement generation and RBC release of hemoglobin can induce acute kidney injury and renal failure, a particularly feared complication of hemolysis.[15] Complement activation can also cause smooth muscle constriction, increased small vessel permeability, and leukocyte activation, contributing to the shocklike symptom often seen in intravascular hemolytic reactions.[16]

In addition to understanding how acute hemolytic reactions cause disease, it is important to consider how these reactions arise from a purely logistic standpoint. Because ABO antigens are strongly expressed throughout life, and because ABO antibodies are induced at an early age and show long detectability in plasma, blood banks do not often encounter problems in identifying a patient's ABO type. Therefore ABO incompatibilities (and the resultant intravascular hemolytic transfusion reactions) most often occur because an error has been made at some point in the *preanalytical* (e.g., mislabeling of a specimen's tube at the bedside), *analytical* (e.g., switching of specimens during testing at the blood bank bench), or *postanalytical* (e.g., administration of an RBC unit to the wrong patient) phase of testing.[17] In fact, it has been estimated that ABO mismatches occur

in about 1 in 40,000 transfusions, with an acute hemolytic transfusion incidence estimated at about 1 in 76,000 transfusions.[18] Therefore rigorous processes of patient identification before, during, and after testing has been performed (and before a unit is administered in clinical wards) are critical in helping to prevent these types of reactions.[17,18]

Extravascular hemolysis. In contrast to intravascular hemolysis, which is typically acute and thunderous at onset, extravascular hemolysis is generally associated with a more subdued, slower RBC clearance, most often with RBCs lysed in the spleen in a non-complement-dependent manner.[15] For this type of hemolytic reaction, RBC clearance occurs because incompatible cells are coated by IgG class antibodies, with antibody-coated cells subsequently phagocytosed. As such, most extravascular reactions are mediated by non-ABO antibodies (e.g., anti-Jk^a, anti-K, and anti-E) since these antibodies are most likely to be IgG in class.[15]

Because of the slower, extravascular nature of these reactions the likelihood of end organ damage and a shocklike symptom is markedly reduced, particularly when compared with intravascular hemolysis. Typically, extravascular RBC clearance results in mild to moderate anemia, low-grade fevers, and occasional jaundice.[2,15] However, the extent of the reaction often depends on the immune competence of the host who received the incompatible transfusion. As such, chronically transfused patients with relatively normal immune systems (e.g., patients with sickle cell disease and thalassemia) have been known to manifest severe extravascular hemolytic reactions with a clinical picture not unlike that seen in patients with acute intravascular lysis.[19] Therefore the severity of the disease process can be highly variable from patient to patient.

Finally, and like intravascular reactions, it is also important to note the unique means by which non-ABO-antibody-mediated extravascular hemolytic reactions arise. Unlike ABO antibodies discussed earlier (which are persistently detectable over decades), antibodies to non-ABO antigens can be quite short lived. In fact, non-ABO antibodies undergo a phenomenon dubbed evanescence, wherein they can disappear from detection over time. Studies have shown that more than 70% of induced non-ABO antibodies can become undetectable, with evanescence typically occurring weeks to months after the antibody is first formed.[20] Given this disappearance phenomenon, the most likely reason underlying extravascular hemolysis is *not* blood bank error, but rather an inability to detect an evanesced non-ABO alloantibody.

The typical scenario giving rise to non-ABO-antibody-mediated extravascular hemolysis has the following pattern:

- A patient with an evanesced antibody is reexposed to the cognate antigen via RBC transfusion (day 0 relative to the day of transfusion).
- The transfusion recipient's immune system encounters this incompatible antigen, which it has previously seen, and an anamnestic (or memory) antibody response is initiated (days 1–3 after transfusion).
- Alloantibodies against the cognate antigen begin to increase in titer with some clearance of the incompatible RBCs (days 3–10 after transfusion).
- As the alloantibody response peaks, increasing numbers of incompatible RBCs are cleared, primarily through extravascular mechanisms (days 11–28 after transfusion).[15]

Because of the time lapse between exposure to the incompatible transfusion and the onset of perceptible hemolysis anywhere from 3 to 21 days later, this phenomenon is also called a delayed hemolytic transfusion reaction (in contrast to the acute nature of most intravascular reactions). Delayed hemolytic reactions are quite common with an estimated incidence of 1:2500 to 1:11,000 transfusions.[18] Despite their frequent occurrence, and as noted earlier, the severity of a delayed hemolytic reaction depends on the immune competence of the transfusion recipient. In some cases, recipients mount only a weak anamnestic response with no evidence of accelerated RBC clearance. In these cases, reactions are dubbed delayed *serologic* transfusion reactions, as the only evidence that a reaction has occurred is a newly detectable blood group antibody.[21]

Diagnostic criteria

As the causes of and pathophysiology for immune-mediated acute and delayed hemolytic reactions are so very different, the CDC has created unique diagnostic criteria for each of these types of adverse events. For acute hemolytic reactions, the CDC indicates that a patient presenting with *any of the following during or within 24 h* of transfusion, back/flank pain, chills, rigors, DIC, fever, hematuria, hypotension, oliguria/anuria, pain at the infusion site, and/or renal failure, *and two or more of the following over that same time frame*, decreased fibrinogen or haptoglobin, elevated bilirubin or lactate dehydrogenase, hemoglobinemia, hemoglobinuria, and/or spherocytes on peripheral smear, has a high suspicion for hemolysis and should undergo direct antiglobulin testing (DAT).[4] Most often this testing will demonstrate positivity for complement and/or

IgG, which would confirm a diagnosis of acute intravascular hemolysis.

For delayed hemolytic reactions, the CDC has somewhat looser criteria indicating that a patient must have a positive DAT associated with a transfusion done 1–28 days previously and either a newly detectable alloantibody or a positive elution study in that time frame.[4] Moreover, such patients should also show either a blunted response to the questionable RBC transfusion, a drop in hemoglobin/hematocrit back to pre-transfusion levels after a recent RBC transfusion, or any unexplained RBC clearance as manifested by increased spherocytes seen on a peripheral smear review following a recent transfusion.[4] Table 7.2 also compares the common signs/symptoms/laboratory tests performed in the setting of acute versus delayed hemolytic transfusion reactions and shows how the results of such testing may differ between these entities.

Treatment

Given the rarity of their occurrence there are no evidence-based recommendations for the treatment of either acute/intravascular or delayed/extravascular hemolytic reactions. Therefore approaches to managing these reactions typically include assessing their severity, providing supportive transfusions to overcome the acute anemia (and coagulation disorders, if they exist), and steps to preserve renal function. We will first tackle the approach to acute hemolytic reactions.

For ongoing RBC transfusion support to overcome anemia, it is imperative that the blood bank identify the problem that caused the acute hemolytic reaction before issuing any additional units. This involves ensuring that the patient's ABO and Rh typing is confirmed as accurate, that any new alloantibodies that may have driven the reaction have been identified, and finally, that the new unit(s) to be administered are fully compatible with the patient using the post-transfusion reaction specimen. In urgent circumstances during which the transfusion of a gravely ill patient cannot be delayed until the completion of a transfusion reaction evaluation, group O, Rh-negative units may be administered until the cause of hemolysis is rectified; obviously, communication between the clinical teams and blood bank is critical to ensure that no unnecessary or potentially dangerous transfusions are performed. Finally, in rare circumstances of massive or large-scale transfusion of incompatible RBCs to individuals, there is growing literature to suggest that RBC exchange with compatible RBC units (when available and feasible to perform) may be useful to prevent or limit hemolysis.[22,23]

In addition to RBC transfusion, there are other important aspects of supportive care in the setting of clinically significant acute hemolysis. Renal function must be closely monitored both clinically and via laboratory assays such as creatinine. Many resources recommend vigorous hydration of patients experiencing significant hemolytic episodes, with one guideline suggesting maintenance of urine output at >1 mL/kg/h for up to 24 h after transfusion.[18] Aggressive monitoring for the onset of DIC is also recommended via testing of fibrinogen as well as measuring the prothrombin time and partial thromboplastin time. Should there be clinical or laboratory evidence of DIC, blood product therapy with plasma, cryoprecipitate, or platelets is advisable.[18] Finally, patients with severe hemolysis may experience shocklike symptoms and such patients benefit from transfer to a monitored setting where intensive pulmonary and cardiovascular support can be adequately provided.

Regarding the approach to delayed hemolytic reactions, in most cases close observation of the patient with supportive care and occasional compatible transfusions to overcome accelerated RBC clearance are more than sufficient to help the patient weather the storm.[18] However, it should be noted that the aforementioned steps of providing aggressive renal, pulmonary, and cardiovascular care apply to the more rare severe delayed reactions, should they be encountered.

Finally, as with many of the adverse events discussed in this chapter, preventative measures are also helpful in mitigating the occurrence of hemolytic transfusion reactions. Since nearly all ABO-related intravascular hemolytic events are associated with human errors, the implementation of rigorous patient identification processes and multiple safety nets in the practice of specimen collection and blood product administration are the key means to minimize the likelihood of mistakes.[17] In light of the unique nature of evanescence and delayed hemolytic reactions, there are not as many readily available approaches to mitigating risks associated with non-ABO antibodies. Nonetheless, actions to increase the portability of antibody information from hospital to hospital (e.g., wallet cards, medical alert bracelets, antibody registries) can help to raise awareness of an alloantibody that is no longer detectable. Obtaining transfusion or pregnancy histories from patients can also be helpful to identify individuals who may be at risk for such reactions, particularly those with multiple past RBC exposures.[23]

Septic Transfusion Reactions

When transfused with a human-derived product, patients are at risk for acquiring numerous infectious

TABLE 7.3
Bacterial Pathogens Commonly Associated With Blood Product Contamination and STRs on a Blood Product Basis

Platelets	RBCs
Staphylococcus aureus	Yersinia enterocolitica
Klebsiella pneumoniae	Pseudomonas fluorescens
Serratia marcescens	Staphylococcus spp.
Staphylococcus epidermidis	Propionibacterium spp.
Group B Streptococcus	Serratia spp.
Escherichia coli	
Bacillus cereus	

Organisms are listed in descending order, with those at the top of the respective columns being the ones most frequently associated with STRs, whereas those listed in the middle and at the bottom of the respective columns being less frequently seen, as collated from various reports.[23a]
RBC, red blood cells; STR, septic transfusion reaction.

diseases, including those mediated by viruses, bacteria, and even parasites. These types of reactions, also referred to as transfusion-transmitted infections (TTIs), can be quite problematic from the blood bank standpoint. STRs in particular (and which will be the focus of this section) occur when a patient is transfused with a bacterially contaminated blood product. Although this is an uncommon occurrence, STRs are responsible for significant morbidity and mortality; between 2011 and 2015, 10% of transfusion-associated fatalities were due to contaminated blood products.[6] The most common blood products implicated in STRs are platelets; this is because platelet units are stored at room temperature, encouraging the growth of any bacteria present.[24] STRs can also result from red cell transfusions, but because RBC units are refrigerated during storage, these typically involve bacteria that thrive at low temperatures.[2] Table 7.3 lists the organisms frequently associated with STRs on a blood component basis.

Pathophysiology

Blood products may be contaminated via several mechanisms. Skin flora may be introduced during collection, or a donor with low-level bacteremia may pass organisms directly into the unit. It is also possible, although uncommon, for blood to be contaminated during processing.[2,24] Many measures have been implemented to reduce the risk of contamination, including more stringent donor health screenings, more rigorous skin disinfection procedures, and the addition of a diversion pouch to collect the first (and most likely to be contaminated) few milliliters of blood taken during a donation.[24–26] Because platelet units carry a higher risk for STRs, specific strategies have been developed to decrease their risk. Platelet units may only be stored for a maximum of 7 days and must be tested for the presence of bacteria at set times.[27] A number of pathogen reduction/pathogen inactivation methods have also been developed with at least one platform available for clinical use in the United States at the time of this writing.[28]

Ultimately, transfusion of a contaminated unit introduces bacteria, and potentially endotoxins, directly into the patient's bloodstream, which can cause rapid and severe septic shock. Because the blood product essentially acts as a culture, a small amount of initial contamination may result in a substantial bacterial load being delivered during transfusion.[2]

Diagnostic criteria

Clinically, a fever with more than 2°C rise from the patient's baseline should raise concern for an STR; other symptoms may include hypotension, rigors/chills, nausea/vomiting, respiratory distress, DIC, or frank shock.[2] The CDC groups STRs with TTIs, which also include parasitic and viral infections. To diagnose a TTI, one only needs "laboratory evidence of a pathogen in the transfusion recipient."[4] Therefore in any suspected STR, blood cultures should be collected from the patient and the blood product (or empty bag or segment, if necessary) should be cultured. An STR is confirmed if the same organism is isolated from the patient's blood and the blood product and there is no other explanation for the recipient's infection.[2,4]

Treatment

As with any suspected transfusion reaction, the transfusion should be immediately stopped. Patients with STRs frequently present in septic shock, so stabilization of the patient is critical.[2] Broad-spectrum antibiotic therapy should be promptly initiated. Once an organism is identified from the patient's blood cultures, antibiotic coverage can be narrowed to optimally treat that organism.[2]

Finally, it is important to note that there are scores of nonbacterial pathogens which can mediate TTIs.[28] A discussion of these is beyond the specific scope of this chapter on noninfectious risks (moreover, these infections rarely manifest as an acute or even delayed transfusion reaction); however, blood donor centers have also taken significant steps to reduce the transmission of such agents including screening donors for high-risk behaviors, testing of products for viruses/pathogens, and the aforementioned processes for inactivating pathogens. Together, these efforts have dramatically reduced the transmission of infectious agents via transfusion.

Anaphylaxis

Anaphylactic transfusion reactions represent the most severe and extreme reactions in the spectrum of allergic transfusion reactions.[3,11] Although allergic transfusion reactions are the most common transfusion reaction, true anaphylactic reactions are thankfully rare, occurring once for every 20,000–47,000 blood products transfused.[29] This section will specifically discuss anaphylactic transfusion reactions; milder allergic transfusion reactions will be discussed later in this chapter in the section titled Low-Morbidity Reactions.

Pathophysiology

Most anaphylactic reactions are associated with platelets or plasma,[2] but they can occur with the transfusion of any blood product. The overarching pathophysiologic theme is complement, mast cell, and basophil activation in response to a specific antigen/allergen.[2] The classic example of anaphylactic transfusion reactions occurs in patients with IgA deficiency who are transfused blood products containing IgA[30,31]; a number of case reports have shown, however, that a wide variety of antigens can trigger anaphylactic transfusion reactions.[2,32] Anaphylaxis may also occur if donor antibodies react with antigens present in the recipient.[29]

Diagnostic criteria

Anaphylactic reactions are characterized by rapid onset of respiratory distress, laryngeal edema, hypotension, and/or gastrointestinal symptoms, often within minutes of starting a transfusion.[2] Other allergic symptoms such as rashes and urticaria may occur in conjunction with these more severe symptoms.[2] The CDC states that the symptoms must appear within 4 h of a transfusion to meet the criteria for an allergic transfusion reaction[4]; apart from this, it does not set forth any specific criteria to define anaphylaxis.

Treatment

Anaphylactic reactions are emergencies and can be fatal if not treated appropriately. The transfusion must be stopped immediately, and the patient must be stabilized as necessary. Epinephrine, intravenous diphenhydramine, and volume resuscitation are often helpful. Respiratory support is vital, and intubation may be required.[2] Patients who have anaphylactic reactions to blood products may require washed products in the future[2,33]; however, the use of washed products does not ensure that the patient will not experience anaphylaxis again. If the culprit antigen can be identified, as in IgA-deficient patients, blood products negative for that antigen should be obtained (if possible).[2,31,33] Any future transfusions in a patient with a history of anaphylactic transfusion reactions should be considered with great caution, and the patient must be closely monitored.

Transfusion-Associated Graft-Versus-Host Disease

Transfusion-associated graft-versus-host disease (TAGVHD) is a highly hazardous transfusion-associated event. As later elaborated on in the subsection Pathophysiology under this section, the risks of TAGVHD vary from population to population because of the diverse HLA haplotype frequencies across the United States and globally. For instance, the risks for TAGVHD range between 1:18,000 and 1:40,000 for Caucasians in the United States, but may be as high as 1:2000–1:8000 for Japanese patients.[34] It is important to note that these risks do not translate to incidences of TAGVHD occurrence per se because in addition to requiring haplotype incompatibility for this reaction to occur, most individuals who experience TAGVHD must be severely immunocompromised. As such, TAGVHD is a relatively rare transfusion reaction to encounter in clinical practice.[2]

Pathophysiology

The primary drivers of TAGVHD are T lymphocytes present in donor units that are infused to transfusion recipients. If an individual is exposed to a donor with a different HLA haplotype, then in most circumstances the recipient's immune system will aggressively attack and eliminate these foreign lymphocytes. However, severely immunocompromised individuals may not be able to mount this attack, allowing donor T lymphocytes to engraft.[35] Alternatively, even in an immunocompetent host, donor T lymphocytes possessing a similar (but not identical) HLA repertoire may evade immune clearance.[35] In either circumstances, the engrafted donor T lymphocytes, particularly CD8+ cytotoxic T cells, mediate substantial tissue and cellular damage including skin lesions (e.g., erythroderma) and multiorgan failure involving the gastrointestinal system, liver, bone marrow, and lymphoid system.[36] The aforementioned manifestations of TAGVHD are not acute in onset and are often encountered days to weeks after the offending transfusion(s), ranging from 2–3 days up to 6 weeks.[35,36] Moreover, virtually any cellular transfusion product can be associated with TAGVHD, including whole blood as well as red cell, platelet, fresh liquid plasma, and granulocyte components.[35,36]

Diagnostic criteria

Per the CDC criteria,[4] TAGVHD must take place between 2 days and 6 weeks after an implicated transfusion. Moreover, patients should present with symptoms discussed previously. Symptoms specifically indicated by the CDC as being consistent with the clinical syndrome of TAGVHD include:[4]

- Characteristic erythroderma rash (with characteristic histologic appearance on biopsy)
- Diarrhea
- Fever
- Hepatomegaly with accompanying hepatic dysfunction
- Marrow failure

Treatment

TAGVHD carries a dismal prognosis, with a reported mortality rate of >90% and death occurring within weeks of onset of the first signs/symptoms of the disorder.[18] Treatment options are highly limited and must also be given rapidly once TAGVHD is recognized given the rapid time course of the disease. There are only scattered reports of overcoming TAGVHD, most referencing the use of either immunosuppressive therapies or stem cell transplant.[18]

Given the high mortality rates associated with TAGVHD and the limited therapeutic options, much emphasis has been placed on the prevention of this reaction.[18,35] Fortunately, there are multiple means by which TAGVHD can be evaded. One common practice is the irradiation of cellular blood components utilizing gamma or x-ray sources. After exposure of a blood product to an irradiation source (typically involving a minimum dose of 2500 cGy to the central part of the product and a minimum dose of 1500 cGy to the noncentral locations),[18] lymphocytes in the product are unable to proliferate after infusion, thereby preventing their engraftment. More recently, pathogen inactivation technologies (where intercalators bind to and disrupt cellular nucleic acids) have also been shown to be effective means of inhibiting lymphocyte proliferation and preventing TAGVHD.[35]

The question remains as to whether all cellular transfusion products should undergo lymphocyte inactivation by irradiation or nucleic acid intercalation. Data would certainly suggest that it is more than just severely immunocompromised individuals who may

TABLE 7.4 Disorders or Scenarios in Which Mitigation Efforts to Prevent TAGVHD Would be Appropriate in US-Based Blood Banks and Transfusion Services	
Lymphocyte inactivation required by AABB Standards regardless of the disease state	Donor is a blood relative of the recipient
	HLA-selected, HLA-matched product
Lymphocyte inactivation recommended based on immunosuppression/disease state	Intrauterine transfusions
	Neonatal transfusions
	Congenital cellular immunodeficiency disorders
	Hodgkin lymphoma
	Treatment with purine analogs, purine antagonists, bendamustine, alemtuzumab, and antithymocyte globulin
	Allogeneic stem cell transplant recipients
	Autologous stem cell transplant recipients
	Recipients of granulocyte products
Lymphocyte inactivation not usually recommended	Human immunodeficiency virus infection
	Primary neutrophil dysfunction disorders
	Solid organ transplantation
Lymphocyte inactivation contraindicated	Stem cell products

AABB, American Association of Blood Banks; *HLA*, human leukocyte antigen; *TAGVHD*, transfusion-associated graft-versus-host disease.

be at risk for TAGVHD.[37] Nonetheless, there are no strict guidelines in place in the United States for universal product irradiation or pathogen inactivation. As such, facilities frequently develop internal policies or procedures indicating when modifications such as irradiation may be most appropriate; such documents are often based on standards established by national accreditation agencies (e.g., the American Association of Blood Banks)[18] as well as on existing literature and guidelines.[38] For a listing of the common indications for the use of irradiated components (or those undergoing pathogen inactivation, as available), please see Table 7.4.

Posttransfusion Purpura

Posttransfusion purpura (PTP) is a relatively uncommon complication of blood transfusion, associated with thrombocytopenia and purpura (as the name of the disorder suggests!). Although this complication is rare, there is a relatively high mortality rate associated with this reaction (up to 15%), with most poor outcomes attributable to intracranial hemorrhage, hence it is critical for providers to be aware of this entity and to recognize its onset. Although PTP can be seen after transfusion of any blood product, it is most commonly encountered after RBC transfusions.[2]

Pathophysiology

PTP can be thought of as a delayed transfusion reaction involving platelets, in which an anamnestic response to a previously encountered foreign platelet antigen leads to an increase in the production of antiplatelet antibodies by the recipient.[39] The antigen most commonly implicated is the human platelet antigen 1a, (HPA-1a), similar to neonatal alloimmune thrombocytopenia and often acquired in the setting of previous pregnancies (hence the female predilection).[2] Unlike the delayed hemolytic reaction, however, these antibodies cause both the destruction of transfused platelets and the bystander destruction of the patient's own platelets, leading to thrombocytopenia.[2,39]

Patients lacking the HPA-1a antigen (or the others implicated in PTP) can be sensitized during pregnancy (women) or through prior transfusion.[2,39] There are three hypotheses that are proposed for the destruction of autologous platelets.[18] In the first theory, immune complexes cause platelet destruction via binding to platelet Fc receptors. Alternatively, some have proposed that a patient's platelets absorb a soluble platelet antigen from the donor plasma, making them "visible" to circulating antibodies. In the third theory, the platelet alloantibody has concomitant autoreactivity that develops when a patient is reexposed to a foreign platelet-specific antigen. Although no one hypothesis has been proven correct, the "allo-auto" concomitant reactivity antibody theory is most supported (at present) by the blood bank community.[18]

The differential diagnosis for PTP can include heparin-induced thrombocytopenia, thrombotic thrombocytopenic purpura, DIC, and drug-induced thrombocytopenia. Patients with PTP can present with severe thrombocytopenia (with platelet count ≤10–20,000/μL), which is sufficient to cause purpura, petechiae, and clinically significant bleeding.[2,18,39] For PTP caused by an alloantigen on the transfused platelets, the onset is approximately 5–10 days following transfusion, and the thrombocytopenia often lasts for days to weeks.

An alternative and even rarer syndrome leading to posttransfusion thrombocytopenia has been reported, in which the recipient of a plasma-rich product (such as FFP) develops severe thrombocytopenia (which may be accompanied by bleeding and an acute transfusion reaction) caused by the *passive transfer* of antiplatelet antibodies (e.g., anti-HPA-1a) from a previously immunized donor.[40] The time course is much more rapid than described for PTP; thrombocytopenia due to passive antibody transfer occurs within hours rather than days, and recovery typically occurs within 5 days (as foreign antibodies are removed from circulation). Implicated donors are typically females with a history of pregnancy, and any such donors should be prevented from subsequent donations.

Diagnostic criteria

As per the CDC criteria,[4] alloantibodies directed against HPAs must be detected at the time of, or after, development of thrombocytopenia (defined as a decrease in platelets to less than 20% of the pretransfusion count) in the patient. As noted previously, circulating alloantibodies to common platelet antigens (most often HPA-1a) are identifiable by a number of platforms, and this is also typically confirmed by the demonstration of the lack of this antigen on the patient's own platelets.

Treatment

The current treatment of choice is intravenous immunoglobulin (IVIG), along with consideration of corticosteroids.[18] Therapeutic plasma exchange may also be considered a therapeutic option in cases in which IVIG cannot be given or does not appear to yield a reasonable platelet response.[18] Regarding preventative efforts, it is very difficult to predict who may develop PTP and therefore prevention may be aimed primarily at those with a history of this adverse event. Fortunately, PTP may not necessarily recur in subsequent transfusions; however, there are case reports of patients with multiple

TABLE 7.5	
Conditions That May be Associated With Fever During Transfusion	
Acute Transfusion-Associated Adverse Events	**Non–Transfusion-Related Events**
Hemolytic transfusion reaction	Underlying infection
Septic transfusion reaction	Tumor- or malignancy-associated fever
TRALI	Postoperative fever
FNHTR	Medication effect

FNHTR, febrile nonhemolytic transfusion reactions; *TRALI*, transfusion-related acute lung injury.

episodes of this disorder.[18] As such, and because there is no meaningful way to predict whether a patient may redevelop PTP, antigen avoidance should be considered. For instance, HPA-1a-negative patients diagnosed with PTP who require subsequent transfusion should receive blood products from an HPA-1a-negative donor; alternatively, RBC and platelet products could be washed to remove contaminating, causative antigens if antigen-negative products are not available.[18]

LOW-MORBIDITY REACTIONS

Febrile Nonhemolytic Transfusion Reactions

Febrile nonhemolytic transfusion reactions (FNHTRs) are among the most common transfusion reactions identified.[1,2,11] As the name implies, these reactions are typically characterized by fever and the absence of hemolysis or other significant symptoms. Notably, FNHTRs may be diagnosed in afebrile patients; the CDC criteria state that rigors are sufficient to diagnose an FNHTR, even in the absence of fever.[4] The key to properly diagnosing FNHTR is ruling out more serious diagnoses.[2] Fever may be a component of many different transfusion reactions, and it is important to perform a thorough review of systems and careful workup to accurately characterize the reaction and rule out a more serious diagnosis. Table 7.5 summarizes the various adverse events, as well as the potential unrelated conditions, which can manifest with fever during transfusion. As such, although FNHTRs are very common, it is imperative that all other reactions associated with fever be excluded before settling on a diagnosis of FNHTR.

Pathophysiology

The pathophysiology of FNHTRs is not completely understood. Historically, FNHTRs were believed to result from antileukocyte antibodies in the recipient.[41] More recently, studies have indicated that FNHTRs associated with platelet transfusions may be due to cytokines that accumulate during product storage and are likely leukocyte derived.[42] Of note, retrospective reviews have linked leukoreduction with a decrease in FNHTR, helping to support the notion that white cell–derived chemo- and cytokines are important drivers of these adverse events.[43,44]

Diagnostic criteria

FNHTRs may be difficult to recognize and diagnose, especially in patients who are febrile at baseline. The CDC guidelines stipulate that to qualify as an FNHTR the fever or chills/rigors must occur within 4 h of completion of the transfusion, and the fever must reflect at least a 1 °C rise (1.8 °F) from the patient's pretransfusion baseline.[4] Confusion may arise when patients present with fever or rigors in addition to other symptoms, or when additional symptoms arise during the course of the reaction workup (Table 7.5). In such instances, one must remember that FNHTR is a diagnosis of exclusion[2]; fever, rigors, and chills are nonspecific and may be seen in a host of other reactions. In addition, the features of FNHTR can be seen concurrently with other defined reactions (i.e., an unrelated fever in a patient meeting criteria for TACO). If more serious reactions are ruled out, it may be appropriate to diagnose the features of FNHTR in addition to the primary reaction; this practice may vary with institution.

Treatment

The transfusion should be stopped as soon as a reaction is suspected. Although there are usually no serious sequelae of FNHTR, there is no way to know that a fever or rigors represent an FNHTR until the reaction workup is complete. In case the symptoms are part of a more serious reaction, continuing the transfusion puts the patient at risk. Acetaminophen and meperidine can be used to treat fever and rigors, respectively[2]; frequently, however, the symptoms of an FNHTR will spontaneously resolve with time. In patients with a history of FNHTR, some clinicians may "premedicate" with acetaminophen before transfusion, although there is some debate over the utility of this practice, with at least one large-scale trial showing no particular benefit of this approach in patients with bone marrow disorders.[45] Washing products may be considered in patients with a history of severe reactions, but this is now strongly discouraged because of the damage the process inflicts on the products and the benign nature of the FNHTRs. Finally, and

as noted earlier, there are ample data suggesting that prestorage leukoreduction of blood products is associated with a reduced incidence of FNHTRs. As such, the implementation of leukoreduced components can be one means to prevent FNHTRs on a large scale at a given facility.

Allergic Reactions (Mild)

Allergic reactions are the most common adverse events associated with transfusion.[1,11] These may range in severity from a single hive or mild pruritus to laryngeal edema or anaphylaxis. Grading the severity of allergic reactions is typically based on the presence and severity of respiratory symptoms. Mild allergic reactions may be characterized by a simple rash, whereas any change in the respiratory function or status automatically raises concern for a moderate or severe allergic reaction. Anaphylaxis is the most extreme manifestation of an allergic transfusion reaction; as it has been discussed previously, this section will focus on less dire allergic reactions.

Pathophysiology

Although one may expect allergic reactions to occur as a result of a recipient reacting to an antigen present in the donor's blood, the pathogenesis is somewhat more complicated. The main factor in allergic transfusion reactions appears to be the transfer of either antigen or antibodies to the recipient via donor plasma. Reactions arising from exposure to antigens from the donor's plasma in patients with preexisting antibodies are well documented.[2,46] The opposite, however, can also occur—donor plasma in the blood product can also transfer antibodies to the recipient, which can then mediate reactions in the recipient.[29] Furthermore, histamine and bradykinins may also be present in blood products and can mediate hypersensitivity reactions in recipients.[2,29]

The role of plasma in mediating allergic transfusion reactions is well known. Data show that products with higher proportions of plasma (i.e., FFP, platelets) are more frequently implicated in allergic reactions.[1] Moreover, studies in which plasma was removed from platelet units and replaced with additive solution showed a decrease in allergic transfusion reactions.[47] Allergic reactions can also occur via other mechanisms. Case reports of patients experiencing allergic reactions to autologous blood products suggest that storage factors such as bag composition and the chemicals involved in processing blood products may be responsible for some allergic reactions.[18,29]

Diagnostic Criteria

Interestingly, although the CDC does *not* require the reporting of minor allergic transfusion reactions, they do set forth criteria for their diagnosis.[4] As described earlier, allergic transfusion reactions may include symptoms such as urticaria, pruritus, maculopapular rash, flushing, erythema of the lips/tongue/uvula, periorbital edema or erythema, conjunctival edema, hypotension, localized angioedema, bronchospasm, and respiratory distress.[4] One of these symptoms presenting within 4 h of completing a transfusion constitutes a probable reaction; two or more within the same time frame are sufficient to definitively diagnose an allergic transfusion reaction.[4] The CDC gives no criteria to grade nonanaphylactic allergic reactions, but as noted previously, respiratory symptoms typically distinguish moderate and severe reactions from milder ones with predominantly mucocutaneous symptoms.[2]

Treatment

Although most minor allergic reactions will typically resolve on their own once the transfusion has been stopped, they are often uncomfortable for patients and necessitate treatment.[2,18] In addition, minor allergic reactions are the only reactions in which a transfusion may be safely restarted with symptom resolution, even if the transfusion reaction evaluation is not complete. Diphenhydramine is the treatment of choice; some patients may also receive famotidine if diphenhydramine is not effective. Patients who have histories of allergic transfusion reactions may benefit from the administration of these medications before transfusion. In patients with histories of multiple severe allergic transfusion reactions, washed products may be necessary, in addition to premedication. However, washing should be reserved as a "last resort." Finally, unlike FNHTRs, leukoreduction has not been shown to decrease the occurrence of allergic transfusion reactions.[43]

Acute Hypotensive Transfusion Reactions

Acute hypotensive transfusion reactions are characterized by a sudden decrease in systolic blood pressure, typically in the absence of other significant signs, symptoms, or changes in vitals. Although listed in the Low-Morbidity Reactions section, it is important to note that there have been rare reports of deaths associated with this type of adverse event per the US FDA.[6]

Pathophysiology

Acute drops in blood pressure during transfusion are most often attributable to increases in bradykinin, a molecule that causes vasodilation. Bradykinin elevations can result from either increased bradykinin generation or accumulation of bradykinin due to the inability to breakdown these molecules.[2] As such, established risk factors for hypotensive reactions include use of negatively charged bedside leukoreduction filters (which increase bradykinin generation), or the administration of angiotensin-converting enzyme inhibitors ([ACEIs], which reduce bradykinin metabolism).[18,48] Notably, not all transfusion recipients of ACEIs experience these reactions for reasons that are not entirely understood. In addition, a small study of hypotensive reactions in patients not on ACEIs found a possible association between this adverse events and polymorphisms in aminopeptidase P, another enzyme responsible for bradykinin degradation.[49]

Diagnostic criteria

As per the CDC criteria,[4] hypotension occurs during or within 1 h after cessation of transfusion and all other adverse reactions presenting with hypotension are excluded. In adults, there should be a decrease in the systolic blood pressure of 30 mm Hg or more and the systolic blood pressure should be 80 mm Hg or less. In the pediatric population (neonates to those aged 18), there should be a drop of at least 25% in the systolic blood pressure from the baseline. There are typically no other signs or symptoms other than blood pressure changes.[4]

Treatment

Once the transfusion is stopped, the hypotension resolves nearly immediately. If a patient on ACEI experiences this reaction, it might be beneficial to stop this medication 24–48 h before the next transfusion, or consider switching the patient to an angiotensin II receptor blocker.[2] A recent case report notes success in the administration of vasopressin following a severe hypotensive reaction that was unresponsive to pressor administration.[50] The risk of these reactions can be reduced by avoiding negatively charged bedside leukoreduction filters. Since most blood products in the United States are leukoreduced prestorage, hypotension due to this cause is uncommonly seen.

SUMMARY

Although the practice of blood transfusion has seen marked improvements in safety over the past several decades, there, nonetheless, remain significant, noninfectious risks to blood component administration. With a knowledge of the incidence, pathophysiology, treatment, and prevention of these disorders, blood bankers and transfusion medicine practitioners can be extremely effective consultants in recognizing, addressing, and even preventing such reactions.

REFERENCES

1. Politis C, Wiersum JC, Richardson C, et al. The international haemovigilance network database for the surveillance of adverse reactions and events in donors and recipients of blood components: technical issues and results. *Vox Sang.* 2016;111:409–417.

2. Torres R, Kenney B, Tormey CA. Diagnosis, treatment and reporting of adverse effects of transfusion. *Lab Med.* 2012;43:217–231.

3. Harvey AR, Basavaraju SV, Chung KW, Kuehnert MJ. Transfusion-related adverse reactions reported to the national healthcare safety network hemovigilance module, United States, 2010 to 2012. *Transfusion.* 2015;55:709–718.

4. Centers for Disease Control. *National Healthcare Safety Network Biovigilance Component Hemovigilance Module Surveillance Protocol.* Available at: https://www.cdc.gov/nhsn/pdfs/biovigilance/bv-hv-protocol-current.pdf.

5. Shaz BH, Stowell SR, Hillyer CD. Transfusion-related acute lung injury: from bedside to bench and back. *Blood.* 2011;117:1463–1471.

6. U.S. Food and Drug Administration (FDA). *Fatalities reported to FDA Following Blood Collection and Transfusion.* Available at: https://www.fda.gov/downloads/Biologics BloodVaccines/SafetyAvailability/ReportaProblem/TransfusionDonationFatalities/UCM518148.pdf.

7. Peters AL, Van Stein D, Vlaar AP. Antibody-mediated transfusion-related acute lung injury; from discovery to prevention. *Br J Haematol.* 2015;170:597–614.

8. Silliman CC, Moore EE, Kelher MR, Khan SY, Gellar L, Elzi DJ. Identification of lipids that accumulate during the routine storage of prestorage leukoreduced red blood cells and cause acute lung injury. *Transfusion.* 2011;51:2549–2554.

9. Bierling P, Bux J, Curtis B, et al. Recommendations of the ISBT Working Party on Granulocyte Immunobiology for leucocyte antibody screening in the investigation and prevention of antibody-mediated transfusion-related acute lung injury. *Vox Sang.* 2009;96:266–269.

10. Goldman M, Webert KE, Arnold DM, et al. Proceedings of a consensus conference: towards an understanding of TRALI. *Transfus Med Rev.* 2005;19:2–31.

11. Hendrickson JE, Roubinian NH, Chowdhury D, et al. Incidence of transfusion reactions: a multicenter study utilizing systematic active surveillance and expert adjudication. *Transfusion.* 2016;56:2587–2596.

12. Li G, Daniels CE, Kojicic M, et al. The accuracy of natriuretic peptides (brain natriuretic peptide and N-terminal pro-brain natriuretic) in the differentiation between transfusion-related acute lung injury and transfusion-related circulatory overload in the critically ill. *Transfusion.* 2009;49:13–20.

13. Roubinian NH, Looney MR, Keating S, et al. Differentiating pulmonary transfusion reactions using recipient and transfusion factors. *Transfusion.* 2017;57:1684–1690.

14. Serious Hazards of Transfusion (SHOT) Steering Group. *SHOT Home Page.* Available at: https://www.shotuk.org/.

15. Hendrickson JE, Tormey CA. The RBC as a target of damage. In: McManus LM, Mitchell RB, eds. *Pathobiology of Human Disease.* San Diego: Elsevier; 2014:3068–3080.

16. Cruvinel Wde M, Mesquita Jr D, Araújo JA, et al. Immune system – part I. Fundamentals of innate immunity with emphasis on molecular and cellular mechanisms of inflammatory response. *Rev Bras Reumatol.* 2010;50:434–461.

17. Bolton-Maggs PH, Wood EM, Wiersum-Osselton JC. Wrong blood in tube - potential for serious outcomes: can it be prevented? *Br J Haematol.* 2015;168:3–13.

18. Mazzei CA, Popovsky MA, Kopko PM. In: Fung MK, et al., eds. *AABB Technical Manual.* 18th ed. Bethesda: AABB Press; 2014:665–696.

19. Danaee A, Inusa B, Howard J, Robinson S. Hyperhemolysis in patients with hemoglobinopathies: a single-center experience and review of the literature. *Transfus Med Rev.* 2015;29:220–230.

20. Tormey CA, Stack G. The persistence and evanescence of blood group alloantibodies in men. *Transfusion.* 2009;49:505–512.

21. Tormey CA, Stack G. Estimation of combat-related blood group alloimmunization and delayed serologic transfusion reactions in U.S. military veterans. *Mil Med.* 2009;174:503–507.

22. Tormey CA, Stack G. Limiting the extent of a delayed hemolytic transfusion reaction with automated red blood cell exchange. *Arch Pathol Lab Med.* 2013;137:861–864.

23. Hendrickson JE, Tormey CA, Shaz BH. Red blood cell alloimmunization mitigation strategies. *Transfus Med Rev.* 2014;28:137–144.

23a. Garraud O, Filho LA, Laperche S, Tayou-Tagny C, Pozzetto B. The infectious risks in blood transfusion as of today – a no black and white situation. *Presse Med.* 2016;45:e303–e311.

24. Eder AF, Goldman M. How do I investigate septic transfusion reactions and blood donors with culture-positive platelet donations? *Transfusion.* 2011;51:1662–1668.

25. Benjamin RJ, Dy B, Warren R, Lischka M, Eder AF. Skin disinfection with a single-step 2% chlorhexidine swab is more effective than a two-step povidone-iodine method in preventing bacterial contamination of apheresis platelets. *Transfusion.* 2011;51:531–538.

26. Eder AF, Kennedy JM, Dy BA, et al. Limiting and detecting bacterial contamination of apheresis platelets: inlet-line diversion and increased culture volume improve component safety. *Transfusion.* 2009;49:1554–1563.

27. Eder AF, Kennedy JM, Dy BA, et al. Bacterial screening of apheresis platelets and the residual risk of septic transfusion reactions: the American Red Cross experience (2004–2006). *Transfusion.* 2007;47:1134–1142.

28. Devine DV, Schubert P. Pathogen inactivation technologies: the advent of pathogen-reduced blood components to reduce blood safety risk. *Hematol Oncol Clin North Am.* 2016;30:609–617.

29. Domen RE, Hoeltge GA. Allergic transfusion reactions: an evaluation of 273 consecutive reactions. *Arch Pathol Lab Med.* 2003;127:316–320.

30. Pineda AA, Taswell HF. Transfusion reactions associated with anti-IgA antibodies: report of four cases and review of the literature. *Transfusion.* 1975;15:10–15.

31. Sandler SG, Mallory D, Malamut D, Eckrich R. IgA anaphylactic transfusion reactions. *Transfus Med Rev.* 1995;9:1–8.

32. Shimada E, Tadokoro K, Watanabe Y, et al. Anaphylactic transfusion reactions in haptoglobin-deficient patients with IgE and IgG haptoglobin antibodies. *Transfusion.* 2002;42:766–773.

33. Anani W, Triulzi D, Yazer MH, Qu L. Relative IgA-deficient recipients have an increased risk of severe allergic transfusion reactions. *Vox Sang.* 2014;107:389–392.

34. Wagner FF, Flegel WA. Transfusion-associated graft-versus-host disease: risk due to homozygous HLA haplotypes. *Transfusion.* 1995;35:284–291.

35. Bahar B, Tormey CA. Prevention of transfusion-associated graft-versus-host disease with blood product irradiation the past, present, and future. *Arch Pathol Lab Med.* 2017 (in press).

36. Fliedner VV, Higby DJ, Kim U. Graft-versus-host reaction following blood product transfusion. *Am J Med.* 1982;72:951–961.

37. Kopolovic I, Ostro J, Tsubota H, et al. A systematic review of transfusion-associated graft-versus-host disease. *Blood.* 2015;126:406–414.

38. Treleaven J1, Gennery A, Marsh J, et al. Guidelines on the use of irradiated blood components prepared by the British Committee for Standards in Haematology blood transfusion task force. *Br J Haematol.* 2011;152:35–51.

39. Padhi P, Parihar GS, Stepp J, Kaplan R. Post-transfusion purpura: a rare and life-threatening aetiology of thrombocytopenia. *BMJ Case Rep.* 2013;2013:bcr2013008860.

40. Ballem PJ, Buskard NA, Decary F, Doubroff P. Post-transfusion purpura secondary to passive transfer of anti-P1A1 by blood transfusion. *Br J Haematol.* 1987;66:113–114.

41. Brubaker DB. Clinical significance of white cell antibodies in febrile nonhemolytic transfusion reactions. *Transfusion.* 1990;30:733–737.

42. Heddle NM. Pathophysiology of febrile nonhemolytic transfusion reactions. *Curr Opin Hematol.* 1999;6:420–426.

43. Paglino JC, Pomper GJ, Fisch GS, Champion MH, Snyder EL. Reduction of febrile but not allergic reactions to RBCs and platelets after conversion to universal prestorage leukoreduction. *Transfusion.* 2004;44:16–24.

44. King KE, Shirey RS, Thoman SK, Bensen-Kennedy D, Tanz WS, Ness PM. Universal leukoreduction decreases the incidence of febrile nonhemolytic transfusion reactions to RBCs. *Transfusion.* 2004;44:25–29.

45. Kennedy LD, Case LD, Hurd DD, Cruz JM, Pomper GJ. A prospective, randomized, double-blind controlled trial of acetaminophen and diphenhydramine pretransfusion medication versus placebo for the prevention of transfusion reactions. *Transfusion.* 2008;48:2285–2291.

46. Gao L, Sha Y, Yuan K, et al. Allergic transfusion reaction caused by the shrimp allergen of donor blood: a case report. *Transfus Apher Sci.* 2014;50:68–70.

47. Tobian AA, Fuller AK, Uglik K, et al. The impact of platelet additive solution apheresis platelets on allergic transfusion reactions and corrected count increment. *Transfusion.* 2014;54:1523–1529.

48. Kalra A, Palaniswamy C, Patel R, Kalra A, Selvaraj DR. Acute hypotensive transfusion reaction with concomitant use of angiotensin-converting enzyme inhibitors: a case report and review of the literature. *Am J Ther.* 2012;19:e90–e94.

49. Hui Y, Wu Y, Tormey CA. The development of a novel molecular assay examining the role of aminopeptidase P polymorphisms in acute hypotensive transfusion reactions. *Arch Pathol Lab Med.* 2013;137:96–99.

50. Pollard R, Boraski M, Block JG. Hypotensive transfusion reaction treated with vasopressin in a patient taking an angiotensin-converting enzyme inhibitor: a case report. *A a Case Rep.* 2017;9:4–8.

CHAPTER 8

Infectious Complications of Transfusion of Blood Components

JOSEPH PETER R. PELLETIER, MD

HISTORY

Early in transfusion compatibility, hemolysis, whether delayed or immediate, was the most life-threatening condition/risk. As blood groups were discovered and avoidance of stimulation of alloantibodies became the norm, transfusion transmissible infections became a greater risk. The risk for acute hemolytic transfusion reaction is reported as 1 in 76,000 and that of bacterial contamination of platelets is 1 in 3000.[1] Most infections were not usually immediately evident, but some came to be recognized as equally fatal as the immediate death from septic transfusions. In the 1940s, testing for syphilis was initiated.[2,3] Syphilis is a disease of direct transfusion.[3] The causal organism is not stable at colder temperatures: after 72 h at 1–6 °C it is not viable and it becomes nonviable immediately at freezing temperatures. During the 1950s, blood was no longer collected from paid donors or inmates to decrease the incidence of transmission of hepatitis.[2] With the development of health questionnaires, which eventually became the universal health questionnaire, the risk for transmission began to decline. In the 1990s, tests were developed to detect antibodies and eventually antigens of hepatitis viruses to further decrease the risk of transfusion transmission.[2] Eventually, nucleic acid testing (NAT) was developed to detect exposure to pathogens by detecting their genetic material in the donor, which has resulted in lower risks for transmission of infection and has created the safest blood products in history. Infection rates for most viruses are very low secondary to screening. Only higher incidence rates can be measured directly; when the rate is less than $1:10^5$, mathematical modeling is required to predict the residual risk. This is a testament to the benefit of the screening questionnaire and serologic testing and NAT in producing the safest transfused blood components to date.[4]

In this chapter, we will explore viruses, bacteria, parasites, and, briefly, prions with some specific examples, mode of detection, risks, and risk mitigation. Finally, what may be done in the future to further reduce the current and potential risks/dangers of these pathogens is discussed.

VIRUSES

Even though the agent of transmission for hepatitis was not known to be viruses, the risk of transfusion transmission of hepatitis has been recognized since the 1940s.[5] Regulations have been in place since the 1950s to decrease the risk of transmission of hepatitis, long before the causative agents were identified.[6] All individuals with hepatitis are screened via the health donor questionnaire with the exception of those who have had hepatitis after the age of 11. In 1998, approximately 13,000 donors were deferred based solely on this questionnaire.[6] Those who are not aware of having this illness have been further screened with an enzymatic immunoassay test to detect the presence of hepatitis B surface antigen, hepatitis B surface antibody, or hepatitis B core antibody and alanine transferase in the 1980's and using NAT since 2012.[7] Historically, hepatitis not caused by hepatitis A or B viruses was called hepatitis non-A non-B. The majority of these was found to be hepatitis C. After screening for hepatitis B, the posttransfusion hepatitis risk was 1 in 400 with 90% of these being due to hepatitis C.[5] Like the hepatitis B virus, the viruses causing hepatitis C typically have an indolent course, which may lead to severe morbidity and eventually mortality through liver failure or hepatitis carcinoma. These viruses are detected in the donor with enzymatic immunoassay (EIA) testing, recombinant immunoblot assay for confirmation, and NAT. The transmission of this infection has decreased from 1:100 to $1:1.9 \times 10^6$.[6,8]

Other viruses that cause hepatitis are not routinely tested. Some of these include transfusion transmitted virus/torque teno virus (TTV); cytomegalovirus (CMV); Epstein-Barr virus (EBV); hepatitis E virus; hepatitis A virus; hepatitis D virus; adenovirus; Lassa fever virus; Rift Valley fever virus; parvovirus B19; Ebola virus; dengue virus; human herpesvirus 6, 7, and 8; influenza virus; echovirus; and Colorado tick virus. Some of these viruses are of unknown clinical significance, even if associated with transfusion transmission. More significant pathogens in this group are discussed later in this chapter.

Other viruses routinely screened for are human T-lymphotrophic virus (HTLV) and human immunodeficiency virus (HIV). HTLV has two copies of single-stranded RNA (ssRNA). HTLV-1 and HTLV-2 were discovered in the 1980s. HTLV can cause lymphoproliferative or demyelinating diseases in those infected, leading to T-cell leukemia or HTLV-associated myelopathy. To prevent the transmission of this virus, serologic testing for antibody against HTLV has been performed since 1988. For this, EIA has a sensitivity and specificity of 99.4% and 98% and Western blot has a sensitivity and specificity of 97% and 65%, respectively. Those receiving seropositive blood products had a 25%–63% conversion rate.[9] Products stored longer were less likely to be infectious. If stored less than 5 days, contaminated units had 75% transmission rate, and if stored longer than 11 days, the risk decreased to 0%. Multiple case reports from around the world demonstrate the transfusion transmissibility of this virus. One case was from a walking donor pool acquired during treatment at military combat operations.[10,11] At present, no NAT is performed for HTLV and none are under development. The prevalence of this infection is 5–10,000,000 worldwide. There is low prevalence in the United States with $1:5.1 \times 10^5$ positive results in first-time tested donors. After screening, there is a $1:2.9 \times 10^6$ chance of transmission of this infection.[10]

HIV has a storied history in the blood community. HIV is a positive-sense ssRNA enveloped virus. Initially, infection and transmission via blood transfusion were thought to be rare events. As time progressed and the seriousness of acquired immunodeficiency syndrome prognosis and ease of transmission via blood transfusion became more appreciated, health questionnaire screening was developed because high-risk populations were identified. In the early 1980's, transfusion transmission of HIV was more recognized and further work on screening testing came to the forefront because screening for history of high risk was not sufficient to protect transfusion recipients. By early 1985, serologic testing for HIV was developed and donor testing was initiated.[2] The questionnaire decreased the risk from $1:100$ to $1:5 \times 10^4$; screening with EIA, antigen testing, and Western blot confirmation decreased the risk to $1:5 \times 10^5$; finally, NAT decreased the risk to $1:1.9 \times 10^6$. Only four cases of transfusion transmission have been reported from 1999–2009. In the United States, the last case of transmission of HIV in via blood transfusion occurred in 2008.[12] Continued formation of new clades will require updating the questionnaires and testing, as was done most recently with clade O, the most recent to arrive, this one from Africa.

Two additional viruses recently included in donor screening testing are the West Nile virus [WNV] and the Zika virus (investigational new drug (IND) testing Phase III at present). WNV is associated with the potentially fatal neurologic disease, meningoencephalitis. This Flavivirus is an ssRNA virus. The natural reservoir is birds, and it is transmitted to incidental hosts, humans, horses, and other mammals, via mosquitoes. It was first seen in New York in 1999, with transfusion transmitted cases noted in 2002 in the United States. Symptoms can be mild to severe (meningoencephalitis), and 80% of those infected are asymptomatic.[13,14] The development of NAT for this virus was rapid. IND research testing went smoothly, and permanent testing was put in place by 2002.[10] Now, the risk from this viral transmission is $1:350,000$.[3,15]

Zika infection is a newly documented transfusion transmissible infection. Zika virus is a positive-sense ssRNA enveloped virus first evident in Africa in 1947. From this time to the 1980s it has spread in Africa and Asia. In 2015, it was found to cause microcephaly in in vivo–infected fetuses of mothers infected with this virus in Brazil. There are at least 56 countries in the world with active Zika infections. Zika viremia may last 1–2 weeks in the primary infection. Since Nov. 2016, NAT is in Phase III testing in the United States. Food and Drug Administration (FDA) approval as a licensed screening test is pending.[16] As with previous NAT risk of transmission should decrease the risk of transfusion transmission to $<1:1 \times 10^6$ as was seen with hepatitis C virus and HIV testing.

CMV is a double-stranded DNA (dsDNA) enveloped virus also called human herpesvirus-5 (HHV-5). Humans are the sole host of this virus, and it is transmitted by person-to-person contact or iatrogenically via blood transfusion or tissue/organ transplantation. After primary infection there is a lifelong viral persistence likely within mononuclear white cells and hematopoietic progenitor cells in the bone marrow.[17] CMV infection during pregnancy can affect the neurodevelopment of the fetus with a 40% vertical transmission rate. In immunocompromised patients, such as those receiving bone marrow/stem cell transplants, infection can cause severe disease in the pulmonary, gastrointestinal, and central nervous systems. Immunocompetent individuals typically have mild flulike symptoms. After primary infection this virus remains in the white cells. Repeat infections can also be seen. Seronegative and prestorage leukocyte-reduced blood products both decrease the risk for CMV transmission.[18,19] There may be additional benefit to having leukodepletion and negative serology together.[17]

There are more recent studies that conclude that CMV-seronegative blood products are safer than leukoreduced blood products.[19] The debate continues. Residual risk after leukocyte reduction for CMV transfusion transmission is 1: 1.3×10^7.[20]

There are other viruses causing viremia with potential for transfusion transmission that are not screened by history or test in the blood donor setting. These viruses may be geographically isolated, produce mild clinical symptoms, and are yet to be identified in transfusion transmission cases. EBV/HHV-4 is a dsDNA enveloped virus with a human reservoir. Blood transfusion transmission is reported rarely. Primary infection can lead to mononucleosis, Burkitt lymphoma, nasopharyngeal carcinoma, and postviral lymphoproliferation. After primary infection this virus remains latent in the lymphocytes. Infection prevalence is 95% by the age of 40 years. Only screening at the time of donation can defer those with hepatitis after the age of 11, no serologic test or NAT is available.[21]

Parvovirus B_{19} is a positive- or negative-sense single-stranded DNA nonenveloped virus. This virus is resistant to pathogen reduction techniques with heat or cold treatment and solvent detergent treatment. This virus was discovered in 1974 and has three genotypes. Parvovirus B_{19} is trophic to red cells and demonstrates a high viremia rate 7–12 days postinfection. There is a 70%–80% prevalence of previous infection by adulthood, and it has been associated with transfusion-associated transmission. Infections can lead to fifth disease in children and fetal hydrops in the unborn. Patients with high red cell turnover rates are susceptible to aplastic anemia following infection with this virus. There are currently no screening tests at blood donor centers. NAT is performed for pooled blood component products produced commercially (albumin, intravenous immunoglobulin (IVIG) anti-D immune globulin, etc.).[22]

Chikungunya is an ssRNA enveloped virus with two genotypes. The vectors for this virus are multiple mosquito species. Birds, humans, mammals, and reptiles are reservoirs for this virus. A high concentration of viremia occurs within the first week of infection. At-risk populations for more severe disease include the elderly, pregnant, and immunocompromised patients. There is at present only theoretical risk of associated transfusion transmission. At present no screening tests are available.[23]

Dengue virus is a positive ssRNA enveloped virus with four serotypes. There are at least two mosquito vectors for this virus. Humans are the main hosts. Viremia may be present 2–12 days postinfection. Infection can lead to dengue or severe dengue fever (also known as dengue hemorrhagic fever). The incidence of infection has increased 30-fold over the last 50 years. This virus is mainly present in the tropics and subtropics of Asia and the Americas. Associated transfusion transmission has been seen in cellular and acellular blood components. Transmission has also been seen with needle sticks and organ transplants. A dengue vaccine has been developed for individuals aged 9–45 years in endemic areas. Blood screening tests are under development and are used in some parts of the world.[22,24,25]

Other emerging viral infections that are transmissible via transfusions include but are not limited to human poxvirus; monkeypox virus; Whitewater Arroyo virus; hantavirus causing hantavirus pulmonary syndrome; viruses causing yellow fever, Marburg hemorrhagic fever, and Ebola hemorrhagic fever; enterovirus 71; Hendra virus; Nipah virus; avian influenza virus (H5N1); viruses causing severe acute respiratory syndrome, Lassa fever, and Rift Valley fever; Hepatitis-G virus (GBV-C); TTV; SEN virus; and HHV-8.[26–28] The risks of transmission for these infections remain relatively low or seasonal. The donor health questionnaire (DHQ) "Are you healthy today," travel history, and temperature measurement ensure that approximately 99.5% potentially infectious donors are screened out. In the future, pathogen reduction technologies should protect against these infectious agents.

BACTERIA

Historically the risks of transfusion transmission of bacteria has been underappreciated. Because we have gained control of the screening out of viruses, the potential clinical sequela of bacteremic/septic transfusion reactions has received more attention. Transmission of these organisms is much more frequent than that of viruses. DHQ and mini-physical examination, puncture site preparation, diversion pouch, and subculturing platelet units have decreased the risks somewhat. Septic reactions occur from bacterial/pathogen-contaminated blood components, usually originating from the blood donor at venipuncture site or during unsuspected bacteremia. Less commonly, it may also result from donor unit processing. Bacterial contamination is more likely to occur in components stored at room temperature than in components stored refrigerated. The risk of transfusion transmission remains relatively high at 1:30,000 for red cells and 1:3000 for platelets as opposed to the residual risk after viral screening.

At the time of collection, bacterial contamination of components is about 10 colony forming units (CFU)/mL, and initially no sepsis occurs when the components are stored for short periods. At the end of the storage time, however, these same components can have 10^7–10^9 CFU/mL. This level of contamination can much more easily lead to sepsis especially in the most at-risk immunocompromised patients. *Staphylococcus* and *Pseudomonas* at optimal conditions can double every 4–8 h without a lag phase.[29]

Even with cold storage bacteremia/sepsis has been associated with transfusion of these components. Red cell components stored longer than 14 days are implicated in bacteremic transfusion. More often still are the red blood cell components stored longer than 25 days. *Yersinia enterocolitica* and *Pseudomonas fluorescens* are the most common agents associated with bacteremic transfusion reactions involving red blood cell components. *Y. enterocolitica* has a 7- to 14-day lag time with an 18- to 20-h doubling time for the remainder of the storage period. Contamination levels can reach 10^9 CFU/mL after 38 days of storage. Prestorage leukoreduction may prevent/inhibit *Yersinia* proliferation. Red cells stored for very short time continue to be associated with *Treponema pallidum* transmissions. Other less common red cell component bacterial contaminants are *Pseudomonas* sp., *Flavobacterium* sp., *Campylobacter jejuni*, *Enterobacter* sp., *Klebsiella* sp., *Escherichia coli*, *Serratia* sp., *Proteus* sp., *Staphylococcus aureus*, and coagulase-negative *Staphylococcus*.[29–31]

Since the 1970's bacterial contamination of platelet components was recognized. Bacteria is the leading cause of death in transfusion transmitted infections. Single-donor platelets (apheresis) and platelet concentrates (3–6 donor pools) are stored at higher temperatures than red cell units. Platelets are stored at 20–24 °C with agitation for up to 5 days. These storage conditions favor aerobic bacterial growth. Organisms typically causing bacterial septicemia more often are skin flora including *Staphylococcus* and *Streptococcus*; however, *Serratia*, *Bacillus*, and *Salmonella* are also among the most common bacterial contaminants in platelet products. *Acinetobacter*, *Proteus*, *Klebsiella*, and *Serratia* have also been implicated in fatal septic transfusion reactions. *Propionibacterium acnes* has been found as a common contaminant of blood products but is usually associated with minimal morbidity and mortality; nonetheless, one fatal reaction with transfusion has been reported. Bacteremic/septic reactions are usually seen at the end of storage of the platelet unit at day 4–5. Higher bacterial septic reactions

secondary to longer stored platelet units in 1985 led the FDA to reverse the 7-day storage to 5 days. In the 2005–08 period 7-day storage was again attempted after subculturing platelets 24 h after collection to try to screen out contaminated units. This reduced the risk slightly but not significantly, and storage was again set for 5 days. Storage is limited to 5 days because longer storage continues to be associated with unacceptable rates of bacterial transmission. When *S. aureus* contaminates platelets, there is a 2-day lag, whereas with *Enterococcus faecalis*, there is no lag in the growth period. The doubling time for these organisms is ≤3 h. By day 3–5 there are 10^8–10^9 CFU/mL of component. Efficacy for removal of bacteria with leukocyte depletion is less clear for platelet products. Risk for bacteremia from platelet transfusion is $1{:}10^3$–3×10^3. Transfusion-related sepsis risk ranges from $1{:}1$–5×10^4 and $1{:}4.7 \times 10^3$, depending on the study; with subculturing, the risk of immediate death from septic transfusion is $1{:}5 \times 10^5$. [29,31–34]

Potential sources of contamination of blood products are improper preparation of the phlebotomy site at donation, donor bacteremia, blood containers used for processing and storage, or equipment used for processing. The risk of transmission from the donor is decreased with the mini-physical examination and clinical, medical, and travel histories. Phlebotomy site risk is reduced by ruling out intravenous drug use, evaluating for skin lesions, and preparing the site with iodine or chlorhexidine and alcohol. Donor bacteremia risk is evaluated with a history of dental procedures, gastrointestinal tract symptoms, and current osteomyelitis. Contamination of blood collection containers is a very rare event with better sterility of the plastics used. When processing (thawing) products, water baths may be a source of contamination and should be cleaned regularly. At the time of issue further steps can be taken. A visual inspection of the unit for color changes, hemolysis, or turbidity is performed. Red cell units tend to be much darker in color because the bacteria use the oxygen stored in the red cells; platelets have lower pH and loose "swirling" when potential contamination is present. These units should be quarantined and not issued to patients. Blood components should be transfused within 4 h of being issued from the blood bank. Proper storage temperature during transport is also recommended. Transfusion administration tubing sets should be changed between blood transfusions per policy: approximately every 4 h. At the time of issue products can be examined to evaluate for contamination. Septic reaction is the fourth leading cause of death as a complication of transfusion. While receiving a transfusion, signs of a septic reaction include temperature greater than 102° F (or higher than 2°F or 3° C above baseline temperature), chills, rigors, tachycardia (heart rate greater than 40 beats over baseline) and shock/falling systolic blood pressure (30 mm Hg below systolic), backache, nausea/vomiting, and unexplained bleeding from mucous membranes or the infusion site. Renal failure may follow later. Once suspected, transfusion is immediately halted and the patient given supportive treatment. Maintain respiratory status, and use mechanical ventilation if indicated. Maintain cardiovascular support with vasopressors as indicated. With the patient stabilized, initiate transfusion reaction workup; send blood (pink or purple tube) and first posttransfusion urine (not from Foley collection bag) to the laboratory. Also send the unit with attached administration set to the laboratory. Perform a gram stain and culture from the implicated blood component and administration set. Draw blood culture from the patient, preferably from two sites. Prompt initiation of intravenous antibiotics as indicated by the gram stain results. Again, future use of pathogen reduction agents will greatly decrease the risk of bacterial transmission of blood products.[29,35]

PARASITES

Leishmania species is an intracellular macrophage/monocyte protozoan that causes leishmaniasis. Sandfly is the vector of this pathogen. A few cases of transmission from blood products have been reported in the United States. Likely leukocyte reduction greatly reduces transfusion transmission because these pathogens are within white blood cells. This protozoan is able to survive for 15 days at erythrocyte storage conditions. Deferral of potential donors with travel history to countries with endemic pathogens likely aids in the prevention of transmission in the United States. There is a 1-year travel history deferral because the incubation for this infection may be weeks to months. Pathogen reduction technology can decrease the viability by a factor of $10^4 - 10^5$.[36]

Plasmodium species is an intracellular erythrocyte protozoan pathogen spending part of its life cycle in hepatocytes. Malaria is a very common disease worldwide caused by this pathogen. *Anopheles* mosquito is the vector for *Plasmodium*. In the universal health donor questionnaire, extensive travel history and questions on exposure/prophylaxis use are included to decrease the risk. There is a 1-year deferral for travel to endemic areas, 3-year deferral for those living in endemic areas, and deferral of 5 or more years for those who had malaria and now are asymptomatic. The Centers for Disease Control and Prevention frequently updates travel exposure risks. These are used by blood donor centers to ensure decreased risk of exposure. There are no FDA-approved screening tests for malaria. Historically, this protozoan can survive 7–10 days in blood containers; there are no new studies on the effect of modern additive solutions on the survival of this organism. Leukocyte reduction is unlikely to decrease the risk of transmission. Ongoing pathogen reduction studies are very promising in reducing transmission via blood transfusion in endemic regions.[36]

Babesia is an intracellular erythrocyte protozoa that causes babesiosis. It is associated with transfusion transmission as shown in at least 162 transfusion events, all red cell components. Freezing red cells did not prevent the transmission of infection. This organism is closely related to *Plasmodium*. The vector of *Babesia* is the ixodid tick with the primary species in the United States being *Babesia microti*. It is most commonly seen in the United States in the New England region and the North Midwest states (e.g., Wisconsin, Minnesota). Humans are an accidental host. Risk of transmission is at $1:10^5$. Patients infected with this organism have a long incubation period, 1–6 weeks after a tick bite and 1–9 weeks after contaminated transfusion, as well as prolonged infectivity. Many are asymptomatic with mild fevers at most. If immunocompromised, the patient may develop hemolysis, disseminated intravascular coagulation, or multiple organ dysfunction syndrome. Travel history is remote to the incidence of inoculation and is a poor screening tool. At present, there are serologic and polymerase chain reaction studies being performed with immunofluorescence assay (IFA)/enzyme-linked immunosorbent assay (ELISA)/NAT; Phase III clinical trials are ongoing to test for this pathogen and screen out potentially infected donors.[2,3,37]

PRIONS

Prions are not infections agents in the classic sense but are proteins that act as infectious particles by recruiting normal cellular isoforms to form disease-causing isoforms. Creutzfeldt-Jakob disease (CJD) may be sporadic, infectious, or inheritable. Even though there is potential for transfusion transmission of this disease, to date there have been no documented human cases of transfusion transmission of this classic form of CJD. There is no donor testing for this, and deferral is permanent to all those with a history of this illness.

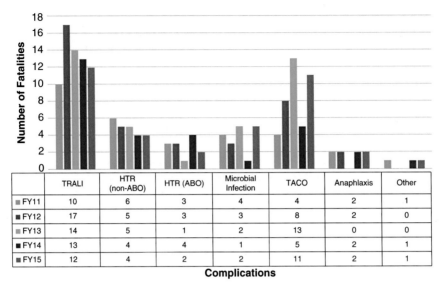

	TRALI	HTR (non-ABO)	HTR (ABO)	Microbial Infection	TACO	Anaphlaxis	Other
■ FY11	10	6	3	4	4	2	1
■ FY12	17	5	3	3	8	2	0
■ FY13	14	5	1	2	13	0	0
■ FY14	13	4	4	1	5	2	1
■ FY15	12	4	2	2	11	2	1

Complications

FIG. 8.1 Transfusion-related fatalities by complication, FY 2010 through FY 2014. *FY*, financial year. (From Food and Drug Administration. *Fatalities Reported to FDA Following Blood Collection and Transfusion Annual Summary for Fiscal Year 2014.* Available at: https://www.fda.gov/downloads/biologicsbloodvaccines/ safetyavailability/reportaproblem/transfusiondonationfatalities/ucm459461.pdf.)

For variant CJD the story is different. This disease first occurred in the United Kingdom in 1994 and was recognized as a distinct disease in 1996 as bovine spongiform encephalopathy (mad cow disease). There is no known vector; cattle and humans serve as reservoirs. Experimentally, in animals a intravascular phase is present before symptoms and there is widespread deposition and replication in the lymphoreticular tissues. Transfusion transmission has been documented. This prion is likely to survive any storage conditions of blood products secondary to the physiochemical characteristics noted in other prions. Incubation of infection is 5–15 years. With transfusion incubation is quicker at 5–8 years. Leukocyte reduction may offer some protection; nanofiltration is effective in experimental model systems. Affinity-based prion removal filters are under development. Pathogen reduction has unknown effect on prions.[38,39]

REDUCING RISK IN THE FUTURE

In the past, the rate of transfusion transmission of infection was over 1% of all transfusions. Now with better screening questions, travel/medical history and screening tests we have decreased the risk of transfusion transmission of infection to many-fold lower levels. Where once the primary cause of death was infection from transfusion, now transfusion transmitted infections may cause only 10% of the transfusion-associated deaths (Fig. 8.1). We have become very good at discovering transfusion transmitted agents and screening for their presence (Fig. 8.2). This, however, takes time and a new virulent pathogen may still await us and we will not be protected by geography. Pathogen reduction technology will soon become routine in the United States as it is in Europe. As this technology becomes easier to use it will become more accepted and utilized first in our most high-risk immunocompromised populations and then universally, as it happened with leukocyte reduction. Commercially developed tests are performed to screen pathogen, but nanofiltration, solvent detergent, and pasteurization reduce the risks of pathogen transmission not detected with screening tests. These processes cannot be used on cellular products. There are processes in place for pathogen reduction in platelets and plasma. For whole blood or red cell components, Phase III studies are ongoing, and in the near future these can be added to our pathogen reduction repertoire.[40]

DISCLOSURE STATEMENT

Research project with Terumo.

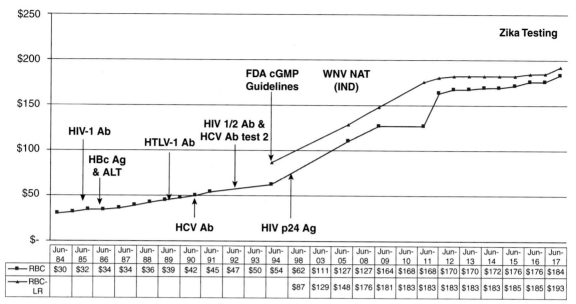

	Jun-84	Jun-85	Jun-86	Jun-87	Jun-88	Jun-89	Jun-90	Jun-91	Jun-92	Jun-93	Jun-94	Jun-98	Jun-03	Jun-05	Jun-08	Jun-09	Jun-10	Jun-11	Jun-12	Jun-13	Jun-14	Jun-15	Jun-16	Jun-17
RBC	$30	$32	$34	$34	$36	$39	$42	$45	$47	$50	$54	$62	$111	$127	$127	$164	$168	$168	$170	$170	$172	$176	$176	$184
RBC-LR												$87	$129	$148	$176	$181	$183	$183	$183	$183	$183	$185	$185	$193

FIG. 8.2 Blood donor center costs from 1994 to 2017. *Ab*, antibody; *Ag*, antigen; *ALT*, alanine transferase; *cGMP*, cyclic guanosine monophosphate; *FDA*, Food and Drug Administration; *HBcAg*, hepatitis B core antigen; *HCV*, hepatitis C virus; *HIV*, human immunodeficiency virus; *HTLV*, human T-lymphotrophic virus; *IND*, investigational new drug; *NAT*, nucleic acid testing; *WNV*, West Nile virus.

REFERENCES

1. Mazzei CA, Popovsky MA, Kopko PM. Noninfectious complications of blood transfusions. In: Fung MK, Grossman BJ, Hillyer CD, et al., eds. *Technical Manual*. 18th ed. Bethesda: AABB; 2014:P665–P696.
2. Dodd RY. Emerging pathogens in transfusion medicine. *Clin Lab Med*. 2010;30(2):499–509. https://doi.org/10.1016/j.cll.2010.02.007. Epub 2010 May 6. PMID: 20513567.
3. Fiebig EW, Busch MP. Emerging infections in transfusion medicine. *Clin Lab Med*. 2004;24(3):797–823, viii. Review. PMID: 15325065.
4. Kleinman SH, Busch MP. The risks of transfusion-transmitted infection: direct estimation and mathematical modelling. *Baillieres Best Pract Res Clin Haematol*. 2000;13(4):631–649. Review. PMID: 11102281.
5. Tobler LH, Busch MP. History of posttransfusion hepatitis. *Clin Chem*. 1997;43(8 Pt 2):1487–1493. Review. PMID: 9265899.
6. Biswas R. History of hepatitis. In: *Blood Products Advisory Committee Meeting*. 2000. Available at: https://www.fda.gov/ohrms/dockets/ac/00/backgrd/3603b1f.pdf.
7. *Guidance for Industry: Use of Nucleic Acid Tests on Pooled and Individual Samples from Donors of Whole Blood and Blood Components, Including Source Plasma, to Reduce the Risk of Transmission of Hepatitis B Virus*. 2012. Available at: https://www.fda.gov/biologicsbloodvaccines/guidancecomplianceregulatoryinformation/guidances/blood/ucm327850.htm.
8. *Guidance for Industry: Nucleic Acid Testing (NAT) for Human Immunodeficiency Virus Type 1 (HIV-1) and Hepatitis C Virus (HCV): Testing, Product Disposition, and Donor Deferral and Reentry*. 2010. Available at: https://www.fda.gov/downloads/biologicsbloodvaccines/guidancecomplianceregulatoryinformation/guidances/blood/ucm210270.pdf.
9. Update: serologic testing for human T-lymphotropic virus type I–United States, 1989 and 1990. *Morb Mortal Wkly Rep Wkly*. 1992;41(15):259–262. Available at: https://www.cdc.gov/mmwr/preview/mmwrhtml/00016579.htm.
10. Murphy EL. Infection with human T-lymphotropic virus types-1 and -2 (HTLV-1 and-2): implications for blood transfusion safety. *Transfus Clin Biol*. 2016;23(1):13–19. https://doi.org/10.1016/j.tracli.2015.12.001.
11. Hakre S, Manak MM, Murray CK, et al. Transfusion-transmitted human T-lymphotropic virus type I infection in a United States military emergency whole blood transfusion recipient in Afghanistan, 2010. *Transfusion*. 2013;53:2176–2182. https://doi.org/10.1111/trf.12101.
12. HIV transmission through transfusion–Missouri and Colorado, 2008. *Morb Mortal Wkly Rep Wkly*. 2010;59(41):1335–1339. Available at: https://www.cdc.gov/mmwr/preview/mmwrhtml/mm5941a3.htm.
13. Qu L, Triulzi DJ. West Nile virus and transfusion. *Transf Med Updates*. 2003;4. Available at: http://www.itxm.org/tmu/tmu2003/issue2003-4.htm.

14. *Guidance for Industry: Use of Nucleic Acid Tests to Reduce the Risk of Transmission of West Nile Virus from Living Donors of Human Cells, Tissues, and Cellular and Tissue-based Products (HCT/Ps).* 2017. Available at: https://www.fda.gov/downlo ads/BiologicsBloodVaccines/GuidanceComplianceRegulat oryInformation/Guidances/Tissue/UCM372084.pdf.

15. Bihl F, Castelli D, Marincola F, et al. Transfusion trans- mitted infections. *J Transl Med.* 2007;5:25–35. https:// doi.org/10.1186/1479-5876-5-25. Available at: https:// translational-medicine.biomedcentral.com/articles/ 10.1186/1479-5876-5-25.

16. *Guidance for Industry: Revised Recommendations for Reducing the Risk of Zika Virus Transmission by Blood and Blood Com- ponents.* 2016. Available at: https://www.fda.gov/downloa ds/biologicsbloodvaccines/guidancecomplianceregulator yinformation/guidances/blood/ucm518213.pdf.

17. Pamphilion DH, Rider JR, Barbara AJ, et al. Prevention of transfusion-transmitted cytomegalovirus infection. *Trans- fus Med.* 1999;9:115–123.

18. Blajchman MA, Goldman M, Freedman JJ, et al. Proceedings of a consensus conference: prevention of post-transfusion CMV in an era of universal leukoreduction. *Transfus Med Rev.* 2001;15:1–20.

19. Vamvakas EC. Is white blood cell reduction equivalent to antibody screening in preventing transmission of cyto- megalovirus by transfusion? A review of the literature and meta-analysis. *Transfus Med Rev.* 2005;19:181–199.

20. Seed CR, Wong J, Polizzotto MN, et al. The residual risk of transfusion-transmitted cytomegalovirus infection as- sociated with leucodepleted blood components. *Vox Sang.* 2015;109:11–17. https://doi.org/10.1111/vox.12250.

21. Stramer SL, Hollinger FB, Katz LM, et al. Emerging infec- tious disease agents and there potential threat to transfu- sion safety. *Transfusion.* 2009;49(Appendix 2):S78–S79. Available at: http://onlinelibrary.wiley.com/doi/10.1111 /j.1537-2995.2009.02281.x/full.

22. Stramer SL, Hollinger FB, Katz LM, et al. Emerging infec- tious disease agents and there potential threat to transfu- sion safety. *Transfusion.* 2009;49(Appendix 2):S107–S109. Updated Jan 2013. Available at: http://www.aabb.org/tm/ eid/Documents/Human-Parvovirus-PARV4.pdf.

23. Stramer SL, Hollinger FB, Katz LM, et al. Emerging infec- tious disease agents and there potential threat to transfu- sion safety. *Transfusion.* 2009;49(Appendix 2):S59–S61. Updated Feb 2014. Available at: http://www.aabb.org/tm/ eid/Documents/chikungunya-virus.pdf.

24. Teo D, Ng LC, Lam S. Is dengue a threat to the blood sup- ply? *Transfus Med.* 2009;19:66–77.

25. WHO website; Media Centre. Dengue and severe dengue fact sheet. Updated Apr 2017. Available at: http://www. who.int/mediacentre/factsheets/fs117/en/.

26. Tapper ML. Emerging viral diseases and infectious disease risks. *Haemophilia.* 2006;12(suppl 1):3–7.

27. Zanetti AR, Zappa A. Emerging and re-emerging infections at the turn of the millennium. *Haemophilia.* 2010;16(suppl 1):7–12.

28. Kitchen AD, Barbara JA. Which agents threaten blood safety in the future? *Baillieres Best Pract Res Clin Haematol.*

December 2000;13(4):601–614. https://doi.org/10.1053/ beha.2000.0102. PMID: 11102279.

29. Wagner SJ, Friedman LI, Dodd RY. Transfusion associated bacterial sepsis. *Clin Microbiol Rev.* 1994;7:290–302.

30. Brecher ME, Hay SN. Bacterial contamination of blood components. *Clin Micrbiol Rev.* 2005;18:195–204.

31. Food and drug Administration. Transfusion/donation fa- talities. Fatalities Reported to FDA Following Blood Col- lection and Transfusion Annual Summary for FY2015. Available at: https://www.fda.gov/downloads/BiologicsB loodVaccines/SafetyAvailability/ReportaProblem/Transfu sionDonationFatalities/UCM518148.pdf.

32. Corash L. Bacterial contamination of platelet compo- nents: potential solutions to prevent transfusion related sepsis. *Expert Rev Hematol.* 2011;4:509–525. https://doi. org/10.1586/ehm.11.53. PMID: 21939419.

33. Blood safety. Available at: https://www.cdc.gov/bloodsafe ty/bbp/bacterial-contamination-of-platelets.html.

34. Ramirez-Arcos S, DiFranco C, McIntyre T, et al. Residual risk of bacterial contamination of platelets: six years of experience in sterility testing. *Transfusion.* 2017;00:1–8. https://doi.org/10.1111/trf.14202.

35. Goodnough LT, Panigrahi AK. Blood transfusion therapy. *Med Clin North Am.* 2017;101(2):431–447. https://doi. org/10.1016/j.mcna.2016.09.012. Epub 2016 Dec 24. Re- view. PMID: 28189180.

36. Stramer SL, Hollinger FB, Katz LM, et al. Emerging infec- tious disease agents and there potential threat to transfu- sion safety. *Transfusion.* 2009;49(Appendix 2):S221–S226. Available at: http://onlinelibrary.wiley.com/doi/10.1111 /j.1537-2995.2009.02281.x/full.

37. Stramer SL, Hollinger FB, Katz LM, et al. Emerging infec- tious disease agents and there potential threat to transfu- sion safety. *Transfusion.* 2009;49(Appendix 2):S215–S218. Updated Jul 2013. Available at: http://www.aabb.org/tm/e id/Documents/babesia-species.pdf.

38. Stramer SL, Hollinger FB, Katz LM, et al. Emerging infec- tious disease agents and there potential threat to transfusion safety. *Transfusion.* 2009;49(Appendix 2):S52–S55. Updated October 2011, Available at: http://www.aabb.org/tm/eid/ Documents/vcjd.pdf.

39. Stramer SL, Hollinger FB, Katz LM, et al. Emerging infec- tious disease agents and there potential threat to transfu- sion safety. *Transfusion.* 2009;49(Appendix 2):S47–S49. updated October 2011, Available at: http://www.aabb.or g/tm/eid/Documents/hpd.pdf.

40. Blajchman MA. Protecting the blood supply from emerg- ing pathogens: the role of pathogen inactivation. *Transfus Clin Biol.* 2009;16:70–74.

FURTHER READING

1. Stramer SL, Hollinger FB, Katz LM, et al. Emerging infec- tious disease agents and there potential threat to transfu- sion safety. *Transfusion.* 2009;49(Appendix 2):S67–S69. Updated Feb 2014, Available at: http://www.aabb.org/tm/ eid/Documents/dengue-viruses.pdf.

CHAPTER 9

Transfusion Support in Emergencies

FAISAL MUKHTAR, MD • JOSEPH PETER R. PELLETIER, MD

During emergency transfusions, we need to decide early on how to best use blood components in a limited quantity with all needed safeguards to transfuse in place (emergent transfusions protocols) or use a large enough supply ready to be delivered for prolonged periods of time, and if shortcuts that potentially decrease the safety of transfusions are required, where the benefits outweigh the inherent risks (massive transfusions protocols). In emergency release, clinicians administer blood components, usually red blood cell (RBC) units, before the completion of standard compatibility testing, and in some cases, before infectious diseases testing. In emergent transfusions, smaller volumes are required more quickly; in this setting, potentially electronic crossmatch may be performed if there is a valid type and antibody screen on file with no alloantibodies noted historically. Emergent release of blood is the fastest means by which a clinical service can receive blood units for patients requiring transfusions. More often than not, these units are uncrossmatched at the time of issue (to be crossmatched later when time allows it) and the risk of death/serious harm to the patient outweighs the risk of adverse reactions. If the clinical situation is critical and massive bleeding is established, a case can easily progress from emergency release to a massive transfusion protocol (MTP) activation. With emergency release, the risk of alloimmunization has been reported to be 3% (with crossmatch this risk is 1%), the risk of incompatibility is 0.3% (0.001% with crossmatching), and the risk of hemolytic reaction is 0.02%.[1] Transfusion of uncrossmatched blood has been reported to have 10.9% positive screens with alloantibodies of which 6.5% were clinically significant.[2]

Trauma is the leading cause of death worldwide in those older than 35 years, causing 5–6 million deaths per year.[3] Likewise, trauma is the third leading cause of death overall, and it is expected to become the second leading cause of death by 2020 across all age groups.[4] Trauma is accountable for more years of life lost than cancer and heart disease combined.[5] Approximately 1 out of every 1000 Americans is hospitalized annually for injuries sustained secondary to trauma, and 1%–3% of these will require a massive transfusion. These patients

receive approximately 10%–15% of the 14.6 million RBC units transfused in the United States.[6,7] From 2000–2008, death from trauma has been increasing even as deaths from cancer and heart disease have decreased over the same period despite improvements in life expectancy. Hemorrhage causes 30%–39% of these deaths, with head trauma causing 42%–52%, and multiorgan failure (MOF) causing 7%–11% of trauma deaths. Exsanguination is an important but reversible cause of mortality in patients with trauma. The successful management of severely injured patients depends in large part on adequate and timely transfusion support. Without a doubt bleeding to death is an acute problem. The majority of deaths from hemorrhage occur in the first 6–12 h of the inciting incident. Of note, 52% of patients die within 12 h of arrival to the emergency department. Additionally, 15% die within 7 days and a further 10% do not survive beyond 10 days.[3,8,9] Death from traumatic brain injury (TBI), MOF, and sepsis occur over much longer periods than hemorrhage in the trauma setting.[10,11] Therefore it is not surprising that in recent years provision of optimal transfusion support for patients with trauma has generated much interest and discussion, especially since new data from both civilian and military settings have been reported.

PREDICTING THE NEED FOR MASSIVE TRANSFUSION/MASSIVE HEMORRHAGE PROTOCOL

Predicting the need for massive transfusion before massive hemorrhage occurs is important to decrease the morbidity and mortality. Many models have been created to predict if a patient will require a massive transfusion. The first of these came from the experiences gained in Operation Iraqi Freedom. In a patient whose systolic blood pressure (SBP) is less than 110 mm Hg, heart rate is greater than 105 beats/min, hematocrit (Hct) is less than 32%, and pH is less than 7.25 there is an 85% risk for requiring a massive transfusion. If three of these parameters are met then the risk is 70%. If two variables are present the risk is 40%, if one variable is present the risk becomes 20%, and if none of these variables are present there is a 10% chance of requiring a massive transfusion. Additional risks to be evaluated are a core body temperature of ≤96°F/34°C, an O_2 saturation on pulse oximeter <75%, an international normalized ratio (INR) of >1.5 for coagulation, lactic acid >2.5 mmol/L, base deficit on blood gas of >6 mEq/L, two positive regions on focused assessment with sonography for trauma (FAST), or an above-the-knee traumatic amputation, multiple traumatic extremity amputation, or penetrating trauma to the chest/abdomen. The receiver-operating characteristic curve (ROC) for this predictive model has an area under the curve (AUC) of 0.839.[12,13] It must be emphasized that there are many other predictive models for massive transfusion. A model easy to use in the emergency department is the Assessment of Blood Consumption (ABC). This ABC score is easy to use because it requires only data obtained in the emergency room and can be applied in real time. No laboratory samples are required. Heart rate over 120 beats per min, SBP under 90 mm Hg, and positive result of FAST examination with a penetrating mechanism of injury are the parameters assessed. If no variables are present, there is less than 10% chance that a massive bleed will occur; with two variables the chance is 40%; and with all four parameters present there is a 100% chance. The ROC for this predictive model has an AUC of 0.859. With massive transfusion predictor models in place, populations can be identified for certain interventions or at least early notice can be provided to the blood bank of the potential need to release blood components quickly and in large quantities. Damage control resuscitation (DCR) involves surgical and medical treatment to ensure concurrent hemorrhage control and blood replacement expediently. DCR minimizes the use of crystalloids, allows permissive hypotension (SBP 80–90 mm Hg when TBI is not present), uses compressive/hemostatic dressings/devices, empirically uses tranexamic acid (TXA), prevents acidosis/hypothermia, provides balanced transfusion of blood components, allows goal-directed correction of coagulopathy, and expedites definitive surgical control of the bleed. Use of DCR with early initiation of MTP has improved survival. In the 1970's, death from trauma requiring MTP was over 90%; by 2005, with the implementation of DCR/MTP death from trauma requiring MTP decreased to 55%–65%, by 2007 it improved to 45%–50%, and by 2013 the mortality was <30%.[11–17]

Massive transfusion is commonly defined as transfusions of 10 or more RBC units within 24 h, which approximates the total blood volume of an adult recipient. Other definitions exist and are quite valuable, including RBC replacement of 50% of total blood volume within 3 h, infusion of four RBC units within an hour, or blood loss exceeding 150 mL/min.[12,13,16,18] Massive transfusion can occur in a variety of clinical settings including cardiovascular, spinal, and liver surgery; trauma; gastrointestinal tract bleeds, and pediatrics and obstetrics. Some centers refer to transfusions in these cases as massive hemorrhagic protocol because they are not waiting until the classic massive transfusion definition is reached.

CLINICAL SIGNIFICANCE

The physiologic response to blood loss is to preferentially maintain tissue oxygenation to the brain and heart by shunting blood from other organs, shifting fluid from intracellular to extracellular space and from interstitial to intravascular space, and conserving water and electrolytes. Loss of less than 10% of the blood volume results in a few symptoms, loss of 20% does not usually cause signs or symptoms when the patient is at rest but will result in tachycardia with exercise, and loss of 30% results in hypotension and tachycardia, especially with exercise. Once the blood loss exceeds 30%, serious signs and symptoms of cardiovascular compromise occur including tachycardia with weak pulse, hyperpnea, hypotension, decreased central venous pressure and cardiac output, and cold clammy skin. At approximately 50% blood loss, severe shock and death occur.[8]

Hemorrhage increases the chance of mortality in trauma. In the severely injured patient with trauma uncontrolled hemorrhage with more than 50% blood loss is one of the most common causes of mortality. From 1970–2000, hemorrhage has remained the ultimate proximal cause of mortality in over 90%, and currently, with new surgical and medical treatments, the mortality ranges from 30% to 39% in trauma fatalities, second only to TBI (52%). Indeed, in a recent large retrospective review the mortality of patients requiring more than 50 units of RBCs was 57%.[3,10,17,19] Other physiologic factors also contribute to make hemorrhage more severe. In surgical circles the lethal triad is often discussed. This triad contributes to death from trauma, makes hemorrhage worse, and is characterized by acidosis, hypothermia, and coagulopathy.[20] Acidosis is considered significantly severe when the pH is less than 7.2, hypothermia is severe when the core temperature is less than 93°F/34°C, and coagulopathy is severe when the prothrombin time (PT) is greater than 19 s or the activated partial thromboplastin time (aPTT) is greater than 60 s. Massive transfusion/trauma also leads to consumptive coagulopathy/disseminated intravascular coagulopathy (DIC) and hyperfibrinolysis. Trauma-induced coagulopathy is found to be distinct from the coagulopathy induced by dilutional factors, hypothermia, and iatrogenic causes. It is found secondary to activation of protein C and exposure of endothelial endocalyx, resulting in endogenous heparin activity.[21,22] Coagulopathy itself is exacerbated by hypothermia and acidosis. A 1°C decrease in the core body temperature will lead to a 10% decrease in coagulation factor activity; at 33°C there is <50% activity of coagulation factors. Decreased coagulation is also demonstrated at lower temperatures with progressive prolongation of PT and aPTT to 50% higher values at 28°C. The coagulopathy of hypothermia is not always recognized because the laboratory warms samples to 37°C when running PT/PTT assays. Due to this well-known and well-described effect, the laboratory test results may appear more normal than what is truly represented in patients with lower temperatures. The activity of von Willebrand factor (vWF) is profoundly reduced in 75% and nonexistent in 50% of individuals with core body temperatures of 30°C. At pH 7.0 the relative rate of factor IIa (thrombin) generation is 25%.[3,23–25] Platelet function is also similarly affected via activation of vWF and lack of thromboxane production in hypothermia. Bleeding time more than doubles when the temperature decreases by 7°C and is reversible. This phenomenon is more often seen in the extremities.[23–27] Acidosis also alters the functions of clotting factors, with a decrease from 50% to 90% of the activity at pH 7.0 when compared with pH 7.4.[3] Likewise, there is much less thrombin generation and fibrinolysis is increased 1.8-fold.[28] However, in the patient with trauma lack of DIC has been confirmed.[22] Derangement of coagulation occurs rapidly after trauma and is related to the injury severity score (ISS). In one study, by the time the patients arrived to the emergency department, 28% had detectable coagulopathy associated with poor outcomes. The incidence of coagulopathy increases with increasing ISS (minor trauma had no or minimal coagulopathy, whereas severe trauma had much higher likelihood of coagulopathy). Mortality is not additive with increase in severity of injury and coagulopathy but exponential because there is a four- to fivefold increase in mortality risk with the presence of coagulopathy compared with its absence at the highest ISS.[29–31] There is also a component of dilution coagulopathy because fibrinogen levels are <100 mg/dL when 142% of the blood volume is replaced and platelet count decreases to <50 × 10⁹/L when 230% of the blood volume is replaced.[22] RBCs are also important in coagulation. When Hct is decreased

by 6% the bleeding time increases 1.5-fold. RBCs are also able to release adenosine diphosphate, which activates platelets. Also they have rheologic effects. At Hct 21%–30% the blood flow is laminar and pushes platelets to the vascular walls where they can interact with the endothelium. Platelet activity is significantly less at Hct <21% and counts <50 × 10⁹/L in the acute bleeding scenario.[28,32]

RESUSCITATION APPROACHES

Maintenance of adequate blood flow and blood pressure by infusing a sufficient volume of crystalloids (defined as a substance that can pass through a semipermeable membrane) such as normal saline or lactated Ringer solution, colloids (defined as a substance that cannot pass through a semipermeable membrane) such as albumin, and/or blood products is paramount to maintaining tissue oxygenation thus helping to ensure survival. RBC transfusion is critical to ensure maximal or near-maximal arterial oxygen content and thus maintain oxygen delivery to tissues, which will depend on the cardiac output and both RBC mass and hemoglobin (Hgb). In this setting, the ability of transfused RBCs to release oxygen optimally depends at least in part on the metabolic status of the patient and the length of RBC unit storage.[8]

Crystalloids distribute quickly into the total body water and can cause peripheral and pulmonary edema, but they are less expensive than colloid solutions. Limit crystalloid use for perfusion. Even though it supports circulatory volume, crystalloids lead to metabolic and physiologic effects that can cause organ dysfunction. Increased volumes (>0.5–1.5 L) are shown to lead to worse outcomes. Hypertonic crystalloids should only be used in incidents in which the TBI has increased intracranial pressures. Colloid solutions primarily remain (at least initially) intravascular but are more expensive and can cause allergic reactions. There is no added benefit to the resuscitation when albumin or artificial colloids are used. Starch colloid solutions may actually worsen coagulopathy. Therefore use blood components as soon as possible for best outcomes. Practice has evolved to earlier use of colloids (especially plasma) and RBC transfusion while simultaneously decreasing the amount of crystalloids administered. This is due to increasing evidence that large-volume crystalloid administration is associated with abdominal compartment syndrome; cardiac, pulmonary, and gastrointestinal tract complications; as well as coagulopathies. In addition, the current goals of volume resuscitation are euvolemia and avoidance of supranormal resuscitation. Euvolemia entails moderate volume resuscitation with possible use of vasopressor agents for hemodynamic support. The use of thromboelastographs (TEGs) also improves survival and aids in evaluating and deciding the best use of blood components.[3,8,11,13,33]

When blood loss is excessive and there is not adequate time for pretransfusion testing, group O RBCs and AB plasma components should be issued until the recipient's blood type is known. Each institution should have well-developed policies for emergency release, issuance, and delivery of blood components; switching blood types (e.g., when to give D-positive RBC products to a D-negative individual); issuing antigen-positive or antigen-untested blood components in a patient with the corresponding alloantibody; and issuing ABO-incompatible plasma (e.g., an AB patient requiring large amounts of plasma). If needed, never frozen plasma can be substituted for thawed plasma. In never frozen (liquid) plasma 85% activity of coagulation factors is retained. In thawed plasma, factors V and VIII quickly lose activity to 65%.[22] Never frozen plasma stored in citrate phosphate dextrose solution expires in 26 days, and plasma stored in citrate phosphate dextrose adenine solution expires in 40 days. These plasma products have much longer shelf life than thawed fresh frozen plasma (FFP) and plasma. Platelets cold-stored for 3 days have been approved for bleeding patients and are used in combat settings. Platelets stored in additive solution and cold-stored retain function for 15 days, and they are the subject of ongoing studies.[13]

D-negative RBCs should be reserved for females of child-bearing age. Use of Rh-negative RBCs prevents formation of alloanti-D, which can result in hemolytic disease of the fetus or newborn. Men and postmenopausal women may be switched to RhD-positive RBCs if the blood inventory is low and there is a need to reserve Rh-negative components for women of child-bearing potential.[8]

Patient samples for blood typing and antibody screen need to be obtained to ensure that the patient receives type-specific components to preserve the often limited group O RBCs and AB plasma supply in the blood bank. Furthermore, transfusion of type-specific blood preserves the patient blood type especially because receiving out of group components may increase the chance for hemolysis.[8]

In the recent past, resuscitation and transfusion protocols would start with significant crystalloid or nonplasma (albumin) colloid infusion and many RBC components. This was followed by a component therapy–type approach to guide blood component choices, volumes, and timing. This component therapy–type approach uses clinical findings and laboratory results and requires that laboratory tests are both timely and reflective enough of the coagulation system to aid in guiding therapy, which is often not the case. An example of using component therapy is to have transfusion thresholds based on laboratory values, such as Hgb ≤8 g/dL, PT≥ 1.5 times the normal, platelet count ≤50 × 10^9/L, and fibrinogen ≤100 g/dL. However, using this type of approach, in the past and at present has not resulted in specific administration ratios of RBC units to plasma, platelets, and cryoprecipitate.[8]

Mortality rates using component therapy–type strategies were unacceptably high, and the value of earlier and more aggressive blood component administration was reconsidered. Thus MTPs were designed to attempt to "recapitulate" or "reconstitute" whole blood. "Recapitulated" whole blood means matching RBC, plasma, platelet, and cryoprecipitate ratios to approximate that of whole blood, whereas "reconstituted" whole blood refers to premixing components to reassemble whole blood into a single product, or to use fresh whole blood. Early reports in the military setting showed significant reduction in mortality (65% reduced to ~20%) with an optimal plasma to RBC component ratio of 1:1.4. The goals of MTP/massive hemorrhage protocol (MHP) are to prevent coagulopathy (hard to catch-up once behind) and to keep coagulation activity ≥40%–60%, platelet count at least 50–100 × 10^9/L or 85 × 10^9/L, and Hgb 8 g/dL or Hct 29%. When transfusion consists of less than five RBC units, typically there will be no requirement for FFP (i.e., small emergent transfusions). This is an important point because overuse of FFP in non-MTP-requiring situations has led to increased incidences of acute respiratory distress syndrome (ARDS).[3,8,18]

MASSIVE TRANSFUSION PROTOCOLS

The chain of events of MTPs can be defined as follows: (1) notification of the transfusion service and laboratory, (2) laboratory testing algorithms (e.g., PT, PTT, platelet count, fibrinogen and Hgb, TEG), (3) blood component preparation (amount of plasma, RBCs, platelets, and cryoprecipitate to prepare and issue at set time intervals), and (4) other patient care needs (e.g., blood warmers).[8]

MTPs are designed to ensure optimal transfusion therapy to prevent and treat the multifactorial coagulopathy that can occur early after injury. Indeed, published reports show that a significantly abnormal PT and PTT upon arrival at the trauma center predicts a high incidence of mortality. When the INR was >1.5 at admission the incidents of mortality increased fivefold.[34]

In 2005, a symposium of surgeons, anesthesiologists, hematologists, transfusion medicine specialists, and epidemiologists, among others, held at the US Army Institute of Surgical Research, recommended a 1:1:1 ratio of RBC:plasma:platelets during massive transfusion. A 2007 retrospective study demonstrated improved survival with more plasma transfused per each RBC component (65% mortality with 1:8 and 19% mortality with 1:1.4 plasma:RBC ratio in DCR). Further analysis found that use of FFP and platelets increased the survival with no decrease in blood component use. In some cases giving FFP in the military trauma setting (penetrating trauma) was beneficial, even though a massive bleed had not occurred. Higher ratio of platelet transfusions were found to have even more beneficial effects than FFP infusions. Additional research will be needed to define the presence of platelet dysfunction in the trauma setting. The higher ratios have also been found to lead to less ARDS and improved survival at 24 h and 30 days postresuscitation.[8,20,34,35]

Based on the dramatic success of MTPs used in combat, studies are underway to show equivalent performance and patient benefit in the nonmilitary setting. Civilian institutions support the clinical benefit in both 24-h and 30-day mortality. The current MTP regimen for blood component administration at one institution is 6 units RBCs, 6 units FFP per cycle, apheresis platelet units every other cycle, and 20 units of cryoprecipitate after the second cycle and 10 units every other cycle thereafter. At our institution, we follow a similar protocol, except we only transfuse 10 units of cryoprecipitate with every fourth cycle of blood components. Initially, we use liquid plasma (never been frozen) to speed the availability of FFP; thereafter we use FFP and keep liquid plasma to FFP ratio 50% or better favoring FFP. The use of TXA has been shown to be useful in trauma scenarios requiring massive transfusion if given within 1 h of the inciting injury. Benefit is still seen when given up to 3 h after injury. With this off-label use in hemorrhagic shock, it is likely that we will see a decrease in the incidence of MOF and all-cause mortality. However, there is no additional benefit after 3 h from the inciting incident and TXA may actually be harmful to the patient at this point. Prothrombin complex concentrate used to reverse warfarin overdose has not been found to be beneficial in the massive transfusion setting, and its use is not standard in MTP/MHP. The use of recombinant factor VII (rFVIIa) is restricted because it has rarely been shown to decrease component usage but has not decreased mortality in military or civilian

settings. Treatment with rFVIIa may have prolonged PT in patients with low Hgb, fibrinogen, or platelet counts. rFVIIa is not to be used when the patient's pH is less than 7.1 (activity is decreased 90%) or the platelet count is less than $50 \times 10^9/L$. With a core body temperature of 33°C there is only 20% activity, rendering the medication ineffective in these conditions.[3,13,25,28,36–39]

Platelets are an essential component in MTP or MHP. Studies have shown that patients with trauma demonstrate an increase in 48-h survival (82% vs. 66%, $P<.001$) and at 30-day survival (62% vs. 50%, $P=.04$) with platelet transfusions versus no platelets. The ratio of platelets transfused to RBCs also has an effect on the outcomes. Low ratio (<1:16), medium ratio (between 1:16 and 1:8), and high ratio (≤1:8) at 24 h show 60%, 85%, and 95% survival, respectively ($P<.001$). Moreover, at 30 days, the survival was 60%, 78%, and 82% respectively ($P<.001$).[40] Giving platelets earlier in the MTP is of benefit. Mortality is increased twofold if the ratio of platelet:RBC of 1:1.5 is not met within the first 4 h of initiation of transfusion; this trend toward mortality is still present when the ratio is not met at the 24-h mark.[41] Hct also has a role in platelet function. In vivo and in vitro Hct below 20% results in less platelet function with less deposition of platelets on the endothelial walls of damaged vessels leading to prolonged bleeding times.[32,40,42]

MTPs require adequate laboratory support to evaluate the patient's Hgb, platelet count, PT, PTT, fibrinogen, ionized calcium, and acidosis status to address and correct these values. Some institutions use TEG technology to provide dynamic and global assessment of the coagulation process including platelet function, coagulation cascade, and fibrinolysis, to guide the transfusion management of patients. Multiple studies have shown the benefit of utilizing TEG in the decision of component support for MTP/MHP. TEG guidance is equivalent to MTP when >6 units RBCs are used or in blunt traumas requiring more the 10 RBC units. TEG guidance has been found to be superior to MTP in patients sustaining penetrating traumas. TEG has been shown to predict the need of MTP better than conventional coagulation assays, resulting in less use of blood components. However, few medical centers are using this tool in managing protocols.[11,17,43–45]

MTP/MHP may be terminated when it is deemed that further care is futile. MTP/MHP are also inactivated when bleeding stops or is controlled and the blood pressure is corrected, when adequate cardiac output is demonstrated via mixed venous saturation of 70% O_2. Resolving lactic acidosis or base deficit are also signs that MTP/MHP can be discontinued.[13,14]

COMPLICATIONS OF MASSIVE RED BLOOD CELL TRANSFUSION

Massive transfusions can lead to complications because large volumes may be transfused over short periods of time (minutes instead of hours). Storage lesion of RBCs may cause the following: (1) hypothermia (components were recently refrigerated and not warmed during reinfusion), increasing tissue oxygen requirements and inducing ventricular arrhythmias; (2) increase in lactic acid causing acidosis; (3) hyperkalemia; (4) decreased oxygen delivery due to decreased 2,3-diphosphoglycerate (2,3-DPG) levels, and (5) abnormal calcium levels secondary to citrate and decreased metabolism.[8]

As RBCs are stored in citrate-containing anticoagulant solutions, administration of large volumes of RBCs (>4 units) may lead to citrate chelation of free calcium and thus hypocalcemia which can cause paresthesias, nausea, hyperventilation, and depressed cardiac function. In addition, citrate is an acid and thus contributes to acidosis. In the trauma setting, citrate is not metabolized quickly by the liver. Severe decreases (<0.84 mmol/L) or elevations (>1.30 mmol/L) in Ca^{++} levels have been shown to be associated with increased mortality. For this reason close monitoring of ionized calcium is important in the trauma stabilization/resuscitation process.[8,46] Last, complications of massive RBC transfusion arise from the transfusion of older RBC units that have undergone changes during storage (termed the storage lesion). The storage lesion includes decreased 2,3-DPG levels, decreased pH, decreased RBC deformability, increased hemolysis, and increased potassium, phosphate, and ammonia concentrations. Microchimerism can develop in up to 10% of those receiving a massive transfusion.[7,8,13] All these changes may adversely affect the recipient during massive transfusion and are the focus of current investigations.

Optimizing Massive Transfusion/Massive Hemorrhage Protocol

In 2007, a military retrospective study showed a 38% absolute and a 62% relative reduction in hemorrhagic death while comparing ratios of FFP:RBC greater than 1:4 with ratios of 1:4–1:2 and ratios lower than 1:2.[47] This study was criticized for its retrospective nature and survival bias. Additional studies have been completed in the civilian setting showing that a ratio close to 1:1 does confer benefit.[3,4,13,18,20,48–51] DCR has given impressive results; however, the appropriate ratio of blood components is yet to be defined. One study showed that patients receiving FFP:RBC at a ratio of 2:3 or greater had a significant reduction in 30-day mortality compared with those receiving less than 2:3 ratio (41% vs. 68%, $P = .008$).

For platelets it was similarly found that a platelet:RBC ratio of 1:5 led to lower mortality than less ratio (38% vs. 61%, $P = .001$).[50] Another study showed that over a 5-year period mortality decreased when the FFP:RBC ratio was changed from greater than 1:5 to 1:2; however, when the ratio approached 1:1 mortality paradoxically increased. In the 2007 study in which data are separated into similar ratios a J-curve is also revealed. This suggests that the most beneficial ratio for greatest survival is somewhere between 1:1 and 1:2 FFP:RBC.[50,51] Separately, a study published in 2009 showed increased survival when FFP:RBC ratio went from 1:8 to 1:2 (90% vs. 25% mortality, $P < .01$).[52] Similarly, a prospective study in a civilian setting also reported that a high FFP:RBC ratio ≥1:1.5 was associated with lower mortality than higher ratios ($P = .002$).[20] In blunt massive trauma the ratio of FFP:RBC of 1:1.5 has also showed improved outcomes. However, there was no improvement with higher ratios of platelet infusions and RBCs in this study.[49] As a result, studies to optimize transfusion ratios should continue to maximize the benefit to patients in a multitude of clinical settings.

In the trauma transfusion triangle, the relative ratios to achieve the desired blood levels are shown (Fig. 9.1). From this example it can be seen that the desired levels are not achieved with FFP:RBC of 1:1 versus 1:1.5 ratio. RBC Hgb levels between 7 and 10 g/dL are adequate for O_2 carrying support. Higher concentrations of RBCs affect rheology, and the flow is less laminar and decreased in capillary beds. PT/INR corrected to ≤1.3 and platelets >50 × 10⁹/L are the desired goals. Having Hgb >7 g/dL also aids platelet function as previously stated.

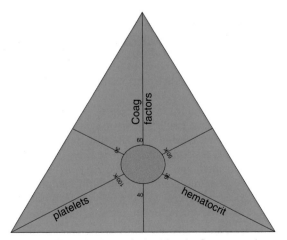

FIG. 9.1 The trauma transfusion triangle. *Coag*, coagulation; *FFP*, fresh frozen plasma; *RBC*, red blood cell. (Courtesy of S. Clayton, MD, Houston, TX.)

The reader must be aware that there is still a continuing argument, among medical professionals, whether longer stored blood is beneficial to patients. Two studies Age of BLood Evaluation (ABLE) (adult critically ill patients) and Age of Red blood cells In Premature Infants (ARIPI) (neonatal patients in the intensive care) demonstrated no increase in multiple organ dysfunction or mortality using blood stored longer. A similar study in the pediatric intensive care population is ongoing. Of interest, a study in patients who underwent liver transplant has shown an increased incidence of acute kidney injury when longer stored RBCs are administered.[53-55] In light of these remaining controversies further studies are warranted.

A multicenter study called Safety of Group A plasma in Trauma Transfusion found it to be safe to use for the initial resuscitation of a patient with unknown ABO group, resulting in no significant difference in in-hospital mortality or length of stay. This was thought to be occurring secondary to the practice of transfusing and replacing patient cells with group O RBCs. Furthermore, the fact that about 80%-85% of individuals are secretors and thus have soluble B and AB antigens that would neutralize out of anti-B antibodies present in A plasma. Of note, platelet transfusions out of type have been found to be safe. Along the same lines, a different study showed that soluble antigens in plasma allow mismatch transfusions without hemolysis, so that soluble B antigens in type B plasma significantly reduced the anti-B titers of type A plasma.[56]

MASSIVE TRANSFUSION PROTOCOL IN OTHER MEDICAL SCENARIOS

Severe hemorrhage accompanying obstetric complications, including placenta previa, uterine atony or rupture, and DIC, can lead to a hysterectomy, loss of future reproductive capacity, and/or loss of the mother, child, or both. Postpartum hemorrhage (PPH) is a leading cause of maternal mortality worldwide with 140,000 deaths per year. PPH is seen in 5%-15% of all births and 3.7/1000 pregnancies. Its incidence has increased two-fold over the last decade with no known increase in risk factors. Massive PPH has been defined as >500 mL blood loss after a vaginal delivery or >1000 mL blood loss following a caesarian delivery. Coagulation factors during pregnancy increase up to 10-fold over the nonpregnant state. However, if fibrinogen were at nonpregnant levels it could be considered critically low in the pregnant state. For each decrease of 100 mg/dL in fibrinogen the risk of PPH increases 2.6-fold. For PPH prevention the use of cryoprecipitate or fibrinogen concentrates is being

studied, and thus far it has been shown to be of benefit. In the obstetric setting, waiting until fibrinogen reaches 150-200 mg/dL, as in most MTP initiations, will essentially guarantee 100% chance of a massive postpartum hemorrhagic bleed in this obstetric setting. The odds ratio for PPH with fibrinogen 200-300 mg/dL is 1.90 (1.16-3.09). This ratio increases to 11.99 (2.56-56.05) for fibrinogen <200 mg/dL. With this information, transfusion of cryoprecipitate when fibrinogen level approaches 200 mg/dL is more protective in the obstetric patient to avoid maternal mortality. When a patient has PPH, initial therapy involves treatment with oxytocin, followed by prostaglandins, and finally intrauterine balloon tamponade. TEG has aided in blood component transfusion support in these emergent cases. In addition, cell savers, fibrinogen concentrates, cryoprecipitate, TXA, and desmopressin have also been used in the treatment of PPH. The goal is to keep Hgb >8 g/dL, platelet count >75 × 10^9/L, PT/PTT <1.5 times the normal, and fibrinogen >200 mg/dL. Optimization of MTP/MHP with early use of cryoprecipitate/fibrinogen concentrates continues to be investigated.[4,28,57-66]

In pediatric patients with trauma most protocols still initially use crystalloids at 20-40 mL/Kg as the preferred dose before instituting blood component infusion. When more than 30 mL/Kg RBCs have been infused emergently, MTP with a 1:1:1 ratio of RBC:FFP:platelets is instituted when the patient is over 30 Kg. On the contrary, when the pediatric patient is less than 30 Kg a ratio of 30:20:20 mL/Kg of RBC:FFP:platelets is recommended. Cryoprecipitate is also infused when fibrinogen is below 100 mg/dL. TXA is used early when a high-risk massive bleed is present at 15 mg/Kg and up to 1 g can be given intravenously. In adults, its use is best within 1 h of injury and no additional benefit is noted if given after 3 h, when it has been shown to be harmful.[33,67] More importantly, predictors of need for MTP in children may need to be modified. The ABC model when applied in the pediatric setting was 29% sensitive. When this model was age adjusted, the sensitivity increased to only 65%. Additional studies will need to be performed to create better predictive models in children.[13,67]

In elderly patients, crystalloid use is limited to 20 mL/Kg. Fluid status can be evaluated with the use of echocardiography and pulse pressure measurements. When there is evidence of cardiac ischemia an Hgb level of 9 g/dL is desirable. A mean arterial pressure of >70 mm Hg to ensure adequate perfusion of the central nervous system (CNS) is also a goal in this scenario.[41]

When there is CNS trauma (i.e., TBI), the goals in MTP/MHP are also different. Instead of tolerating lower blood pressures to stabilize clots, a higher SBP is the goal. SBP lower than 90 mm Hg can lead to further CNS damage, and as a result, a goal of at least 90 mm Hg is more desirable. Moreover, due to the potential for end organ ischemia at lower RBC concentrations an Hgb goal of 9 g/dL is also set.[3,13]

In other surgical/medical scenarios various successes have been seen with MTP. In patients with ruptured abdominal aortic aneurysms (rAAA) the mortality decreased from 66% to 44%.[22] Separately, another study of rAAA showed increased survival with cell saver technology and no increased benefit in reducing mortality with use of FFP.[68] In the operating room, repair of rAAA using massive transfusion support improved the survival by decreasing the mortality from 80% to 30%. In these patients, repair of rAAA using endovascular aneurysm repair required less blood, but 55% of patients needed massive transfusions. Importantly, the ratio of blood components used in this repair process did not change the mortality of the procedure.[69] Patients who have pelvic ring fractures had no additional benefit from MTP over standard component transfusion.[70] Patients requiring transfusions in cardiothoracic, gastrointestinal tract, and hepatopancreaticobiliary bleeds tolerated higher ratio of FFP:RBC with no increase in 30-day mortality. High RBC:platelet ratio decreased the 48-h mortality, and at 30 days, no increased mortality was seen. Interestingly, cardiopulmonary patients who were on cardiobypass for greater than an hour benefited from platelet transfusions. Gastrointestinal tract bleeds requiring ≤5 units RBCs receive no additional benefit with concomitant FFP transfusion. Based on the aforementioned data it becomes clear that additional research is still needed to establish guidelines for appropriate blood component ratios in patients without trauma.[22,71]

DISCLOSURE STATEMENT

Research is being conducted with Terumo.

REFERENCES

1. Mulay SB, Jaben EA, Johnson P, et al. Risks and adverse outcomes associated with emergency-release red blood cell transfusion. *Transfusion.* 2013;53:1416–1420.
2. Goodell PP, Uhl L, Mohammed M, et al. Risk of hemolytic transfusion reactions following emergency-release RBC transfusion. *Am J Clin Pathol.* 2010;134:202–206.
3. Elmer J, Wilcox SR, Raja AS. Massive transfusion in traumatic shock. *J Emer Med.* 2013;44:829–838.
4. Griffee MJ, DeLoughery TG, Thorborg PA. Coagulation management in massive bleeding. *Curr Opin Anesthesiol.* 2010;23:263–268.
5. Stephens CT, Gumbert S, Holcombb JB. Trauma-associated bleeding: management of massive transfusion. *Curr Opin Anesthesiol.* 2016;29:250–255.
6. Yuan S, Ziman A, Anthony MA, et al. How do we provide blood products to trauma patients? *Transfusion.* 2009;49:1045–1049.
7. Perkins JG, Cap AP, Weiss BM, et al. Massive transfusion and nonsurgical hemostatic agents. *Crit Care Med.* 2008;36:S325–S339.
8. Shaz BH, Hillyer CD. Massive transfusion. In: *Transfusion Medicine and Hemostasis: Clinical and Laboratory Aspects.* 1st ed. New York: Elsevier; 2009:287–291.
9. Stewart RM, Myers JG, Dent DL, et al. Seven hundred fifty-three consecutive deaths in a level I trauma center: the argument for injury prevention. *J Trauma.* 2003;54:66–71.
10. Oyeniyi BT, Fox EE, Scerbo M, et al. Trends in 1029 trauma deaths at a level 1 trauma center: impact of a bleeding control bundle of care. *Inj Int J Care Inj.* 2017;48:5–12.
11. Chang R, Holcomb JB. Optimal fluid therapy for traumatic hemorrhagic shock. *Crit Care Clin.* 2017;33:15–36.
12. McLaughlin DF, Niles SE, Salinas J, et al. A predictive model for massive transfusion in combat casualty patients. *J Trauma.* 2008;64:S57–S63.
13. Cap AP, Reade M, Pidcoke HF, et al. Damage control resuscitation. In: *Joint Trauma System Clinical Practice Guidelines.* 2017. Available at: http://www.usaisr.amedd.army.mil/cpgs/DamageControlResuscitation_03Feb2017.pdf.
14. Cantle PM, Cotton BA. Prediction of massive transfusion in trauma. *Crit Care Clin.* 2017;33:71–84.
15. Nunez TC, Voskresensky IV, Dossett LA, et al. Early prediction of massive transfusion in trauma: simple as ABC (assessment of blood consumption)? *J Trauma.* 2009;66:346–352.
16. Hayter MA, Pavenski K, Baker J. Massive transfusion in the trauma patient: continuing professional development. *Can J Anesth.* 2012;59:1130–1145.
17. Tapia NM, Chang A, Norman M, et al. TEG-guided resuscitation is superior to standardized MTP resuscitation in massively transfused penetrating trauma patients. *J Trauma Acute Care Surg.* 2013;74:378–386.
18. Malone DL, Hess JR, Fingerhut A. Massive transfusion practices around the globe and a suggestion for a common massive transfusion protocol. *J Trauma.* 2006;60:S91–S96.
19. Vaslef SN, Knudsen NW, Neligan PJ, et al. Massive transfusion exceeding 50 units of blood products in trauma patients. *J Trauma.* 2002;53:291–295.
20. Sperry JL, Ochoa JB, Gunn SR, Alarcon LH, et al. An FFP:PRBC transfusion ratio >1:1.5 is associated with a lower risk of mortality after massive transfusion. *J Trauma.* 2008;65:986–993.
21. Cohen MJ, Christie SA. Coagulopathy of trauma. *Crit Care Clin.* 2017;33:101–118.
22. Callum JL, Nascimento B, Alam A. Massive haemorrhagic protocol: what's the best protocol? *ISBT Sci Ser.* 2016;11:297–306.
23. Rohrer MJ, Natale AM. Effect of hypothermia on coagulation cascade. *Crit Care Med.* 1992;20:1402–1405.

24. Kermonde JC, Zheng Q, Milner EP. Marked temperature dependence of the platelet calcium signal induced by human von Willebrand factor. *Blood.* 1999;94:199–207.

25. Meng ZH, Wolberg AS, Monroe DM, et al. The effect of temperature and pH on the activity of factor VIIa: implications for the efficacy of high-dose factor VIIa in hypothermic and acidotic patients. *J Trauma.* 2003;55:886–891.

26. Gubler KD, Gentilello LM, Hassantash SA, et al. The impact hypothermia dilutional coagulopathy. *J Trauma.* 1994;36:847–851.

27. Valeri CR, Cassidy G, Khuri AS, et al. Hypothermia-induced reversible platelet dysfunction. *Ann Surg.* 1987;205:175–181.

28. Gando S, Hayakawa M, et al. Pathophysiology of trauma-induced coagulopathy and management of critical bleeding requiring massive transfusion. *Semin Thromb Hemost.* 2016;42:155–165.

29. Macleod JB, Lynn M, McKenney MG, et al. Early coagulopathy predicts mortality in trauma. *J Trauma.* 2003;55:39–44.

30. Niles SE, McLaughlin DF, Perkins JG, et al. Increase mortality associated with the early coagulopathy of trauma in combat casualties. *J Trauma.* 2008;64:1459–1465.

31. Brohi K, Singh J, Heron M, et al. Acute traumatic coagulopathy. *J Trauma.* 2003;54:1127–1130.

32. Valeri CR, Cassidy G, Pivacek LE, et al. Anemia-induced increase in the bleeding time: implications for treatment of nonsurgical blood loss. *Transfusion.* 2001;41:977–983.

33. Wise R, Faurie M, Malbrain MLNG, et al. Strategies for intravenous fluid resuscitation in trauma patients. *World J Surg.* 2017;41:1170–1183.

34. Pidcoke HF, Aden JK, Mora AG, et al. Ten-year analysis of transfusion in Operation Iraqi Freedom and Operation Enduring Freedom: increased plasma and platelet use correlates with improved survival. *J Trauma Acute Care Surg.* 2012;73:S445–S452.

35. Spinella PC, Perkins JG, Grathwohl KW, et al. Effect of plasma and red blood cell transfusions on survival in patients with combat related traumatic injuries. *J Trauma.* 2008;64:S69–S78.

36. McMullin NR, Wade CE, Holcomb JB, et al. Prolonged prothrombin time after recombinant activated factor VII therapy in critically bleeding trauma patients is associated with adverse outcomes. *J Trauma.* 2010;69:60–69.

37. Wade CE, Eastridge BJ, Jones JA, et al. Use of recombinant factor VIIa in US military casualties for a five-year period. *J Trauma.* 2010;69:353–359.

38. Nishida T, Kinoshita T, Yamakawa K. Tranexamic acid and trauma-induced coagulopathy. *J Intensive Care.* 2017;5:5–12.

39. Alburaih A. Tranexamic acid (TXA) in trauma patients: barriers to use among trauma surgeons and emergency physicians. *Emerg Med Int.* 2017. Available at: https://doi.org/10.1155/2017/4235785.

40. Perkins JG, Andrew CP, Spinella PC, et al. An evaluation of the impact of apheresis platelets used in the setting of massively transfused trauma patients. *J Trauma.* 2009;66:S77–S85.

41. Peralta R, Vijay A, El-Menyer A, et al. Early high ratio platelet transfusion in trauma resuscitation and its outcomes. *Int J Crit Illn Inj Sci.* 2016;6:188–193.

42. Escolar G, Mazzara R, Castillo R, et al. The role of the Baumgartner technique in transfusion medicine: research and clinical applications. *Transfusion.* 1994;34:542–549.

43. Etchill E, Sperry J, Zuckerbraun B, et al. The confusion continues: results from an American Association for the Surgery of Trauma survey on massive transfusion practices among United States trauma centers. *Transfusion.* 2006;56:2478–2486.

44. Kashuk JL, Moore EE, Wohlauer M, et al. Initial experiences with point-of-care rapid thrombelastography for management of life-threatening postinjury coagulopathy. *Transfusion.* 2012;52:23–33.

45. Gonzalez E, Moore EE, Moore HB. Management of trauma-induced coagulopathy with thromboelastography. *Crit Care Clin.* 2017;33:119–134.

46. MacKay EJ, Stubna MD, Holena DN, et al. Abnormal calcium levels during trauma resuscitation are associated with increased mortality, increase blood product use and greater hospital resource consumption: a pilot investigation. *Anesth Analg.* 2017;125:895–901.

47. Borgman MA, Spinella PC, Perkins JG, et al. The ratio of blood products transfused affects mortality in patients receiving massive transfusions at a combat support hospital. *J Trauma.* 2007;63:805–813.

48. Johansson PI, Hansen MB, Sørensen H. Transfusion practice in massively bleeding patients: time for a change? *Vox Sang.* 2005;89:92–96.

49. Lustenberger T, Frischknecht A, Brüesch M, et al. Blood component ratios in massively transfused, blunt trauma patients – a time-dependent covariate analysis. *J Trauma.* 2011;71:1144–1151.

50. Gunter Jr OL, Au BK, Isbell JM, et al. Optimizing outcomes in damage control resuscitation: identifying blood product ratios associated with improved survival. *J Trauma.* 2008;65:527–534.

51. Kashuk JL, Moore EE, Johnson JL, et al. Postinjury life threatening coagulopathy: is 1:1 fresh frozen plasma: packed red blood cells the answer? *J Trauma.* 2008;65:261–271.

52. Teixeira PGR, Inaba K, Shulman I, et al. Impact of plasma transfusion in massively transfused trauma patients. *J Trauma.* 2009;66:693–697.

53. Wang Y, Li Q, Ma T, et al. Transfusion of older red blood cells increases the risk of acute kidney injury after orthotopic liver transplantation: a propensity score analysis. *Anesth Analg.* 2017. Available at: https://www.ncbi.nlm.nih.gov/pubmed/28863026.

54. Lacroix J, Hébert PC, Fergusson DA, et al. Age of transfused blood in critically ill adults. *N Engl J Med.* 2015;372:1410–1418.

55. Fergusson DA, Hébert P, Hogan DL, et al. Effect of fresh red blood cell transfusions on clinical outcomes in premature, very low-birth-weight infants: the ARIPI randomized trial. *JAMA.* 2012;308:1443–1451.

56. Dunbar NM, Yazen MH, Biomedical Excellence for Safer Transfusion (BEST) Collaborative and the STAT Study Investigators. Safety of the use of group A plasma in trauma: the STAT study. *Transfusion*. 2017;57:1879–1884.

57. Sentilhes L, Vayssière C, Deneux-Tharaux C, et al. Postpartum hemorrhage: guidelines for clinical practice from the French College of Gynaecologists and Obstetricians (CNGOF) in collaboration with the French Society of Anesthesiology and Intensive Care (SFAR). *Eur J Obstet Gynecol Reprod Biol*. 2016;198:12–21.

58. Butwick AJ, Goodnough LT. Transfusion and coagulation management in major obstetric hemorrhage. *Curr Opin Anaesthesiol*. 2015;28:275–284.

59. Gutierrez MC, Goodnough LT, Druzin M, et al. Postpartum hemorrhage treated with a massive transfusion protocol at a tertiary obstetric center: a retrospective study. *Int J Obstet Anesth*. 2012;21:230–235.

60. Ducloy-Bouthors AS, Mignon A, Huissoud C, et al. Fibrinogen concentrate as a treatment for postpartum haemorrhage-induced coagulopathy: a study protocol for a randomised multicentre controlled trial. The fibrinogen in haemorrhage of DELivery (FIDEL) trial. *Anesth Crit Care Pain Med*. 2015;35:293–298.

61. Seto S, Itakura A, Okagaki R, et al. An algorithm for the management of coagulopathy from postpartum hemorrhage, using fibrinogen concentrate as first-line therapy. *Int J Obstet Anesth*. 2017. Available at: https://doi.org/10.1016/j.ijoa.2017.03.005.

62. Belaouchi M, Romero E, Mazzinari G, et al. Management of massive bleeding in a Jehovah's Witness obstetric patient: the overwhelming importance of a pre-established multidisciplinary protocol. *Blood Transfus*. 2016;14:541–544.

63. Dahlke JD, Mendez-Figueroa H, Maggio L, et al. Prevention and management of postpartum hemorrhage: a comparison of 4 national guidelines. *Am J Obstet Gynecol*. 2015;213:76.e1–76.e10. Available at: https://doi.org/10.1016/j.ajog.2015.02.023.

64. Kramer MS, Berg C, Abenhaim H, et al. Incidence, risk factors, and temporal trends in severe postpartum hemorrhage. *Am J Obstet Gynecol*. 2013;209:449.e1–449.e7.

65. Carillo AP, Chandraharan E. Postpartum haemorrhage and haematological management. *Obstet Gynecol Reprod Med*. 2014;24:291–295.

66. Muirhead B, Weiss ADH. Massive hemorrhage and transfusion in the operating room. *Can J Anesth*. 2017;64:962–978.

67. Misir A. Fluid and medication considerations in the traumatized patient. *Curr Pediatr Rev*. 2017;13. Available at: http://www.eurekaselect.com/154922/article.

68. Kauvar DS, Sarfati MR, Kraiss LW. Intraoperative blood product resuscitation and mortality in ruptured abdominal aortic aneurysm. *J Vasc Surg*. 2012;55:688–692.

69. Montan C, Hammar U, Wikman A, et al. Massive blood transfusion in patients with ruptured abdominal aortic aneurysm. *Eur J Vasc Surg*. 2016;52:597–603.

70. Söderlund T, Ketonen T, Handolin L. Bleeding pelvic fracture patients: evolution of resuscitation protocols. *Scand J Surg*. 2017;106:255–260.

71. Etchill EW, Myers SP, McDaniel LM, et al. Should all massively transfused patients be treated Equally? An analysis of massive transfusion ratios in the nontrauma setting. *Crit Care Med*. 2017;45:1311–1316.

FURTHER READING

1. Acker SN, Hall B, Hill L, et al. Adult-based massive transfusion protocol activation criteria do not work in children. *Eur J Pediatr Surg*. 2017;27:32–35.

CHAPTER 10

Transfusion Medicine in Pediatric Settings

HOLLIE M. REEVES, DO

TRANSFUSION IN NEONATES (YOUNGER THAN 4 MONTHS)

Neonatal Red Blood Cell Transfusion

Neonates are one of the most transfused patient populations. It is reported that 90% of extremely low-birth-weight (ELBW, <1000 g) infants receive at least one red blood cell (RBC) transfusion during their neonatal intensive care unit (NICU) stay.[4]

A full-term infant has a normal hemoglobin value of 14–20 g/dL in the first few days of life.[5] This hemoglobin gradually decreases over 10–12 weeks to a nadir of 10–12 g/dL and then gradually increases; this is termed physiologic anemia of infancy.[4] There are many factors that contribute to this physiologic anemia, including a switch from fetal to adult hemoglobin and downregulation of erythropoietin (EPO) production leading to suppressed erythropoiesis. For most full-term infants, this change is well tolerated.[4]

This physiologic anemia can be exaggerated in premature infants who often have lower hemoglobin concentrations at birth and experience a lower and earlier nadir of 8–10 g/dL at 1–2 months.[6] Premature babies weighing less than 1200 g can display even more rapid and severe anemia, with a nadir at 4–8 weeks and hemoglobin concentration of 6.5–9 g/dL.[4] This can lead to anemia of prematurity (AOP), which is defined as anemia in a preterm infant <32 weeks of gestation with inappropriately low reticulocyte count for the severity of anemia and an inappropriately low circulating EPO concentration for the degree of anemia.[4] This AOP coupled with other factors, such as iatrogenic blood loss, iron deficiency, and chronic illness, may lead to the need for RBC transfusion in these patients.

RBC transfusion indications and thresholds

The decision to transfuse RBCs should take into consideration the clinical status and laboratory findings of the patient for both full-term and premature infants. Although several large, prospective, randomized trials have concluded that RBC transfusions given at a lower hemoglobin threshold are safe in adults and may even lead to better clinical outcomes,[7–9] these results are not necessarily able to be extrapolated to pediatric patients, particularly neonates.[3]

Previous studies

Two previously published randomized controlled trials (RCTs) have evaluated RBC transfusion thresholds in very-low-birth-weight (VLBW, <1500 g) infants. [10,11] The first study by Bell and colleagues[10] randomized 100 hospitalized preterm infants with birth weights of 500–1300 g to either a restrictive hematocrit or a liberal hematocrit RBC transfusion threshold group. They found that, although both transfusion programs were well tolerated, infants in the restrictive group were significantly more likely to have major adverse neurologic events, including grade 4 intraventricular hemorrhage (IVH) and periventricular leukomalacia. Interestingly, follow-up studies of these same infants as school-aged children found that those from the liberal transfusion threshold group had worse neurocognitive outcomes and smaller brain volumes.[12,13]

The second study evaluated RBC transfusion thresholds in ELBW infants and was published in 2006 by Kirpalani and colleagues.[11] In this study, 451 infants weighing less than 1000 g at birth were randomized to high (liberal) or low (restrictive) hemoglobin transfusion thresholds based on patient age and respiratory status. The researchers found no statistically or clinically significant difference between the two treatment groups in the primary composite outcome of death or neonatal morbidity, which included severe retinopathy, bronchopulmonary dysplasia, or brain injury on cranial ultrasonography.[11] In a follow-up study of these patients at 18–21 months' corrected age, however, a post hoc analysis found a significant difference favoring the liberal threshold group, with more patients in the restrictive group having cognitive delay.[14]

Given the conflicting data of the previous studies, there are no current evidence-based RBC transfusion thresholds in neonates but guidelines using laboratory and clinical parameters are available. (Table 10.1).

TABLE 10.1
RBC Transfusion Guidelines in Patients Younger Than 4 months

Laboratory Parameters	Accompanying Clinical Parameters
Hgb <7 g/dL (Hct <20%) in a neonate with:	• Symptomatic anemia (tachycardia, tachypnea, poor feeding) and low reticulocyte count
Hgb <10 g/dL (Hct <30%) in a neonate with:	• Hood O₂ <35% • O₂ by nasal cannula • CPAP and/or IMV with mechanical ventilation with mean airway pressure of <6 cm water • Significant apnea or bradycardia[a] • Significant tachypnea or tachycardia[b] • Low weight gain of <10 g/day observed over 4 days while receiving ≥100 kcal/kg/day
Hgb <12 g/dL (Hct <35%) in a neonate with:	• Hood O₂ >35% • CPAP/IMV with mean airway pressure of ≥6–8 cm water
Hgb <15 g/dL (Hct <45%) in a neonate with:	• ECMO support • Congenital cyanotic heart disease

CPAP, continuous positive airway pressure; *ECMO*, extracorporeal membrane oxygenation; *Hct*, hematocrit; *Hgb*, hemoglobin; *IMV*, intermittent mandatory ventilation; *RBC*, red blood cell.
[a]More than six episodes in a 12-h period or two episodes in a 24-h period requiring bag and mask ventilation and therapeutic doses of methylxanthines.
[b]Respiratory rate >80 breaths/min for 24 h; heart rate >180 beats/min for 24 h.
Adapted from Roseff SD, Luban NL, Manno CS. Guidelines for assessing appropriateness of pediatric transfusion. *Transfusion.* 2002;42(11):1398–1413; with permission.

Current studies

The National Institute of Child Health and Human Development is sponsoring a trial entitled Transfusion of Prematures (TOP) (NCT01702805) to try and help answer the question of the most appropriate RBC transfusion threshold in premature infants. This multicenter trial began enrolling infants in 2012, and the goal is to enroll 1824 infants weighing less than 1000 g with gestational ages between 22 and 29 weeks. The infants are randomized into high or low hemoglobin threshold groups depending on patient age and respiratory support. The study is designed to detect an absolute difference in the proportion of patients who

died or had serious neurodevelopmental impairment at 22–26 months.[3]

In Germany, a multicenter trial is ongoing to study the Effects of Transfusion Thresholds on Neurocognitive Outcome of Extremely Low Birth-Weight Infants (ETTNO) (NCT01393496). In a similar protocol to the TOP trial, ETTNO plans to enroll 920 ELBW infants to receive RBC transfusions at either restrictive or liberal transfusion trigger thresholds.[15] The primary outcome is death or neurodevelopmental impairment determined at (corrected) 24 months of age.

Dosing

Small-volume transfusions are generally defined as 5–15 mL/kg, with transfusion of 10 mL/kg generally raising the hemoglobin by 2–3 g/dL depending upon the storage solution.[16]

Pretransfusion Testing in Neonates

Before RBC transfusion, testing is commonly performed using the recipient's plasma or serum and donor RBCs to prevent incompatible transfusions that may lead to hemolytic reactions.[17] In neonates or infants younger than 4 months any RBC antibodies in the serum or plasma, including ABO isoagglutinins, are presumed to be of maternal origin. This is largely based on early studies showing the failure of alloantibody production in response to transfusion in patients younger than 4 months.[18,19] Current AABB *Standards for Blood Banks and Transfusion Services*, therefore, has special considerations for neonatal pretransfusion testing.[20] For example, on ABO typing, the neonate's red cells need to be tested only with anti-A and anti-B reagents. Neonatal or maternal serum or plasma may be used for the initial detection of unexpected red cell antibodies. If the initial antibody screen is negative for unexpected red cell antibodies, repeat testing may be omitted for the remainder of the neonate's hospital admission or until the neonate reaches 4 months of age, whichever comes first. If non-group-O RBCs are transfused to a non-group-O neonate or infant, then there must be additional testing performed to evaluate for the presence of maternally derived incompatible ABO isoagglutinins depending on the maternal ABO type. Therefore, transfusion services may choose to transfuse only patients younger than 4 months exclusively with group O RBCs. If the initial antibody screen for unexpected red cell antibodies is positive in a neonate, the crossmatch can be omitted as long as antigen-negative blood is transfused.[20]

Special Considerations and Processing of RBCs Transfused to Neonates

Anticoagulant-preservative and additive solutions

RBCs are stored in an anticoagulant preservative, and some have additional additive solutions (AS) that extend the shelf life of the RBC unit. The safety of these AS for use in neonatal transfusion has been questioned, specifically the amount of adenine and mannitol in AS and the potential for nephrotoxicity and fluctuations in cerebral blood flow/increased intracranial pressure.[21] Most studies suggest, however, that for small-volume transfusions the use of AS RBCs is safe in neonates.[22-24]

Safety of AS in large-volume transfusion, such as exchange transfusion, cardiac surgery, and extracorporeal membrane oxygenation (ECMO), for neonates has not been adequately studied, and they should be used with caution.[24,25]

Storage age of RBCs

In addition to no clear optimal RBC transfusion threshold for this very vulnerable population, there is controversy regarding the effect of RBC unit storage age on clinical outcomes. Because premature infants may receive many RBC transfusions during their first few weeks of life,[26,27] there has been agreement that minimizing donor exposures is beneficial.[22,28,29] In fact, methods for aliquoting from one dedicated RBC unit assigned to a neonate have been described.[16] However, concerns regarding transfusing older stored aliquots, particularly those stored for greater than 14 days, remain.[30] The RBC "storage lesion" is characterized by red cell shape and rheologic change, metabolic derangements, changes in oxygen affinity and delivery, and loss of membrane proteins and carbohydrates, including a decrease in 2,3-diphosphoglycerate, accumulation of extracellular potassium and free hemoglobin, increased adherence to vascular endothelium, and changes in nitric oxide bioactivity.[31]

The Age of Red Blood Cells in Premature Infants (ARIPI) trial was a multicenter trial to investigate the effect of stored RBCs in neonates.[32] A total of 377 premature infants weighing less than 1250 g at birth were randomized to receive RBCs stored less than or equal to 7 days or standard issue RBCs stored up to 42 days. The mean age of transfused blood in the fresh RBC group was 5.1 days versus 14.6 days in the standard group. Patients in both groups received a similar number of transfusions (median four transfusions). They found that the use of fresh RBCs compared with standard issue RBCs did not improve outcomes of death

or major neonatal morbidities, including necrotizing enterocolitis (NEC), retinopathy of prematurity, bronchopulmonary dysplasia, or IVH, in premature, VLBW infants requiring RBC transfusion. However, three issues with the external validity of the ARIPI trial have been raised: (1) the transfusion threshold, (2) the RBC preparation method, and (3) the average duration of RBC storage in the standard care group, indicating that additional studies in neonates are needed.[33]

Leukocyte Reduced and Cytomegalovirus Seronegative

Transfusing cellular blood components that have been leukocyte reduced have the reported benefits of reducing febrile nonhemolytic transfusion reactions, human leukocyte antigen (HLA) alloimmunization, and transmission of transfusion-associated cytomegalovirus (CMV).[16] The prevention of transfusion-transmitted CMV infection is of particular importance in neonatal patients, especially those VLBW premature infants born to CMV-seronegative mothers. In donated blood, the primary vector of CMV is the latently infected white blood cells; therefore studies have shown that reduction in the number of white blood cells is an effective way of reducing the risk of transfusion-transmitted CMV.[34-36]

An alternative strategy is to transfuse high-risk patient populations with cellular blood components collected only from CMV seronegative donors.[37,38] With either strategy, however, there is still a 1%–3% residual risk of CMV transmission.[35] A prospective study showed no cases of transfusion-transmitted CMV in 539 VLBW infants who received a total of 2061 transfusions that were both leukocyte reduced and from CMV seronegative donors.[39] The difficult logistics of this "belt and suspenders" approach, however, is the ability to maintain a large enough CMV-seronegative donor pool given the high seroprevalence of CMV.[39] In a systematic review and meta-analysis, the authors concluded that, "at present, the scientific evidence does not favor a single strategy for reducing the risk of transfusion-related CMV infection in high-risk patients."[40] Therefore, wide variability in transfusion practices to reduce the risk of transfusion-transmitted CMV exists.[41,42] An emerging alternative approach to reduce the risk of transfusion-transmitted CMV infection is to use pathogen reduction/inactivation technology.[43]

Irradiation

Transfusion-associated graft versus host disease (TA-GVHD) results when immunocompetent transfused lymphocytes engraft in blood transfusion recipients whose immune system is unable to reject them.[44] This may occur in an immune-compromised host or if there are HLA similarities between the donor and recipient. Neonates, and in particular premature neonates weighing less than 1200 g at birth, are thought to be at increased risk for TA-GVHD.[36] Other at-risk populations include those with known or suspected T-lymphocyte immunodeficiency, those with certain hematologic malignancies, patients who have undergone hematopoietic stem cell transplant (HSCT), and any transfusion recipient receiving HLA-matched blood components or components from first- or second-degree relatives.[45] Irradiation of cellular blood components can minimize this risk. Therefore, some institutions provide irradiated cellular blood components to all or some of their neonatal patient population.

Irradiation of RBCs increases the level of extracellular potassium in the supernatant[46] and reports of adverse transfusion reactions due to high potassium levels have been published.[47,48] The concern for transfusion-associated hyperkalemia may be greater in infants with high plasma potassium levels and/or impaired renal function or those receiving large-volume transfusions, generally >20–25 mL/kg.[49] In these situations, washing may be performed to remove the excess potassium before transfusion,[50] but indications for this may vary from institution to institution.[21]

Alternatives to Neonatal RBC Transfusion

In addition to the well-known infectious and noninfectious risks associated with transfusion, there are some entities, such as NEC and IVH that may follow RBC transfusion in neonates, although causal relationships have not been established.[51] With this in mind, it becomes imperative to avoid unnecessary transfusion in this patient population. Some alternatives to RBC transfusion or ways to minimize transfusion have been recommended. These include delayed cord clamping or cord milking, use of fetal cord blood at delivery for initial laboratory tests, programs to limit phlebotomy losses, appropriate test utilization and obtaining appropriate volumes, and the selected use of erythropoiesis-stimulating agents.[51,52]

Transfusion-Associated Necrotizing Enterocolitis/Transfusion-Related Acute Gut Injury

NEC is a common cause of morbidity and mortality in premature infants. One study found an increase in NEC-related deaths among very premature infants in the United States from 2000 to 2011.[53] In 1987 McGrady and colleagues published a single-center

NICU's outbreak of NEC and raised the question of a possible association with RBC transfusion.[54] Some propose using the term transfusion-related acute gut injury to characterize a severe gastrointestinal reaction associated with RBC transfusion in VLBW neonates, likening it to TRALI (transfusion-related acute lung injury).[55] Others have looked at the degree to which RBC transfusion may affect mesenteric blood flow or oxygenation of tissues.[56] Marin et al. measured the mesenteric tissue oxygenation of preterm infants up to 48 h following RBC transfusion and found decreased postprandial mesenteric tissue oxygenation patterns in infants fed during RBC transfusion compared with those who were not.[57] Some institutions have implemented policies in which infants are not fed during or near transfusion, showing possible protective effects.[58,59] However, to date, there have been no RCTs confirming that withholding feeds during RBC transfusion leads to a decrease risk of NEC.

In a meta-analysis of the available observational data (11 case-control studies and 1 cohort study), the authors concluded that recent exposure to RBC transfusion was associated with NEC in neonates, but additional studies adjusting for confounders were needed.[60] However, data from a limited number of RCTs do not support a causal relationship between RBC transfusion and NEC.[61] Experts call for more research in this area before recommendations on feeding and transfusion practices can be made.[3,62]

Neonatal Exchange Transfusion

Neonates may undergo whole-blood exchange transfusion for hyperbilirubinemia. In these cases, the primary purpose of the exchange transfusion is to remove the high levels of unconjugated bilirubin from the neonate. Owing to the immature liver physiology and poor ability to conjugate bilirubin, both full-term and preterm infants can be susceptible to high concentrations of bilirubin. This bilirubin can cross the immature blood-brain barrier, concentrate in the cerebellum and basal ganglia, and lead to neurotoxicity (kernicterus).[63] For most neonates with hyperbilirubinemia, the first-line treatment is phototherapy, or the use of fluorescent ultraviolet lights. However, if the infant does not respond to phototherapy, exchange transfusion can be performed.[16] Exchange transfusion for hyperbilirubinemia is often a double-volume exchange, with estimated full-term infant blood volume of ~85 mL/kg and preterm/VLBW infant blood volume of ~100 mL/kg.[16] Performing a double-volume exchange removes approximately 70%–90% of the circulating red cells and approximately 50% of the total bilirubin.[16]

The RBCs used for the exchange are often reconstituted with ABO-compatible plasma to the desired hematocrit, usually 45%–60%. Traditionally, the RBCs are fresh, less than 5 or 7 days, stored in non-AS, and group O/Rh(D) compatible. If AS RBCs are used, some blood banks will volume-reduce or wash to remove the additive-containing plasma.[16] Additional RBC attributes for neonatal exchange also often include CMV reduced risk (leukocyte reduced and/or CMV seronegative), irradiated, and hemoglobin S negative.[16] If the hyperbilirubinemia is due to hemolytic disease of the fetus and newborn (HDFN), in which there is a maternal red cell alloantibody or antibodies to antigen(s) present on the neonate's red cells causing hemolysis, the RBCs used for the exchange must lack that antigen(s) and/or be antiglobulin cross-match compatible.[20]

Exchange transfusion may also be used to eliminate certain drugs, toxins, or other chemicals that may have been administered to the mother near the time of delivery or to the infant in toxic doses or that may have accumulated owing to inborn errors of metabolism.[64,65]

Neonatal Platelet Transfusion

Among neonates, preterm infants have the highest risk of thrombocytopenia and intracranial hemorrhage (ICH). Neonatal platelets have differences in production, function, and hemostatic capabilities versus those in older pediatric patients and adults.[66] In terms of platelet production, researchers have found that healthy neonates have higher levels of thrombopoietin (TPO) than healthy adults, are more sensitive to low TPO concentrations, have more proliferative megakaryopoiesis, but have megakaryocytes of smaller size and ploidy.[67] Neonatal platelets are hyporeactive to several known platelet agonists; however, this appears to be compensated for with factors in neonatal blood that enhance the platelet-vessel wall interaction, leading to increased primary hemostasis.[67]

Neonatal thrombocytopenia, a platelet count of less than 150×10^9/L is not uncommon, occurring in up to a third of neonates admitted to the NICU.[68] The incidence in ELBW (<1000 g) infants is even higher.[69] Causes of neonatal thrombocytopenia can be congenital or acquired and can reflect increased platelet destruction, decreased platelet production, or a combination of the two. Platelet transfusion is a common therapy for thrombocytopenic patients with evidence of bleeding; however, the role of prophylactic platelet transfusions in neonates is more controversial and significant variability in transfusion practices exist.

Platelet transfusion indications and thresholds

Previous studies. Over the years several studies have analyzed platelet transfusion practice in neonates in an attempt to define transfusion triggers and thresholds. In an early multicenter, RCT, Andrew and colleagues studied whether early use of platelet transfusions would reduce the incidence or extension of ICH or both in thrombocytopenic sick infants of less than 33 weeks gestational age.[70] They randomized 152 neonates with a birth weight of 500–1500 g to maintain a platelet count either greater than 150×10^9/L or greater than 50×10^9/L for the first week of life. Both groups had similar numbers of new ICH, ICH extension, or both. Unfortunately, this study did not include infants with severe thrombocytopenia (initial platelet counts of less than 50×10^9/L). Therefore, focusing on the management of severe thrombocytopenia in NICU patients, Murray et al. conducted a retrospective observational cohort study of their NICU and found that none of the neonates with platelet counts of less than 50×10^9/L who were not transfused had major hemorrhage, suggesting that a lower platelet count may be safe in stable infants.[71] Two additional retrospective studies[68,72] found that the use of a restrictive platelet threshold compared with a more liberal one did not increase the incidence or severity of ICH but did lead to a significantly lower rate of platelet transfusions.[68]

Although these studies are helpful in guiding neonatal platelet transfusion practice, to date an optimal, evidence-based platelet transfusion threshold has not been determined. See Table 10.2 for a summary of available guidelines on neonatal platelet transfusion.

TABLE 10.2
Platelet Transfusion Guidelines in Neonates

Platelet Count	Accompanying Clinical Parameters
Less than 20×10^9/L to 30×10^9/L	• Stable, nonbleeding, term infant
30×10^9/L to 50×10^9/L	• Unstable[a] infant, not bleeding, not on ECMO
Less than or equal to 50×10^9/L	• Active bleeding or invasive procedure
Less than 100×10^9/L	• On ECMO, not bleeding • Immediately before or after surgery

ECMO, extracorporeal membrane oxygenation.
[a]More likely to have spontaneous hemorrhage.
Adapted from Roseff SD, Luban NL, Manno CS. Guidelines for assessing appropriateness of pediatric transfusion. *Transfusion*. 2002;42(11):1398–1413; with permission.

Current study

A multicenter European trial, the Platelets for Neonatal Transfusion Study 2, began enrolling patients in 2011.[73] The study is designed as a two-stage, randomized, parallel-group, superiority trial comparing clinical outcomes in neonates of less than 34 weeks' gestation who are randomized to either receive prophylactic platelet transfusion to maintain platelet counts at or above either 25×10^9/L or 50×10^9/L. The primary outcome is to detect an 8% difference in mortality or major bleeding.

Platelet mass

Researchers have considered using platelet mass rather than platelet count as a threshold for transfusion. Platelet mass is calculated by multiplying the platelet count by the mean platelet volume. The rationale behind this is that if there is normal platelet and endothelial function, the platelet mass may influence the efficacy of platelet plug formation and hemostasis more than the platelet count.[74] In a prospective, two-centered, before versus after design study, Gerday and colleagues found that the use of platelet mass–based NICU transfusion guidelines were associated with fewer platelet transfusions and no increase in hemorrhagic events, including IVH.[75] A more recent feasibility study was conducted and found that using platelet mass rather than platelet count as a transfusion trigger in neonates is feasible; however, they found no differences in the number of platelet transfusions, bleeding events, or mortality. Therefore, they concluded that a definitive comparative-effectiveness trial would likely require a very large sample size to detect any reduction in transfusion rates using platelet mass as the trigger versus platelet count.[76]

Components

There are a variety of platelet products available for transfusion, including apheresis platelets (single-donor platelets) and whole-blood–derived platelet concentrates (random donor platelets), which can be pooled before or after storage. ABO-identical or ABO-compatible platelets are preferred for transfusion in pediatric patients, especially neonates, to avoid large amounts of incompatible plasma. If the transfusion of incompatible platelets is necessary, volume reduction or washing can be considered. As a cellular component, platelets can also be irradiated to minimize the risk of transfusion-associated graft versus host disease (TA-GVHD) and leukocyte reduced or CMV seronegative.

Dose

A platelet transfusion dose of 5–10 mL/kg has been reported to raise the platelet count by 50,000–100,000/µL in an average full-term infant.[77] However, most neonatologists routinely order a platelet transfusion dose of 10 mL/kg.[78]

Neonatal Alloimmune Thrombocytopenia

Neonatal alloimmune thrombocytopenia or fetal and neonatal alloimmune thrombocytopenia (FNAIT) is similar to hemolytic disease of the fetus and newborn (HDFN) in that it is due to an incompatibility between mother and fetus, but of platelets, not red cells. In FNAIT, the mother makes platelet-specific IgG antibodies to paternally inherited platelet antigens that she lacks and are expressed on fetal cells. These antibodies, because they are IgG in nature, can cross the placenta, bind to fetal platelets, and cause thrombocytopenia. The platelet antigen implicated in up to 80% of cases in women of European ancestry is the human-platelet-antigen 1a (HPA-1a).[79] FNAIT affects approximately 1 in 1000 to 1 in 2000 pregnancies.[79] FNAIT, unlike HDFN, typically affects the first pregnancy, and the severity increases with subsequent pregnancies.

Not all infants born to women with anti-HPA-1a have thrombocytopenia, but about 20% have severe thrombocytopenia associated with bleeding.[80,81] FNAIT should be suspected in an otherwise healthy neonate with isolated thrombocytopenia. Maternal platelet count is generally normal. ICH represents the most severe bleeding complication and can occur in utero.[82] FNAIT may be diagnosed prenatally if ICH is seen on fetal ultrasound scan or if the mother has a history of a previously affected pregnancy. In this case, prenatal testing to identify maternal platelet alloantibodies can be performed.[80]

Part of the difficulty in managing FNAIT is that 40%–60% of cases present unexpectedly during the first pregnancy.[80] FNAIT is often a diagnosis of exclusion, as other causes of neonatal thrombocytopenia, such as sepsis, should be ruled out. Maternal platelet alloantibody detection and newborn platelet antigen typing can aid in the diagnosis postnatally; however, treatment including platelet transfusion may be necessary before the results are available. In cases of severe thrombocytopenia or bleeding, platelet transfusion is appropriate. Although current guidelines recommend antigen-negative platelets,[83] these products may not be readily available. In that case, there are reports to support the use of platelets from the general blood bank inventory (most likely antigen positive).[82,83] Antigen-negative platelets can be obtained from the mother or from specially selected blood bank donors whose platelets lack the corresponding antigen. If maternal platelets are transfused, they must be volume reduced or washed to limit the amount of antibody-containing plasma and irradiated to minimize risk of TA-GVHD. In prenatal or postnatal cases of FNAIT, a multidisciplinary approach to diagnosis and treatment is important. This often involves several departments, such as maternal-fetal medicine, pediatric and adult hematology-oncology, neonatology, and transfusion medicine.

Neonatal Plasma Transfusion
Indications
Plasma transfusion has been reported to occur in up to 12%–15% of NICU patients,[84,85] with the most common deciding factor for its use being an abnormal coagulation test result, specifically either abnormal prothrombin time (PT) or activated partial thromboplastin time (aPTT). However, in neonates it has been documented that coagulation test abnormalities are poor predictors of bleeding[86-88] and that transfusing a nonbleeding neonate with plasma does not reduce the risk of future hemorrhage.[89,90] Therefore it has been recommended that the most appropriate plasma use is in the treatment of a bleeding neonate with a laboratory-confirmed coagulopathy (PT or aPTT significantly above the normal gestational and postnatal age-related reference range).[86,91] Plasma may be indicated in the setting of disseminated intravascular coagulation (DIC) with overt hemorrhage or as replacement fluid in certain disease entities treated with therapeutic plasma exchange, such thrombotic thrombocytopenic purpura (TTP).[85] Plasma should not be used for volume expansion or for the replacement of a single coagulation factor if a specific factor concentrate exists.

Dosing and administration
A dose of 10–15 mL/kg should be effective in increasing factor levels by 15%–20%, assuming there is not an ongoing consumptive coagulopathy.[16] Volume status of the patient should be taken into consideration when dosing. Transfused plasma should be ABO compatible with the recipient, particularly neonates, given their small overall total blood volumes.

PEDIATRIC TRANSFUSION (INFANTS AND CHILDREN OLDER THAN 4 MONTHS)
This section focuses on the transfusion needs of pediatric patients that are older than 4 months.

RBC Transfusion
Indications
RBC transfusions are often performed to increase the oxygen-carrying capacity in patients with anemia or hemoglobinopathies or acute blood loss of 15%–20% of their blood volume.[92,93] The decision to transfuse should take into consideration not only the laboratory values in the patient but also their clinical status.[92] Evidence of hypoperfusion, such as tachycardia, hypotension, pallor, and decreased mentation, may also indicate the need for RBC transfusion, particularly in cases of acute blood loss, as laboratory parameters may not be reflective of the degree of anemia.[5]

RCTs evaluating transfusions and their outcomes in many pediatric populations are lacking. One trial randomly assigned pediatric intensive care unit patients to either a restrictive-strategy group in which the patients were transfused RBCs at a hemoglobin threshold of 7 g/dL or a liberal-strategy group with a hemoglobin threshold of 9.5 g/dL.[93] The investigators concluded that in stable, critically ill children a restrictive RBC transfusion strategy can decrease transfusion requirements without increasing adverse outcomes. The authors did note, however, that this restrictive strategy may not apply to children with severe hypoxemia, hemodynamic instability, active blood loss, or cyanotic heart disease.[93]

Another pediatric patient population that frequently undergoes transfusion is those with hematologic malignancies or HSCT. Most pediatric oncologists and physicians overseeing pediatric patients with HSCT use RBC transfusion thresholds of 7–8 g/dL as reported in two separate surveys.[94,95] A survey of hematologists taking care of patients with aplastic anemia reported that 50% transfuse to maintain a hemoglobin greater than 6–8 g/dL and approximately 30% transfuse only when symptomatic.[96] An RCT evaluating high (12 g/dL) versus low (7 g/dL) hemoglobin thresholds in pediatric patients undergoing HSCT was stopped early because of an increase in severe venoocclusive disease in the high-hemoglobin arm.[97]

Dosing, administration, and special considerations
A dose of 10–15 mL/kg is appropriate for small-volume transfusion and should increase the hemoglobin by 2–3 g/dL.[16] Larger-volume transfusions may be needed in certain situations such as exchange transfusion, cardiopulmonary bypass, and ECMO. Red cells should be ABO and Rh(D) antigen compatible with the recipient, and an antibody screen for unexpected RBC antibodies should be performed. A crossmatch should be performed to ensure that the donor unit is compatible with the recipient. The RBC unit may be leukocyte reduced and irradiated, if applicable.

RBC Transfusion in Pediatric Patients With SCD

Sickle cell disease (SCD) is the most common inherited blood disorder in the United States, affecting 1 in every 500 African American births.[98] The pathophysiology is complex, involving changes in red cell membrane structure and function, increased adherence to vascular endothelium, hypoxia-reperfusion injury, nitric oxide depletion, and hemolysis.[98] RBC transfusion has been a mainstay of therapy for patients with SCD for decades, often times beginning early in childhood.[99]

Long-term RBC transfusion can be associated with iron overload, red cell alloimmunization, delayed transfusion reactions, and hyperhemolysis.[100] Rates of RBC alloimmunization in children with SCD range from 18% to 47% compared with 5%–11% in patients with thalassemia who undergo long-term transfusion and 0.2%–2.6% in the general population.[5] This is largely attributed to differences in red cell antigen expression in the patient population with SCD and that of the general donor population. To minimize this risk, most institutions have developed protocols for transfusing patients with SCD. Many of these protocols include early RBC phenotyping or genotyping and prophylactic phenotype matching transfused red cells for the C, E, and K antigens. Some institutions perform extended phenotype matching of RBC units to include Kidd, Duffy, and MNSs blood group antigens,[100-102] but this can be logistically challenging and may not be feasible in emergent situations.

Over time, red cell alloantibodies can evanesce, putting the patient at risk for a delayed hemolytic transfusion reaction (DHTR) during subsequent transfusion. DHTRs are characterized by hemolysis and alloantibody formation, either de novo or anamnestic response, and generally occur 4–10 days after transfusion.[103] Patients with SCD are at a higher risk of DHTR. In one study, greater than 90% of patients with SCD with evanesced alloantibodies visited multiple hospitals for RBC transfusion and of those, nearly 30% were admitted for transfusion after the antibody was no longer detected.[104] There is currently no centralized database to keep track of alloimmunization in patients with SCD, making it difficult to avoid transfusion of incompatible units. Hyperhemolysis is a rare but potentially fatal complication of RBC transfusion seen in patients with SCD that can be considered a subset of DHTR. In the case of hyperhemolysis, however, there may not always be alloantibody formation identified and there is hemolysis of the patient's own RBCs in addition to

the transfused cells.[103] In this setting, additional transfusion should be avoided, as it can exacerbate the hemolysis. Intravenous immunoglobulin and steroids have been used with some success.[105]

RBC transfusion may be indicated to help manage acute and chronic complications of SCD.[99] Red cell administration, via either simple transfusion or exchange transfusion, can be effective in decreasing the level of sickle hemoglobin (HbS) while maintaining an adequate hemoglobin concentration. Current evidence-based recommendations are to avoid transfusing to a target hemoglobin level of greater than 10 g/dL owing to concerns for hyperviscosity and in children with SCD receiving chronic transfusion therapy to maintain a HbS level of less than 30% before the next transfusion[99] (Box 10.2).

Platelet Transfusion

Indications

Platelet transfusion is second only to RBC transfusion in pediatric patients, making up approximately 19% of transfusions in children's hospitals.[106] Outside of the neonatal period, the most platelet transfusions are to pediatric hematology/oncology patients with

---

BOX 10.1
Plasma Transfusion Guidelines

- Replacement therapy in a bleeding patient or in need of invasive procedure with coagulopathy
- DIC with bleeding
- Coagulation factor replacement *only* if specific factor concentrate not available
- Warfarin reversal in emergent situations, such as hemorrhage or invasive procedure
- Replacement fluid in TPE when plasma is indicated (e.g., ADAMTS13 replacement in TTP)
- Reconstitution of whole blood for neonatal exchange transfusion
- Circuit priming for ECMO or cardiopulmonary bypass

ADAMTS13, a disintegrin and metalloprotease with thrombospondin type 1 domain 13; *DIC*, disseminated intravascular coagulation; *ECMO*, extracorporeal membrane oxygenation; *TPE*, therapeutic plasma exchange; *TTP*, thrombotic thrombocytopenic purpura.
Data from Keir AK, Stanworth SJ. Neonatal plasma transfusion: an evidence-based review. *Transfus Med Rev.* 2016;30(4):174–182, Motta M, Del Vecchio A, Chirico G. Fresh frozen plasma administration in the neonatal intensive care unit: evidence-based guidelines. *Clin Perinatol.* 2015;42(3):639–650, Roseff SD, Luban NL, Manno CS. Guidelines for assessing appropriateness of pediatric transfusion. *Transfusion.* 2002;42(11):1398–1413.

BOX 10.2
RBC Transfusion Guidelines in Pediatric Patients Older Than 4 months

- Acute blood loss of ≥15% total blood volume
- Hemoglobin <7 g/dL with symptomatic anemia perioperatively
- Hemoglobin <7 g/dL in stable, critically ill children[a,93]
- Hemoglobin between 7 and 8 g/dL in nonbleeding pediatric HPC transplant patients[94,95]
- Preoperative anemia when other corrective therapy is not available or surgery is emergent
- Hemoglobin <13 g/dL on ECMO or with severe pulmonary disease
- Management of acute complications in SCD[99]
- Patients with hemoglobinopathies or other types of chronic anemia/disorders of RBC production on chronic transfusion programs

---

ECMO, extracorporeal membrane oxygenation; *HPC*, hematopoietic progenitor cell; *RBC*, red blood cell; *SCD*, sickle cell disease.
[a]This threshold may not be appropriate for children with severe hypoxemia, hemodynamic instability, active blood loss, or cyanotic heart disease.
Adapted from Roseff SD, Luban NL, Manno CS. Guidelines for assessing appropriateness of pediatric transfusion. *Transfusion*. 2002;42(11):1398–1413; with permission.

TABLE 10.3
Platelet Transfusion Guidelines in Pediatric Patients Older Than 4 months

Platelet Count	Accompanying Clinical Parameters
<10 × 10⁹/L	• Failure of platelet production
<50 × 10⁹/L	• Active bleeding • Invasive procedure or surgery
<100 × 10⁹/L	• CNS bleeding or surgery • On ECMO[a]
Variable	• Patients with qualitative platelet disorders and bleeding

CNS, central nervous system; *ECMO*, extracorporeal membrane oxygenation.
[a]If bleeding, may require platelet transfusion at higher platelet counts.
Adapted from Roseff SD, Luban NL, Manno CS. Guidelines for assessing appropriateness of pediatric transfusion. *Transfusion*. 2002;42(11):1398–1413; with permission.

thrombocytopenia related to malignancy, therapy, and/or HSCT or those with surgery-related bleeding.[107] The current pediatric platelet transfusion practice is largely based on adult studies or expert opinion; however, pediatric patients may be at a higher bleeding risk over a wide range of platelet counts.[108] Prophylactic platelet transfusions are generally given when the platelet count is less than 10 × 10⁹/L and there is a platelet production problem.[107] Prophylactic platelet transfusions may also be given in thrombocytopenic patients who are to undergo an invasive procedure or surgery.[107] Platelet transfusion may also be indicated in patients with qualitative platelet disorders, such as Glanzmann thrombasthenia or Bernard-Soulier syndrome, to treat bleeding, but this is not universally accepted.[107] See Table 10.3 for general platelet transfusion guidelines for older children. Platelet transfusions are associated with higher odds of arterial thrombosis and mortality among patients with consumptive disorders, such as TTP and heparin-induced thrombocytopenia (HIT), and are therefore contraindicated.[109] In immune thrombocytopenic purpura there is no such association, but it is recommended that platelet transfusions be reserved only for catastrophic hemorrhage or surgery.[110]

Dosing and administration

A dose of 5–10 mL/kg of either an apheresis platelet unit or a whole-blood-derived platelet unit is appropriate for a pediatric patient.[16] This dose should result in an increase in the platelet count of 50,000 to 100,000 × 10⁹/L but may be reduced in the setting of comorbid conditions, such as sepsis, DIC, or other platelet consumptive disorders.[16] Some patients may have an inappropriate increment following transfusion owing to alloimmunization in which they develop class I HLA antibodies or platelet-specific antibodies and therefore may require additional evaluation or specially matched products for transfusion. For these patients, it is best to coordinate with the transfusion service. For patients on volume restriction, volume reduction of the platelet product can be performed; however, this is not routine practice. Volume reduction can lead to activation of the platelets and is associated with a decreased platelet count post transfusion.[111–113]

If an Rh(D)-negative patient receives an Rh(D)-positive platelet unit or units, it may be necessary to provide Rh immune globulin (RhIG) to minimize the risk of sensitization and formation of anti-D resulting from the residual RBCs in the platelet product. This practice is not well standardized, however, and several studies have shown very low to no rates of anti-D formation after Rh(D)-positive platelet transfusion.[114–116] One 300-µg dose should provide coverage for 15 mL of Rh(D)-positive RBCs or 30 mL of Rh(D)-positive whole blood.[5]

Plasma and Cryoprecipitate Transfusion
Indications
Indications for plasma transfusion in pediatric patients include treatment of coagulopathies associated with massive hemorrhage, DIC and liver failure, and sepsis.[117] Plasma may also be used for extracorporeal circuit priming and in cases in which a specific factor concentrate is not available. Plasma is also indicated as replacement fluid in therapeutic plasma exchange for certain disease entities, such as TTP. See Box 10.1 for plasma transfusion guidelines. Plasma is not indicated for volume expansion or in patients with a single-factor deficiency for which a specific replacement exists.

Cryoprecipitated antihemophilic factor (Cryo) is a product that is derived from plasma and contains fibrinogen, factor VIII, factor XIII, von Willebrand factor (vWF), and fibronectin. The current primary use for cryoprecipitate is to replace fibrinogen in the setting of a patient with hypofibrinogenemia and bleeding or need for an invasive procedure. Historically, it was used for factor VIII or vWF replacement in patients with hemophilia A or von Willebrand disease, respectively, but this is no longer standard practice, as there are specific factor concentrates available.[117] Fibrinolytic states associated with bleeding, either localized as a result of plasminogen activators produced during surgery of the prostatic bed, urothelium, or salivary gland tissue or systemic in the setting of wide-spread amyloidosis or L-asparaginase chemotherapy in acute lymphoblastic leukemia, may benefit from cryoprecipitate transfusion.[118] See Box 10.3 for guidelines. Concentrations of fibrinogen in the range of 50–100 mg/dL are often adequate to maintain hemostasis; however, routine coagulation tests can become abnormal when fibrinogen concentrations fall below 100 mg/dL.[118]

Dosing and administration
A plasma dose of 10–15 mL/kg (20 mL/kg in the setting of liver disease) should be effective in increasing factor levels by 15%–20% immediately after infusion.[16,117] Of course, this response may be blunted in settings of marked consumptive coagulopathies and is based on the steady-state volume of distribution.[117] The biological half-lives of the various clotting proteins differ and should be considered when attempting to correct a coagulopathy with plasma transfusion.[118] Volume status of the patient should be taken into consideration when dosing. As in neonates, transfused plasma should be ABO compatible with the recipient.

Cryoprecipitate units are of small volume, generally 5–15 mL, and often are pooled to facilitate transfusion. About 1–2 units/10 kg should increase the fibrinogen by 60–100 mg/dL and 1 unit is generally sufficient for infants.[16] When dosing cryoprecipitate to correct hypofibrinogenemia, a common calculation can be used in which often the target fibrinogen is at least 200 mg/dL. See Box 10.4 for calculation.[118]

Granulocyte Transfusion
Indications
Despite advances in antimicrobial therapy and granulocyte stimulating factors, patients with prolonged disease- or therapy-induced neutropenia or defective granulocyte function still suffer morbidity and/or mortality associated with bacterial and fungal infections.[119] Therapeutic granulocyte transfusion in these patients has been reported, although with varying degrees of

---

BOX 10.3
Cryoprecipitate Transfusion Guidelines

- Hypofibrinogenemia or dysfibrinogenemia with bleeding or invasive procedure
- Replacement of factor VIII, vWF, or factor XIII *only* if specific factor concentrate not available and is clinically indicated
- Fibrinolysis, either localized or systemic, associated with bleeding

vWF, von Willebrand factor.
Data from Roseff SD, Luban NL, Manno CS. Guidelines for assessing appropriateness of pediatric transfusion. *Transfusion.* 2002;42(11):1398–1413, Goldenberg NA, Manco-Johnson MJ. Pediatric hemostasis and use of plasma components. *Best Pract Res Clin Haematol.* 2006;19(1):143–155, Theresa Nester, Shweta Jain, Poisson J. *Hemotherapy Decisions and Their Outcomes.* 18th ed. Bethesda, Maryland: AABB; 2014.

BOX 10.4
Calculation for Replacing Fibrinogen With Cryoprecipitate

1. Calculate patient's total blood volume (TBV)
   a. Weight (kg) × 70 mL/kg[a]
2. Calculate patient's plasma volume (PV)
   a. TBV × (1 − hematocrit)
3. Determine fibrinogen deficiency
   a. Target fibrinogen − current fibrinogen
4. Mg of fibrinogen needed
   a. Fibrinogen deficiency × PV/100
5. Number of cryoprecipitate units needed
   a. Mg fibrinogen needed/250 mg[b]

[a]Average conversion factor for adult.
[b]Usual content of fibrinogen/unit.

success, including posttransfusion increment and survival.[120–123] To date, an RCT in children has not been performed, but some would argue that the current evidence supports the early use of granulocyte transfusion, especially in patients with bacterial infections.[119] Most institutions have guidelines for initiating granulocyte transfusion, see Box 10.5. It is important to consult a transfusion medicine physician regarding the decision to transfuse granulocytes and for help in coordinating the logistics of such. Owing to improvements in antimicrobials available, granulocyte transfusion is not commonly used to treat neonatal sepsis.

Regarding prophylactic granulocyte transfusion, a Cochrane review concluded that there is low-grade evidence to support the use of prophylactic granulocyte transfusion to reduce the risk of bacterial or fungal infection in neutropenic patients due to myelosuppressive chemotherapy or HSCT, low-grade evidence that the effect of prophylactic granulocyte transfusions may be dose dependent, and currently insufficient evidence to determine any difference in mortality rates due to infection, all-cause mortality, or serious adverse events.[125]

Dose and administration

Granulocyte concentrates are mainly collected via apheresis from blood donors who are stimulated with steroids, granulocyte-colony stimulating factor, or both. Accreditation standards indicate that granulocyte products must contain at least 1×10^{10} granulocytes.[20] For infants, the suggested dose is 10–15 mL/kg or $1–2 \times 10^9$ cells/kg.[16] For larger pediatric patients, a dose of $4–8 \times 10^{10}$ granulocytes is recommended or one-half or a whole unit if > 20 kg.[5] A trial of three to five daily doses is common.[120,123] Once collected, granulocyte viability is labile, and the product should be transfused within 24 h, ideally sooner if possible. Granulocytes

---

BOX 10.5
Guidelines for Granulocyte Transfusion

- Severe neutropenia (ANC $<0.5 \times 10^9$/L) or granulocyte dysfunction (congenital or acquired)
- Expected duration of neutropenia for at least 5 days
- Documented or suspected bacterial or fungal infection unresponsive to appropriate antimicrobial therapy
- Neutrophil recovery anticipated

ANC, absolute neutrophil count.
From Averbuch D, Engelhard D, Pegoraro A, et al. Review on efficacy and complications of granulocyte transfusions in neutropenic patients. *Curr Drug Targets*. 2016.

---

should be ABO compatible with the recipient, antigen negative for any corresponding clinically significant alloantibodies that the recipient has, and RBC crossmatch compatible. Granulocytes should also be irradiated and preferably from a CMV-seronegative donor if the recipient is CMV seronegative, as the product cannot be leukocyte reduced.

Risks

It is not uncommon for the granulocyte transfusion recipient to experience reactions such as fever, chills, allergic reactions, and hypotension.[126] However, more serious pulmonary complications have been reported with symptoms such as dyspnea, hypoxemia, and pulmonary edema.[121,127,128] It may be recommended that there be a time gap of at least 4 h between granulocyte transfusion and amphotericin B administration in patients receiving both therapies because of reports of severe pulmonary reactions when administered within 4 h of each other.[129] However, this observation has not been supported in subsequent studies.[130]

Extracorporeal Membrane Oxygenation

ECMO is a modified form of cardiopulmonary bypass and is used to support patients with reversible cardiac and/or pulmonary disease or as a bridge to transplant. There are two types of ECMO, venovenous or venoarterial. Although the initial application for ECMO was in neonates with severe respiratory failure, it is now used in the supportive care of patients of all ages.[131]

Patients on ECMO often require multiple blood components because of the large extracorporeal volume of the circuit, required priming of the ECMO circuit, and severity of the patient's clinical status. Therefore ECMO programs are often dependent on the blood bank for support, and close communication between the ECMO team and the blood bank is important.[16]

Currently there are no standard guidelines for the transfusion of blood components to patients undergoing ECMO, and protocols may vary. The ECMO circuit and tubing can lead to platelet activation and thrombosis, and therefore patients are often heparinized. In turn, the use of heparin, in addition to possible platelet dysfunction and/or loss and other coagulation defects, increases the bleeding risks in these patients. Platelet counts are generally maintained between 80,000 and 150,000, hemoglobin is maintained between 10 and 12 g/dL, and plasma and cryoprecipitate may be used to replace clotting factors.[5]

Before placing a patient on ECMO, the circuit requires priming with RBCs and plasma. Institutions may have protocols regarding ordering blood for

ECMO priming and transfusion. ABO- and Rh(D)-compatible RBCs should be used for priming in pediatric ECMO cases and are often leukocyte reduced (or CMV seronegative), less than 5-7 days old, irradiated, and hemoglobin S negative.[16] Washing of red cell units may be performed if there is concern for hyperkalemia or AS use in neonates. Once the patient is established on the ECMO circuit, transfusion of blood components is often of smaller volumes, and therefore some of the above-mentioned recommendations may not apply. Platelet, plasma, and cryoprecipitate thresholds and use may vary, and it is important to refer to your institutional protocol.

Therapeutic Apheresis in Pediatric Patients

Therapeutic apheresis in pediatric patients may require modifications to accommodate their smaller size, blood volume, and developmental age.[132] Because of their smaller total blood volume, an RBC prime may be needed to prevent dilution of the hematocrit from the normal saline prime. Anticoagulants commonly used during apheresis procedures include heparin, anticoagulant citrate dextrose (ACD), or a combination of both. Pediatric patients may be more sensitive to the hypocalcemic effects of ACD and therefore may require calcium supplementation to prevent or treat low ionized calcium levels, scheduled monitoring of ionized calcium levels throughout the procedure, or a change in anticoagulant.[132] Despite these considerations, therapeutic apheresis can be a safe and efficacious therapy in children.[133-137]

REFERENCES

1. Hillyer CD, Mondoro TH, Josephson CD, Sanchez R, Sloan SR, Ambruso DR. Pediatric transfusion medicine: development of a critical mass. *Transfusion.* 2009;49(3):596-601.
2. Strauss RG. 2008 Emily Cooley Memorial Lecture: lessons learned from pediatric transfusion medicine clinical trials... a little child shall lead them. *Transfusion.* 2009;49(9):1996-2004.
3. Nickel RS, Josephson CD. Neonatal transfusion medicine: five major unanswered research questions for the twenty-first century. *Clin Perinatol.* 2015;42(3):499-513.
4. Colombatti R, Sainati L, Trevisanuto D. Anemia and transfusion in the neonate. *Semin Fetal Neonatal Med.* 2016;21(1):2-9.
5. AABB. *Pediatric Transfusion: A Physician's Handbook.* 4th ed. Bethesda, Maryland: AABB; 2015.
6. Strauss RG. How I transfuse red blood cells and platelets to infants with the anemia and thrombocytopenia of prematurity. *Transfusion.* 2008;48(2):209-217.
7. Hebert PC, Wells G, Blajchman MA, et al. A multicenter, randomized, controlled clinical trial of transfusion requirements in critical care. Transfusion Requirements in Critical Care Investigators, Canadian Critical Care Trials Group. *N Engl J Med.* 1999;340(6):409-417.
8. Carson JL, Terrin ML, Noveck H, et al. Liberal or restrictive transfusion in high-risk patients after hip surgery. *N Engl J Med.* 2011;365(26):2453-2462.
9. Villanueva C, Colomo A, Bosch A, et al. Transfusion strategies for acute upper gastrointestinal bleeding. *N Engl J Med.* 2013;368(1):11-21.
10. Bell EF, Strauss RG, Widness JA, et al. Randomized trial of liberal versus restrictive guidelines for red blood cell transfusion in preterm infants. *Pediatrics.* 2005;115(6):1685-1691.
11. Kirpalani H, Whyte RK, Andersen C, et al. The Premature Infants in Need of Transfusion (PINT) study: a randomized, controlled trial of a restrictive (low) versus liberal (high) transfusion threshold for extremely low birth weight infants. *J Pediatr.* 2006;149(3):301-307.
12. McCoy TE, Conrad AL, Richman LC, Lindgren SD, Nopoulos PC, Bell EF. Neurocognitive profiles of preterm infants randomly assigned to lower or higher hematocrit thresholds for transfusion. *Child Neuropsychol.* 2011;17(4):347-367.
13. Nopoulos PC, Conrad AL, Bell EF, et al. Long-term outcome of brain structure in premature infants: effects of liberal vs restricted red blood cell transfusions. *Arch Pediatr Adolesc Med.* 2011;165(5):443-450.
14. Whyte RK, Kirpalani H, Asztalos EV, et al. Neurodevelopmental outcome of extremely low birth weight infants randomly assigned to restrictive or liberal hemoglobin thresholds for blood transfusion. *Pediatrics.* 2009;123(1):207-213.
15. Investigators E. The 'effects of transfusion thresholds on neurocognitive outcome of extremely low birth-weight infants (ETTNO)' study: background, aims, and study protocol. *Neonatology.* 2012;101(4):301-305.
16. Josephson CDME. *Neonatal and Pediatric Transfusion Practice.* 18th ed. Bethesda, Maryland: AABB; 2014.
17. Downes KASI. *Pretransfusion Testing.* 18th ed. Bethesda, Maryland: AABB; 2014.
18. Ludvigsen Jr CW, Swanson JL, Thompson TR, McCullough J. The failure of neonates to form red blood cell alloantibodies in response to multiple transfusions. *Am J Clin Pathol.* 1987;87(2):250-251.
19. Floss AM, Strauss RG, Goeken N, Knox L. Multiple transfusion fail to provoke antibodies against blood cell antigens in human infants. *Transfusion.* 1986;26(5):419-422.
20. *Standards for Blood Banks and Transfusion Services.* 30th ed. Bethesda, MD: AABB; 2015.
21. Fung MK, Roseff SD, Vermoch KL. Blood component preferences of transfusion services supporting infant transfusions: a University Health System Consortium benchmarking study. *Transfusion.* 2010;50(9):1921-1925.

22. Strauss RG, Burmeister LF, Johnson K, et al. AS-1 red cells for neonatal transfusions: a randomized trial assessing donor exposure and safety. *Transfusion.* 1996;36(10): 873–878.

23. Strauss RG, Burmeister LF, Johnson K, Cress G, Cordle D. Feasibility and safety of AS-3 red blood cells for neonatal transfusions. *J Pediatr.* 2000;136(2):215–219.

24. Luban NL, Strauss RG, Hume HA. Commentary on the safety of red cells preserved in extended-storage media for neonatal transfusions. *Transfusion.* 1991;31(3): 229–235.

25. Rock G, Poon A, Haddad S, Romans R, St Louis P. Nutricel as an additive solution for neonatal transfusion. *Transfus Sci.* 1999;20(1):29–36.

26. Crowley M, Kirpalani H. A rational approach to red blood cell transfusion in the neonatal ICU. *Curr Opin Pediatr.* 2010;22(2):151–157.

27. Strauss RG. Transfusion therapy in neonates. *Am J Dis Child.* 1991;145(8):904–911.

28. Wang-Rodriguez J, Mannino FL, Liu E, Lane TA. A novel strategy to limit blood donor exposure and blood waste in multiply transfused premature infants. *Transfusion.* 1996;36(1):64–70.

29. Liu EA, Mannino FL, Lane TA. Prospective, randomized trial of the safety and efficacy of a limited donor exposure transfusion program for premature neonates. *J Pediatr.* 1994;125(1):92–96.

30. Collard KJ. Transfusion related morbidity in premature babies: possible mechanisms and implications for practice. *World J Clin Pediatr.* 2014;3(3):19–29.

31. Remy KE, Natanson C, Klein HG. The influence of the storage lesion(s) on pediatric red cell transfusion. *Curr Opin Pediatr.* 2015;27(3):277–285.

32. Fergusson DA, Hebert P, Hogan DL, et al. Effect of fresh red blood cell transfusions on clinical outcomes in premature, very low-birth-weight infants: the ARIPI randomized trial. *JAMA.* 2012;308(14):1443–1451.

33. Patel RM, Josephson CD. Storage age of red blood cells for transfusion of premature infants. *JAMA.* 2013; 309(6):544–545.

34. Eisenfeld L, Silver H, McLaughlin J, et al. Prevention of transfusion-associated cytomegalovirus infection in neonatal patients by the removal of white cells from blood. *Transfusion.* 1992;32(3):205–209.

35. Bowden RA, Slichter SJ, Sayers M, et al. A comparison of filtered leukocyte-reduced and cytomegalovirus (CMV) seronegative blood products for the prevention of transfusion-associated CMV infection after marrow transplant. *Blood.* 1995;86(9):3598–3603.

36. Strauss RG. Data-driven blood banking practices for neonatal RBC transfusions. *Transfusion.* 2000;40(12):1528–1540.

37. Nichols WG, Price TH, Gooley T, Corey L, Boeckh M. Transfusion-transmitted cytomegalovirus infection after receipt of leukoreduced blood products. *Blood.* 2003;101 (10):4195–4200.

38. Vamvakas EC. Is white blood cell reduction equivalent to antibody screening in preventing transmission of cytomegalovirus by transfusion? A review of the literature and meta-analysis. *Transfus Med Rev.* 2005;19(3): 181–199.

39. Josephson CD, Caliendo AM, Easley KA, et al. Blood transfusion and breast milk transmission of cytomegalovirus in very low-birth-weight infants: a prospective cohort study. *JAMA Pediatr.* 2014;168(11):1054–1062.

40. Mainou M, Alahdab F, Tobian AA, et al. Reducing the risk of transfusion-transmitted cytomegalovirus infection: a systematic review and meta-analysis. *Transfusion.* 2016;56(6 Pt 2):1569–1580.

41. Smith D, Lu Q, Yuan S, Goldfinger D, Fernando LP, Ziman A. Survey of current practice for prevention of transfusion-transmitted cytomegalovirus in the United States: leucoreduction vs. cytomegalovirus-seronegative. *Vox Sang.* 2010;98(1):29–36.

42. Aabb CTMC, Heddle NM, Boeckh M, et al. AABB Committee Report: reducing transfusion-transmitted cytomegalovirus infections. *Transfusion.* 2016;56(6 Pt 2): 1581–1587.

43. Roback JD, Conlan M, Drew WL, Ljungman P, Nichols WG, Preiksaitis JK. The role of photochemical treatment with amotosalen and UV-A light in the prevention of transfusion-transmitted cytomegalovirus infections. *Transfus Med Rev.* 2006;20(1):45–56.

44. Gokhale SG, Gokhale SS. Transfusion-associated graft versus host disease (TAGVHD)–with reference to neonatal period. *J Matern Fetal Neonatal Med.* 2015;28(6): 700–704.

45. Treleaven J, Gennery A, Marsh J, et al. Guidelines on the use of irradiated blood components prepared by the British Committee for Standards in Haematology blood transfusion task force. *Br J Haematol.* 2011;152(1):35–51.

46. Moroff G, Holme S, AuBuchon JP, Heaton WA, Sweeney JD, Friedman LI. Viability and in vitro properties of AS-1 red cells after gamma irradiation. *Transfusion.* 1999;39(2):128–134.

47. Dani C, Perugi S, Benuzzi A, et al. Effects of red blood cell transfusions during the first week of life on acid-base, glucose, and electrolytes in preterm neonates. *Transfusion.* 2008;48(11):2302–2307.

48. Smith HM, Farrow SJ, Ackerman JD, Stubbs JR, Sprung J. Cardiac arrests associated with hyperkalemia during red blood cell transfusion: a case series. *Anesth Analg.* 2008;106(4):1062–1069 (table of contents).

49. Strauss RG. RBC storage and avoiding hyperkalemia from transfusions to neonates & infants. *Transfusion.* 2010;50(9):1862–1865.

50. Ohto H, Anderson KC. Posttransfusion graft-versus-host disease in Japanese newborns. *Transfusion.* 1996; 36(2):117–123.

51. Del Vecchio A, Franco C, Petrillo F, D'Amato G. Neonatal transfusion practice: when do neonates need red blood cells or platelets? *Am J Perinatol.* 2016;33(11):1079–1084.

52. Christensen RD, Carroll PD, Josephson CD. Evidence-based advances in transfusion practice in neonatal intensive care units. *Neonatology.* 2014;106(3):245–253.

53. Patel RM, Kandefer S, Walsh MC, et al. Causes and timing of death in extremely premature infants from 2000 through 2011. *N Engl J Med.* 2015;372(4):331–340.

54. McGrady GA, Rettig PJ, Istre GR, Jason JM, Holman RC, Evatt BL. An outbreak of necrotizing enterocolitis. Association with transfusions of packed red blood cells. *Am J Epidemiol.* 1987;126(6):1165–1172.

55. Blau J, Calo JM, Dozor D, Sutton M, Alpan G, La Gamma EF. Transfusion-related acute gut injury: necrotizing enterocolitis in very low birth weight neonates after packed red blood cell transfusion. *J Pediatr.* 2011;158(3):403–409.

56. Banerjee J, Leung TS, Aladangady N. Blood transfusion in preterm infants improves intestinal tissue oxygenation without alteration in blood flow. *Vox Sang.* 2016;111(4):399–408.

57. Marin T, Josephson CD, Kosmetatos N, Higgins M, Moore JE. Feeding preterm infants during red blood cell transfusion is associated with a decline in postprandial mesenteric oxygenation. *J Pediatr.* 2014;165(3):464–471. e461.

58. El-Dib M, Narang S, Lee E, Massaro AN, Aly H. Red blood cell transfusion, feeding and necrotizing enterocolitis in preterm infants. *J Perinatol.* 2011;31(3):183–187.

59. Derienzo C, Smith PB, Tanaka D, et al. Feeding practices and other risk factors for developing transfusion-associated necrotizing enterocolitis. *Early Hum Dev.* 2014;90(5):237–240.

60. Mohamed A, Shah PS. Transfusion associated necrotizing enterocolitis: a meta-analysis of observational data. *Pediatrics.* 2012;129(3):529–540.

61. Hay S, Zupancic JA, Flannery DD, Kirpalani H, Dukhovny D. Should we believe in transfusion-associated enterocolitis? Applying a GRADE to the literature. *Semin Perinatol.* 2017;41(1):80–91.

62. La Gamma EF, Blau J. Transfusion-related acute gut injury: feeding, flora, flow, and barrier defense. *Semin Perinatol.* 2012;36(4):294–305.

63. Porter ML, Dennis BL. Hyperbilirubinemia in the term newborn. *Am Fam Physician.* 2002;65(4):599–606.

64. Ballard RA, Vinocur B, Reynolds JW, et al. Transient hyperammonemia of the preterm infant. *N Engl J Med.* 1978;299(17):920–925.

65. Leonard JV. The early detection and management of inborn errors presenting acutely in the neonatal period. *Eur J Pediatr.* 1985;143(4):253–257.

66. Sola-Visner M. Platelets in the neonatal period: developmental differences in platelet production, function, and hemostasis and the potential impact of therapies. *Hematol Am Soc Hematol Educ Program.* 2012;2012:506–511.

67. Ferrer-Marin F, Stanworth S, Josephson C, Sola-Visner M. Distinct differences in platelet production and function between neonates and adults: implications for platelet transfusion practice. *Transfusion.* 2013;53(11):2814–2821. quiz 2813.

68. von Lindern JS, Hulzebos CV, Bos AF, Brand A, Walther FJ, Lopriore E. Thrombocytopaenia and intraventricular haemorrhage in very premature infants: a tale of two cities. *Arch Dis Child Fetal Neonatal Ed.* 2012;97(5):F348–F352.

69. Christensen RD, Henry E, Wiedmeier SE, et al. Thrombocytopenia among extremely low birth weight neonates: data from a multihospital healthcare system. *J Perinatol.* 2006;26(6):348–353.

70. Andrew M, Vegh P, Caco C, et al. A randomized, controlled trial of platelet transfusions in thrombocytopenic premature infants. *J Pediatr.* 1993;123(2):285–291.

71. Murray NA, Howarth LJ, McCloy MP, Letsky EA, Roberts IA. Platelet transfusion in the management of severe thrombocytopenia in neonatal intensive care unit patients. *Transfus Med.* 2002;12(1):35–41.

72. Borges JP, dos Santos AM, da Cunha DH, Mimica AF, Guinsburg R, Kopelman BI. Restrictive guideline reduces platelet count thresholds for transfusions in very low birth weight preterm infants. *Vox Sang.* 2013;104(3):207–213.

73. Curley A, Venkatesh V, Stanworth S, et al. Platelets for neonatal transfusion - study 2: a randomised controlled trial to compare two different platelet count thresholds for prophylactic platelet transfusion to preterm neonates. *Neonatology.* 2014;106(2):102–106.

74. Christensen RD, Paul DA, Sola-Visner MC, Baer VL. Improving platelet transfusion practices in the neonatal intensive care unit. *Transfusion.* 2008;48(11):2281–2284.

75. Gerday E, Baer VL, Lambert DK, et al. Testing platelet mass versus platelet count to guide platelet transfusions in the neonatal intensive care unit. *Transfusion.* 2009;49(10):2034–2039.

76. Zisk JL, Mackley A, Clearly G, Chang E, Christensen RD, Paul DA. Transfusing neonates based on platelet count vs. platelet mass: a randomized feasibility-pilot study. *Platelets.* 2014;25(7):513–516.

77. Poterjoy BS, Josephson CD. Platelets, frozen plasma, and cryoprecipitate: what is the clinical evidence for their use in the neonatal intensive care unit? *Semin Perinatol.* 2009;33(1):66–74.

78. Josephson CD, Su LL, Christensen RD, et al. Platelet transfusion practices among neonatologists in the United States and Canada: results of a survey. *Pediatrics.* 2009;123(1):278–285.

79. Davoren A, Curtis BR, Aster RH, McFarland JG. Human platelet antigen-specific alloantibodies implicated in 1162 cases of neonatal alloimmune thrombocytopenia. *Transfusion.* 2004;44(8):1220–1225.

80. Strong NK, Eddleman KA. Diagnosis and management of neonatal alloimmune thrombocytopenia in pregnancy. *Clin Lab Med.* 2013;33(2):311–325.

81. Bertrand G, Kaplan C. How do we treat fetal and neonatal alloimmune thrombocytopenia? *Transfusion.* 2014;54(7):1698–1703.

82. Bakchoul T, Bassler D, Heckmann M, et al. Management of infants born with severe neonatal alloimmune thrombocytopenia: the role of platelet transfusions and intravenous immunoglobulin. *Transfusion.* 2014;54(3):640–645.

83. Kiefel V, Bassler D, Kroll H, et al. Antigen-positive platelet transfusion in neonatal alloimmune thrombocytopenia (NAIT). *Blood.* 2006;107(9):3761–3763.

84. Puetz J, Darling G, McCormick KA, Wofford JD. Fresh frozen plasma and recombinant factor VIIa use in neonates. *J Pediatr Hematol Oncol.* 2009;31(12):901–906.

85. Keir AK, Stanworth SJ. Neonatal plasma transfusion: an evidence-based review. *Transfus Med Rev.* 2016;30(4): 174–182.

86. Motta M, Del Vecchio A, Chirico G. Fresh frozen plasma administration in the neonatal intensive care unit: evidence-based guidelines. *Clin Perinatol.* 2015;42(3):639–650.

87. Motta M, Del Vecchio A, Perrone B, Ghirardello S, Radicioni M. Fresh frozen plasma use in the NICU: a prospective, observational, multicentred study. *Arch Dis Child Fetal Neonatal Ed.* 2014;99(4):F303–F308.

88. Christensen RD, Baer VL, Lambert DK, Henry E, Ilstrup SJ, Bennett ST. Reference intervals for common coagulation tests of preterm infants (CME). *Transfusion.* 2014;54(3):627–632. quiz 626.

89. Van de Bor M, Briet E, Van Bel F, Ruys JH. Hemostasis and periventricular-intraventricular hemorrhage of the newborn. *Am J Dis Child.* 1986;140(11):1131–1134.

90. Tran TT, Veldman A, Malhotra A. Does risk-based coagulation screening predict intraventricular haemorrhage in extreme premature infants? *Blood Coagul Fibrinolysis.* 2012;23(6):532–536.

91. Gibson BE, Todd A, Roberts I, et al. Transfusion guidelines for neonates and older children. *Br J Haematol.* 2004;124(4):433–453.

92. Roseff SD, Luban NL, Manno CS. Guidelines for assessing appropriateness of pediatric transfusion. *Transfusion.* 2002;42(11):1398–1413.

93. Lacroix J, Hebert PC, Hutchison JS, et al. Transfusion strategies for patients in pediatric intensive care units. *N Engl J Med.* 2007;356(16):1609–1619.

94. Wong EC, Perez-Albuerne E, Moscow JA, Luban NL. Transfusion management strategies: a survey of practicing pediatric hematology/oncology specialists. *Pediatr Blood Cancer.* 2005;44(2):119–127.

95. Bercovitz RS, Quinones RR. A survey of transfusion practices in pediatric hematopoietic stem cell transplant patients. *J Pediatr Hematol Oncol.* 2013;35(2):e60–e63.

96. Williams DA, Bennett C, Bertuch A, et al. Diagnosis and treatment of pediatric acquired aplastic anemia (AAA): an initial survey of the North American Pediatric Aplastic Anemia Consortium (NAPAAC). *Pediatr Blood Cancer.* 2014;61(5):869–874.

97. Robitaille N, Lacroix J, Alexandrov L, et al. Excess of veno-occlusive disease in a randomized clinical trial on a higher trigger for red blood cell transfusion after bone marrow transplantation: a canadian blood and marrow transplant group trial. *Biol Blood Marrow Transpl.* 2013;19(3):468–473.

98. Wahl S, Quirolo KC. Current issues in blood transfusion for sickle cell disease. *Curr Opin Pediatr.* 2009;21(1): 15–21.

99. Yawn BP, Buchanan GR, Afenyi-Annan AN, et al. Management of sickle cell disease: summary of the 2014 evidence-based report by expert panel members. *JAMA.* 2014;312(10):1033–1048.

100. Yazdanbakhsh K, Ware RE, Noizat-Pirenne F. Red blood cell alloimmunization in sickle cell disease: pathophysiology, risk factors, and transfusion management. *Blood.* 2012;120(3):528–537.

101. Vichinsky EP, Luban NL, Wright E, et al. Prospective RBC phenotype matching in a stroke-prevention trial in sickle cell anemia: a multicenter transfusion trial. *Transfusion.* 2001;41(9):1086–1092.

102. Lasalle-Williams M, Nuss R, Le T, et al. Extended red blood cell antigen matching for transfusions in sickle cell disease: a review of a 14-year experience from a single center (CME). *Transfusion.* 2011;51(8):1732–1739.

103. Aragona E, Kelly MJ. Hyperhemolysis in sickle cell disease. *J Pediatr Hematol Oncol.* 2014;36(1):e54–e56.

104. Harm SK, Yazer MH, Monis GF, Triulzi DJ, Aubuchon JP, Delaney M. A centralized recipient database enhances the serologic safety of RBC transfusions for patients with sickle cell disease. *Am J Clin Pathol.* 2014;141(2):256–261.

105. Win N, Sinha S, Lee E, Mills W. Treatment with intravenous immunoglobulin and steroids may correct severe anemia in hyperhemolytic transfusion reactions: case report and literature review. *Transfus Med Rev.* 2010;24(1):64–67.

106. Slonim AD, Joseph JG, Turenne WM, Sharangpani A, Luban NL. Blood transfusions in children: a multiinstitutional analysis of practices and complications. *Transfusion.* 2008;48(1):73–80.

107. Sloan SR, Parker RI. Current status of platelet transfusion in pediatric patients. *Transfus Med Rev.* 2016;30(4):230–234.

108. Josephson CD, Granger S, Assmann SF, et al. Bleeding risks are higher in children versus adults given prophylactic platelet transfusions for treatment-induced hypoproliferative thrombocytopenia. *Blood.* 2012;120(4): 748–760.

109. Goel R, Ness PM, Takemoto CM, Krishnamurti L, King KE, Tobian AA. Platelet transfusions in platelet consumptive disorders are associated with arterial thrombosis and in-hospital mortality. *Blood.* 2015;125(9):1470–1476.

110. Neunert C, Lim W, Crowther M, et al. The American Society of Hematology 2011 evidence-based practice guideline for immune thrombocytopenia. *Blood.* 2011;117(16):4190–4207.

111. Holme S, Sweeney JD, Sawyer S, Elfath MD. The expression of p-selectin during collection, processing, and storage of platelet concentrates: relationship to loss of in vivo viability. *Transfusion.* 1997;37(1):12–17.

112. Pineda AA, Zylstra VW, Clare DE, Dewanjee MK, Forstrom LA. Viability and functional integrity of washed platelets. *Transfusion.* 1989;29(6):524–527.

113. Schoenfeld H, Muhm M, Doepfmer UR, Kox WJ, Spies C, Radtke H. The functional integrity of platelets in volume-reduced platelet concentrates. *Anesth Analg.* 2005;100(1):78–81.

114. Molnar R, Johnson R, Sweat LT, Geiger TL. Absence of D alloimmunization in D-pediatric oncology patients receiving D-incompatible single-donor platelets. *Transfusion*. 2002;42(2):177–182.

115. Cid J, Carbasse G, Pereira A, et al. Platelet transfusions from D+ donors to D- patients: a 10-year follow-up study of 1014 patients. *Transfusion*. 2011;51(6):1163–1169.

116. O'Brien KL, Haspel RL, Uhl L. Anti-D alloimmunization after D-incompatible platelet transfusions: a 14-year single-institution retrospective review. *Transfusion*. 2014;54(3):650–654.

117. Goldenberg NA, Manco-Johnson MJ. Pediatric hemostasis and use of plasma components. *Best Pract Res Clin Haematol*. 2006;19(1):143–155.

118. Nester Theresa, Jain Shweta, Poisson J. *Hemotherapy Decisions and Their Outcomes*. 18th ed. Bethesda, Maryland: AABB; 2014.

119. Cugno C, Deola S, Filippini P, Stroncek DF, Rutella S. Granulocyte transfusions in children and adults with hematological malignancies: benefits and controversies. *J Transl Med*. 2015;13:362.

120. Atay D, Ozturk G, Akcay A, Yanasik M, Anak S, Devecioglu O. Effect and safety of granulocyte transfusions in pediatric patients with febrile neutropenia or defective granulocyte functions. *J Pediatr Hematol Oncol*. 2011;33(6):e220–e225.

121. Diaz R, Soundar E, Hartman SK, Dreyer Z, Teruya J, Hui SK. Granulocyte transfusions for children with infection and neutropenia or granulocyte dysfunction. *Pediatr Hematol Oncol*. 2014;31(5):425–434.

122. Price TH, Boeckh M, Harrison RW, et al. Efficacy of transfusion with granulocytes from G-CSF/dexamethasone-treated donors in neutropenic patients with infection. *Blood*. 2015;126(18):2153–2161.

123. Seidel MG, Minkov M, Witt V, et al. Granulocyte transfusions in children and young adults: does the dose matter? *J Pediatr Hematol Oncol*. 2009;31(3):166–172.

124. Averbuch D, Engelhard D, Pegoraro A, Cesaro S. Review on efficacy and complications of granulocyte transfusions in neutropenic patients. *Curr Drug Targets*. 2016.

125. Estcourt LJ, Stanworth S, Doree C, et al. Granulocyte transfusions for preventing infections in people with neutropenia or neutrophil dysfunction. *Cochrane Database Syst Rev*. 2015;(6):CD005341.

126. Bercovitz RS, Josephson CD. Transfusion considerations in pediatric hematology and oncology patients. *Hematol Oncol Clin North Am*. 2016;30(3):695–709.

127. Peters C, Minkov M, Matthes-Martin S, et al. Leucocyte transfusions from rhG-CSF or prednisolone stimulated donors for treatment of severe infections in immunocompromised neutropenic patients. *Br J Haematol*. 1999;106(3):689–696.

128. Lee JJ, Chung IJ, Park MR, et al. Clinical efficacy of granulocyte transfusion therapy in patients with neutropenia-related infections. *Leukemia*. 2001;15(2):203–207.

129. Wright DG, Robichaud KJ, Pizzo PA, Deisseroth AB. Lethal pulmonary reactions associated with the combined use of amphotericin B and leukocyte transfusions. *N Engl J Med*. 1981;304(20):1185–1189.

130. Bow EJ, Schroeder ML, Louie TJ. Pulmonary complications in patients receiving granulocyte transfusions and amphotericin B. *Can Med Assoc J*. 1984;130(5):593–597.

131. Maslach-Hubbard A, Bratton SL. Extracorporeal membrane oxygenation for pediatric respiratory failure: history, development and current status. *World J Crit Care Med*. 2013;2(4):29–39.

132. Galacki DM. An overview of therapeutic apheresis in pediatrics. *J Clin Apher*. 1997;12(1):1–3.

133. Kim HC. Therapeutic pediatric apheresis. *J Clin Apher*. 2000;15(1–2):129–157.

134. McLeod BC. Therapeutic apheresis: history, clinical application, and lingering uncertainties. *Transfusion*. 2010;50(7):1413–1426.

135. Carter CE, Benador NM. Therapeutic plasma exchange for the treatment of pediatric renal diseases in 2013. *Pediatr Nephrol*. 2014;29(1):35–50.

136. Maitta RW, Vasovic LV, Mohandas K, Music-Aplenc L, Bonzon-Adelson A, Uehlinger J. A safe therapeutic apheresis protocol in paediatric patients weighing 11 to 25 kg. *Vox Sang*. 2014;107(4):375–380.

137. Cortina G, Ojinaga V, Giner T, et al. Therapeutic plasma exchange in children: one center's experience. *J Clin Apher*. 2017.

FURTHER READING

1. Stanworth SJ, Clarke P, Watts T, et al. Prospective, observational study of outcomes in neonates with severe thrombocytopenia. *Pediatrics*. 2009;124(5):e826–e834.

2. Venkatesh V, Khan R, Curley A, New H, Stanworth S. How we decide when a neonate needs a transfusion. *Br J Haematol*. 2013;160(4):421–433.

CHAPTER 11

Transfusion Medicine in Obstetrics and Prenatal Patients

HOLLIE M. REEVES, DO • HONG HONG, MD, PHD

RED CELL ANTIBODIES IN PREGNANCY AND HEMOLYTIC DISEASE OF THE FETUS AND NEWBORN

Pregnant patients may become alloimmunized (make antibodies) to red cell antigens that they lack on their red cell surfaces. This can occur following transfusion, transplant, or pregnancy. In pregnancy, these antibodies usually result from exposure to fetal red cells that express paternally derived antigens that the mother lacks. This exposure to fetal red blood cells (RBCs) can occur during a fetomaternal hemorrhage (FMH). FMH can occur spontaneously during pregnancy or at the time of delivery. The likelihood of FMH increases with gestational age[1,2] and with any trauma or invasive procedures during pregnancy.[2] Therefore it is important to obtain a baseline ABO/Rh(D) type and antibody screen for unexpected red cell antibodies early in the prenatal care of a pregnant patient.

Many factors influence the likelihood of a patient becoming alloimmunized. Some of these factors are patient specific and some are related to the specific antigen or antibody. For example, Rh(D) is the most potent immunogen. In fact, it can take as little as 0.1–1 mL of Rh(D) antigen–positive blood to stimulate the production of anti-D in an Rh(D) negative patient.[3] Interestingly though, only approximately 85% of Rh(D)-negative patients will make an anti-D if exposed to antigen-positive blood.[4] Fortunately, the overall rates of alloimmunization in pregnancy are low.[3]

Pregnant patients may also have or can make antibodies to other red cell antigens besides anti-D that can cause hemolytic disease of the fetus and newborn (HDFN). The most common of these antibodies are anti-K and anti-c.[5] Several other antibodies have been implicated in HDFN (see Table 11.1). It has also been reported that pregnant patients with multiple antibodies are more likely to develop HDFN.[6–8]

Pathophysiology of Hemolytic Disease of the Fetus and Newborn

In the United States, it has been reported that 35 per 10,000 live births are at risk for HDFN due to RBC alloimmunization.[6] HDFN is caused when there is either hemolysis of fetal RBCs or impaired erythropoiesis due to a maternal-fetal red cell antigen incompatibility.[10] The mother makes an antibody or antibodies to red cell antigens on the fetal red cells that were inherited from the father. If these antibodies are IgG in nature, they can cross the placenta, bind to fetal red cell antigen, and cause hemolysis.[10] This early red cell destruction can lead to fetal anemia, resulting in increased erythropoiesis and release of immature red cells into the fetal circulation or erythroblastosis fetalis. As the anemia worsens, extramedullary erythropoiesis can occur causing organomegaly and portal hypertension. Decreased oncotic pressure from reduced albumin production can lead to generalized edema or hydrops fetalis, which can be associated with high-output cardiac failure and even fetal death.

Hemolysis of the fetal red cells causes release of hemoglobin, which gets broken down into bilirubin. In utero, this bilirubin is passed into the maternal circulation where it gets conjugated by the maternal liver. However, once the baby is delivered and no longer shares circulation with the mother, this resulting bilirubin cannot efficiently be conjugated by the newborn liver and can build up in the neonatal circulation. This increased level of unconjugated bilirubin can cross the blood-brain barrier and lead to permanent damage, known as kernicterus.[11]

Laboratory Testing

Prenatal studies should include an ABO and Rh(D) type on the patient as well as an antibody screen for unexpected red cell antibodies. If a clinically significant red cell antibody or antibodies (i.e., are capable of causing decreased RBC survival, either hemolytic transfusion reaction or HDFN) are identified in the mother's plasma, then antibody titration studies may be performed. Antibody titration is a semiquantitative test to measure the relative concentration of antibody, performed using serial dilutions, and compared with a previous titer from the patient (if available) while

TABLE 11.1
Alloantibodies in Hemolytic Disease of the Fetus and Newborn

Common	Rare	Never
Anti-D	Anti-Fy[a]	Anti-Le[a]
Anti-D+C	Anti-s	Anti-Le[b]
Anti-D+E	Anti-M	Anti-I
Anti-C	Anti-N	Anti-IH
Anti-E	Anti-S	Anti-P₁
Anti-c	Anti-Jk[a]	
Anti-e		
Anti-K		

From Kennedy MS. Hemolytic disease of the fetus and newborn (HDFN). In: Harmening DM, ed. *Modern Blood Banking & Transfusion Practices*, 6th ed. Philadelphia: F. A. Davis Company; 2012; with permission.

BOX 11.1
Characteristics of RBCs for IUT

- Type O, Rh(D) negative
- Negative for cognate antigen(s) to which maternal antibody(ies) are directed
- Irradiated
- CMV reduced risk
- Hemoglobin S negative
- Collected <7 days before transfusion, if possible

CMV, cytomegalovirus; *IUT*, intrauterine RBC transfusion; *RBC*, red blood cell.
Data from Kennedy MS, Delaney M, Scrape S. Perinatal issues in transfusion practice. In: Fung MK, Grossman BJ, Hillyer CD, Westhoff CM, eds. *Technical Manual*, 18th ed. Bethesda: AABB; 2014 and Hendrickson JE, Delaney M. Hemolytic disease of the fetus and newborn: modern practice and future investigations. *Transfus Med Rev*. 2016;30(4):159–164.

she is being monitored during pregnancy. Most pregnant patients with clinically significant antibodies will be monitored with monthly titers,[12] the frequency of which may increase near the end of gestation or if otherwise clinically indicated. A critical titer for most antibodies in pregnant females is 16 (1:16) in the anti-human globulin phase.[4] However, certain antibodies, such as those directed at antigens in the Kell system, generally have a lower critical titer value of 8. Kell system antigens are expressed on early red cell precursors, and antibodies to these antigens can cause destruction of fetal RBC precursors, producing a reticulocytopenia and severe anemia.[13]

Determination of paternal zygosity if a sample is available may be part of the management of an alloimmunized pregnancy.[14] This can be done serologically for most common red cell antibodies implicated in HDFN; one notable exception is Rh(D). *RHD* zygosity testing is performed using molecular methods to assess the genotype. If the father is homozygous for the cognate antigen to which the mother has made an antibody, then the fetus is 100% at risk for developing HDFN and may require closer monitoring. If the father is heterozygous for the cognate antigen, then there would be a 50% chance that the fetus is antigen positive and therefore at risk of HDFN.[14] In this scenario, evaluation of the fetal antigen status can be performed. Previously, this was performed on a fetal sample obtained via amniocentesis; however, with the development of noninvasive prenatal tests using cell-free fetal DNA, it may be possible to perform on a maternal sample.[10,14,15]

Patient Monitoring and Management

In addition to antibody titration studies in these patients with clinically significant red cell alloantibodies, noninvasive ultrasound Doppler studies are also performed to assess for fetal anemia. Fetal middle cerebral artery peak systolic velocities above 1.5 times the median for gestational age can predict moderate or severe fetal anemia.[16] If fetal Doppler studies indicate moderate to severe anemia, depending upon the gestational age, periumbilical blood testing may be indicated followed by intrauterine RBC transfusion (IUT).[17,18] See Box 11.1 for general characteristics of the RBCs used for IUT. The red cells are usually irradiated to minimize the risk of transfusion-associated graft-versus-host disease and cytomegalovirus (CMV) reduced-risk either by leukocyte reduction or by CMV-seronegative donor status to minimize the risk of transfusion transmitted CMV.

The volume for IUT can be calculated by (1) multiplying the ultrasound-estimated fetal weight in grams by 0.14 mL/g (this provides the fetal and placental total blood volume), (2) then multiplying this amount by the difference in the desired posttransfusion hematocrit and the pretransfusion hematocrit, and (3) then dividing the resulting amount by the hematocrit of the RBC unit.[4] Generally the goal of IUT is to maintain the hematocrit of the fetus at or above 30%.[18] Alternative or adjunctive therapies include the use of therapeutic plasma exchange (TPE) and/or intravenous immunoglobulin (IVIG) for high-titer RBC antibodies and HDFN. This therapy may be indicated in rare cases in which there is a high risk of fetal demise or signs of hydrops at gestational age less than 20 weeks, before IUT can be administered. The American Society for Apheresis (ASFA) gives TPE in this situation a Category III indication, meaning that the optimum role for apheresis is not established and decision making should be on a case-by-case basis.[19]

Prevention

Three different categories of maternal alloimmunization prevention have been described: primary, secondary, and tertiary.[18] Primary prevention focuses on reducing the exposure (mainly during transfusion) to non-self RBC antigens. In times of medical emergency when RBC transfusion is needed urgently, universal donor type O blood is routinely given. In most institutions, there are policies in place to provide women of childbearing age/potential with Rh(D)-negative products in addition to group O. This is done to minimize the risk of becoming alloimmunized and forming an anti-D that may affect future pregnancies. This may not be feasible 100% of the time. In more routine settings, some European nations provide additional prophylactic phenotype matching for the K antigen and/or E and c antigens to female patients of childbearing age.[5] However, in the 2017 multinational study of 293 mothers who had at least one pregnancy affected by severe HDFN, the authors concluded that a previous pregnancy was the predominant stimulus of alloimmunization, not previous transfusion.[20]

Secondary prevention focuses on the administration of Rh immune globulin (RhIG) to Rh(D)-negative pregnant females.[18] The use of RhIG prophylaxis has dramatically reduced the prevalence of HDFN due to anti-D, decreasing the incidence from 16% to less than 0.1%.[21] Rh(D)-negative pregnant patients who have not already made an anti-D should receive RhIG antenatally at approximately 28 weeks' gestation or in the event of possible FMH and at delivery of an Rh(D)-positive or Rh(D)-unknown newborn.[22]

Some women may be a variant of Rh(D), which may lead to discrepancies on serologic testing. Some of these variants may be at risk for forming anti-D, and therefore practice often includes giving RhIG. Maternal red cell genotyping (molecular testing) may be useful in these situations to determine the variant and assist with RhIG treatment decision making and has been advocated by several professional organizations.[23]

Tertiary prevention pertains to the use of extended antigen matching of RBC units used for IUT.[18] However, this practice is not standardized across institutions, and it can be difficult to obtain the necessary RBC units.[24] Additional research is needed to determine the efficacy of this approach in alloimmunized patients.

BOX 11.2
How to Calculate RhIG Dose

1. Calculate volume of FMH (in mL) = % of fetal cells determined either by Kleihauer-Betke test or flow cytometry/100 × maternal blood volume[a]
2. Volume of FMH in mL/30 mL[b] = # of RhIG vials to give *once rounding rules have been applied*
3. Rounding rules:
   a. If calculated dose to the right of the decimal point is ≥0.5, then round up to the next whole number and add one vial
   b. If calculated dose to the right of the decimal point is <0.5, then round down to the next whole number and add one vial

FMH, fetomaternal hemorrhage; RhIG, Rh immune globulin.
[a] Maternal blood volume = maternal weight (kg) × 70 mL/kg or estimated at 5000 mL.
[b] One 300 μg vial of RhIG protects against 30 mL fetal whole blood.
Data from Kennedy MS, Delaney M, Scrape S. Perinatal issues in transfusion practice. In: Fung MK, Grossman BJ, Hillyer CD, Westhoff CM, eds. *Technical Manual*, 18th ed. Bethesda: AABB; 2014.

Rh Immune Globulin

In the United States, RhIG (anti-D immune globulin) is available in a 300 μg (1500 IU) or 50 μg dose. The current antepartum immunoprophylaxis regimen is one 300 μg dose of RhIG given at 28 weeks' gestation.[22] A 300 μg dose of RhIG should suppress immunization by 15 mL fetal red cells or 30 mL fetal whole blood.[25] In the event of a suspected FMH or at the time of delivery additional testing should be performed to determine if one dose (300 μg) is appropriate. This additional testing consists of a screen to assess for the presence of Rh(D)-positive fetal cells in the maternal circulation. If the screen is negative, then one dose is appropriate. If the screen is positive (indicating a larger FMH) then a quantitative test such as the Kleihauer-Betke test or flow cytometry to measure fetal hemoglobin and/or Rh(D) positive RBCs should be performed to establish the dose.[25] Postpartum RhIG should ideally be administered within 72 h of delivery.[22] See Box 11.2 for RhIG dose calculation.

Hemolytic Disease of the Fetus and Newborn due to ABO Incompatibility

Maternal-fetal ABO incompatibility is now the most common cause of HDFN as opposed to anti-D because of the routine use of RhIG prophylaxis.[4] Naturally occurring IgG anti-A,B in the serum of type O mothers can cross the placenta and bind to fetal RBCs expressing

A antigen, B antigen, or both. This can lead to a positive direct antiglobulin test (DAT) on the cord blood. Fortunately, the resulting anemia/hyperbilirubinemia, if any, is mild because of poor expression of the A and B antigens on fetal RBCs and antibody neutralization that occurs due to tissue and soluble antigens.[4] Often these newborns, if they have hyperbilirubinemia, can be managed with phototherapy and rarely require exchange transfusion.[4]

RED BLOOD CELL AUTOANTIBODIES IN PREGNANCY

RBC autoantibodies are produced in response to self-antigens as opposed to alloantibodies that are made in response to foreign antigens. Autoantibodies may have a detectable specificity on serologic testing but more commonly do not.[26] They are often associated with a positive DAT with either IgG or complement positivity, or both. Some individuals make autoantibodies that readily attach to their own RBCs but do not cause any decreased red cell survival or clinically apparent hemolysis but may cause interference with routine blood bank serologic testing and detection of alloantibodies. Others may have clinically relevant autoantibodies, causing decreased red cell survival, or autoimmune hemolytic anemia (AIHA).[27]

There have been reports of an association of increased autoantibody production and pregnancy.[28,29] One study found that autoantibodies were approximately five times as frequent in pregnant patients than in nonpregnant females of childbearing age.[28] However, none of these patients or their infants needed a blood transfusion or developed clinically significant anemia. Rarely these autoantibodies can be associated with clinically significant hemolysis. A few cases of AIHA in pregnancy have been reported in the literature.[30] The autoantibodies in AIHA are classified based on the thermal amplitude at which they optimally bind patient RBCs. The most common type is warm AIHA in which the autoantibody binds at body temperature and is often of IgG isotype.[30] Because these antibodies are often IgG they can cross the placenta and bind to fetal RBCs. Corticosteroids are generally the first-line therapy for warm AIHA. Other therapies can include splenectomy, IVIG, rituximab, and other immunosuppressants; however, their safety in pregnancy needs to be considered.

The second most common type is cold agglutinin disease (CAD) in which the antibodies bind optimally at colder temperatures and are often of IgM subtype. The typical treatment modalities used in warm AIHA are less effective in CAD.[31] IgM antibodies do not cross the placenta, and therefore hemolysis in the newborn is not seen.[29,30] In both warm AIHA and CAD, RBC transfusion may be necessary. Autoantibodies can make the serologic identification of alloantibodies difficult, often requiring additional testing with specialized techniques, and can result in an incompatible crossmatch. It is generally recommended that if transfusion in these patients cannot be avoided small amounts should be transfused slowly with close monitoring for signs and symptoms of hemolysis. In CAD, a blood warmer at the time of transfusion may be beneficial, if available.

TRANSFUSION MANAGEMENT IN PREGNANT PATIENTS WITH HEMOGLOBINOPATHIES

Pregnancy can pose a significant clinical risk for patients with hemoglobinopathies, specifically sickle cell disease (SCD).[32,33] Patients with homozygous SCD (hemoglobin SS) are at increased risk for maternal complications, such as preterm labor, premature rupture of membranes, antepartum hospitalization, and postpartum infection, compared with those with normal hemoglobin.[33] These patients may also be at increased risk for fetal complications, including intrauterine growth restriction (IUGR), low birth weight, and preterm delivery.[34,35] Patients with hemoglobin SC may also be at risk for the aforementioned complications but usually to a lesser degree.[35]

Transfusion, via simple transfusion or exchange transfusion, is a mainstay of therapy for many patients with SCD and other hemoglobinopathies. The need for transfusion during pregnancy in SCD is common.[34,36] The American College of Obstetricians and Gynecologists (ACOG) recommends that pregnant patients should be transfused for hemoglobin values less than 6 g/dL[37]; currently there are not specific guidelines addressing transfusion thresholds in pregnant patients with SCD.

In 2015, a meta-analysis demonstrated that prophylactic transfusion in pregnant patients with SCD may reduce maternal mortality, vaso-occlusive pain crises, pulmonary complications, perinatal mortality, neonatal death, and preterm birth. However, this was based on a relatively small number of studies with limitations.[38] If prophylactic transfusion occurs, the goal is to maintain the hemoglobin level at 10–11 g/dL and the hemoglobin S level at less than or equal to 30%. This is generally accomplished with transfusions every 3–4 weeks.[39] Some suggest potential benefit from prophylactic RBC exchange in those with severe complications, twin pregnancy, or chronic organ injury.[39–41] The ASFA lists RBC exchange in nonacute pregnant patients with SCD as a Category III indication, with Grade 2C recommendation.[19]

When looking at pregnant patients with other hemoglobin variants, such as hemoglobin SC, some have found that these patients also have higher rates of maternal and fetal complications[42] and may benefit from prophylactic automated or manual exchange transfusion.[43] Currently, however, there is no consensus on the use of prophylactic transfusion therapy, either simple or exchange transfusion, to minimize complications in this patient population.[39,44]

In patients with β-thalassemia major transfusion goals are similar to those outside of pregnancy, with a hemoglobin target of >9–10 g/dL and a potential for increase in transfusion requirements with anemia of pregnancy.[45,46] In pregnant patients with β-thalassemia intermedia the transfusion practice is quite variable, with some centers transfusing to maintain hemoglobin values >10 g/dL[45–47] but at a risk of alloimmunization, particularly in those who were only minimally or never transfused prepregnancy.[46]

High rates of alloimmunization have been reported in patients with SCD and thalassemia.[48,49] In pregnant patients with SCD, up to 30% have detectable alloantibodies before conception and another 5%–20% develop new antibodies during pregnancy.[45] Previously formed or new alloantibodies can contribute to increased morbidity during pregnancy with both delayed hemolytic transfusion reactions and HDFN.[46,47,50] Obtaining a complete transfusion and alloimmunization history and relaying this information to the blood bank before transfusion is important. It is recommended that transfusions to patients with SCD be RBC phenotype matched for the E, C, and Kell antigens, in addition to ABO and Rh(D).[48] Some advocate for extended phenotype matching in heavily alloimmunized patients requiring RBC transfusion[45]; however, such a protocol may be impractical because of the low prevalence of such phenotypes among random blood donors compared with the SCD population.[51]

THROMBOCYTOPENIA IN PREGNANCY

Thrombocytopenia, defined as a platelet count of less than 150×10^9/L, is common during pregnancy. Diagnoses and management of thrombocytopenia during pregnancy may be challenging because there are many potential causes, related or unrelated to the pregnancy. Some causes of thrombocytopenia are serious and have the potential for maternal and fetal morbidity. Table 11.2 summarizes the common causes of pregnancy-associated thrombocytopenia.

TABLE 11.2
Causes of Pregnancy-Associated Thrombocytopenia

Isolated Thrombocytopenia	Thrombocytopenia Associated With Systemic Disorders
Gestational (incidental)	Microangiopathic • Preeclampsia • HELLP syndrome • HUS • TTP • Disseminated intravascular coagulation • Acute fatty liver of pregnancy
Immune (ITP)	Collagen vascular diseases • Systemic lupus erythematosus • Antiphospholipid syndrome • Others
Drug induced • HIT (with or without thrombosis)	Viral infections • HBV • EBV • CMV
Inherited • Type IIb von Willebrand disease	Nutritional deficiencies • Hypersplenism • Bone marrow dysfunction

CMV, cytomegalovirus; *EBV*, Epstein-Barr virus; *HBV*, hepatitis B virus; *HELLP*, hemolysis, elevated liver enzymes, low platelets; *HIT*, heparin-induced thrombocytopenia; *HUS*, hemolytic uremic syndrome; *ITP*, immune thrombocytopenia; *TTP*, thrombotic thrombocytopenic purpura.
From Stavrou E, McCrae KR. Immune thrombocytopenia in pregnancy. *Hematol Oncol Clin North Am*. 2009;23(6):1300; with permission.

Immune Thrombocytopenia

Immune thrombocytopenia (ITP) is an autoimmune disease in which antiplatelet autoantibodies interfere with platelet production and cause the destruction of circulating platelets. The incidence is approximately 1–3 in 10,000 pregnancies, approximately 10-fold greater than the incidence of ITP in the general population, and accounts for 5% of the cases of pregnancy-associated thrombocytopenia.[53] ITP may occur anytime during the pregnancy, but it remains the most common cause of isolated thrombocytopenia during the first and early second trimesters.[54]

The presentation of ITP in pregnancy is much like that in the nonpregnant individual. Most commonly the patient presents with asymptomatic thrombocytopenia detected by routine testing. Less commonly the patient presents with severe thrombocytopenia accompanied by bruising, bleeding, and petechiae. The degree of thrombocytopenia can vary during pregnancy; for some the platelet count may decline even more during pregnancy and improve after delivery, but for many the platelet count remains stable.[52,55]

IgG antiplatelet antibodies may cross the placenta and cause fetal thrombocytopenia. However, in one study of pregnant patients with ITP, there was no relationship observed between maternal platelet count at delivery and infant platelet count at birth. Also, no serious bleeding event was seen in either the mother or their infants.[56] Most women with ITP have uncomplicated pregnancies, and even those with severe thrombocytopenia have good outcomes with the strict care of a hematologist and gynecologist.[56] For most pregnant women with ITP, there is no indication to monitor fetal platelet counts during pregnancy.[57]

The management of ITP during pregnancy is generally the same as that in a nonpregnant patient. Bleeding, and not platelet count, is the rationale for treatment. It is generally not necessary to maintain platelet count within the normal range during pregnancy. The goal of treatment is to minimize the risk of bleeding complications associated with thrombocytopenia at times of regional anesthesia and delivery.[58] It has been accepted that treatment is indicated for patients with platelet counts less than $20–30 \times 10^9/L$ since bleeding risks are significantly higher in such patients. For patients with platelet counts of $30–50 \times 10^9/L$, treatment may be indicated when accompanied by substantial mucous membrane bleeding.[59] For pregnant women with ITP, the mode of delivery should be based on obstetric indications.[58] At the time of delivery, management of ITP is also based on the assessment of maternal bleeding risks associated with delivery, epidural anesthesia, and the minimum platelet counts recommended to undergo those procedures ($80 \times 10^9/L$ for epidural placement and $50 \times 10^9/L$ for cesarean delivery).[60]

That being said, the majority of pregnant women with a history of ITP do not require treatment. However, if prenatal treatment is indicated, corticosteroids or IVIG are the initial choice.[58] Neonatal outcomes were comparable for mothers who received IVIG or corticosteroids.[61] Other potential treatments include high-dose dexamethasone, intermittent anti-D immunoglobulin infusions, and rituximab, but they are not currently recommended as their efficacy and safety remain unclear.[59]

Hemolysis, Elevated Liver Enzymes, Low Platelets Syndrome

The name "HELLP" syndrome was given by Dr. Louis Weinstein in 1982 as an abbreviation of the three main features of the syndrome: H (*h*emolysis), EL (*e*levated

liver enzymes), and LP (*l*ow *p*latelet count).[62] HELLP syndrome is a life-threatening pregnancy complication, occurring in 0.5%–0.9% of all pregnancies and in 10%–20% of cases with severe preeclampsia.[63] It usually occurs during the later stages of pregnancy, or sometimes postpartum.[63,64] HELLP syndrome has been associated with higher incidences of cesarean section, disseminated intravascular coagulation (DIC), and need for transfusion.[65,66] The presence of this syndrome can be associated with increased risk of adverse outcome for both the mother and the fetus.[67]

The pathogenesis of HELLP syndrome is unclear. Most obstetricians presume that HELLP derives from an autoimmune reaction, leading to a maternofetal imbalance, with accompanying aggregation of platelets, endothelial malfunction, and inborn errors of fatty acid oxidative metabolism.[64] Combinations of multiple gene variants, each with a moderate risk, with contributing effects of maternal and environmental factors are the probable etiologic mechanisms.[68]

HELLP syndrome can have a variable presentation with symptoms including proteinuria, hypertension, right upper quadrant/epigastric pain, nausea, vomiting, headache, visual changes, and jaundice. The most commonly reported symptom is abdominal pain with tenderness in the midepigastrium, right upper quadrant, or below the sternum.[66] Patients who present with nausea, vomiting, and malaise may be mistaken to have a nonspecific viral illness or viral hepatitis, particularly if the serum aspartate aminotransferase (AST) and lactate dehydrogenase (LDH) are markedly elevated.[69,70] Up to 85% of HELLP cases may present with hypertension and proteinuria, but either or both may be absent in women with otherwise severe HELLP syndrome.[67] This syndrome may also be associated with serious liver manifestations, including infarction, hemorrhage, and rupture.[62]

The diagnosis of HELLP syndrome requires the presence of hemolysis based on examination of the peripheral smear, elevated indirect bilirubin levels, or low serum haptoglobin levels in association with significant elevation in liver enzymes and a platelet count $<100 \times 10^9/L$ after ruling out other common causes of hemolysis and thrombocytopenia.[67]

The severity of HELLP syndrome is measured according to the maternal platelet count and is divided into three categories, according to a system called "the Mississippi classification"[71]:

- Class I (severe thrombocytopenia): platelets under $50 \times 10^9/L$
- Class II (moderate thrombocytopenia): platelets between 50 and $100 \times 10^9/L$

- Class III (AST > 40 IU/L, mild thrombocytopenia): platelets between 100 and 150×10^9/L

Laboratory and clinical indices of disease severity in patients with severe preeclampsia or eclampsia were generally the highest with class I HELLP syndrome. Class III HELLP syndrome is considered as a transitional stage or a progression phase of the HELLP syndrome.[72]

The definitive treatment of HELLP syndrome is delivery. Many patients with HELLP syndrome may require blood component transfusion, including red cells, platelets, and plasma. Patients with HELLP with an intrapartum platelet count maintained above 40×10^9/L are unlikely to have clinically significant postpartum bleeding.[73] Corticosteroids can be used in early pregnancy to help the fetal lungs mature. Some healthcare providers may also use steroids to improve maternal outcome.[64,67] In severe cases of postpartum HELLP syndrome, TPE may be utilized when the patient fails to show improvement within 48–72 h following delivery (ASFA Category III indication with grade 2C recommendation).[19] TPE is usually performed until platelet counts are greater than 100×10^9/L or LDH has normalized.

The outcome for mothers with HELLP syndrome is generally good, but serious complications may occur. In a serial study of 437 women with HELLP syndrome, the following complications were observed: DIC (21%), abruptio placentae (16%), acute renal failure (8%), pulmonary edema (6%), subcapsular liver hematoma (1%), and retinal detachment (1%).[66] The most prominent neonatal outcomes associated with HELLP syndrome were antenatal fetal death, IUGR, and prematurity. The overall perinatal mortality from HELLP syndrome ranges from 7.7% to 60%. Most of these deaths are attributed to abruptio placentae, placental failure with intrauterine asphyxia, and extreme prematurity.[74,75]

Acute Fatty Liver of Pregnancy

Acute fatty liver of pregnancy (AFLP) is a rare potentially fatal liver disorder unique to pregnancy, reported to occur in 1 in 7000–15,000 deliveries.[76] It is characterized by microvesicular fatty infiltration of hepatocytes and is more common with multiple gestations and possibly in women who are underweight.[77,78] Other risk factors for AFLP include multigravida state, male sex of fetus, coexistence of other liver diseases during pregnancy, and previous episode of AFLP.[78]

AFLP always presents before delivery, typically in the third trimester, although it is not always diagnosed before delivery. The clinical presentation is broad and can range from asymptomatic elevations in aminotransferases to fulminant hepatic failure with jaundice, profound coagulopathy, hepatic coma, and hypoglycemia, requiring maximum supportive care.[78]

Laboratory studies usually reveal additional liver dysfunction, not just elevated liver enzymes, which is rarely seen in other obstetric liver diseases.[79] Approximately 50% of patients do not have thrombocytopenia at presentation, and AFLP was exclusively associated with pregnancy-induced antithrombin deficiency.[79] Hemostatic dysfunction with AFLP may persist 4–5 days postpartum, resulting from substantive ongoing DIC with reduced procoagulant synthesis and clinically significant hemolysis.[80] Serial monitoring of the patient's platelet count, international normalized ratio, partial thromboplastin time (aPTT), and fibrinogen levels should be done for overt or evolving coagulopathy.

Treatment of AFLP is by a combination of maternal stabilization and prompt delivery of the fetus, regardless of the gestational age. Early administration of appropriate blood components, such as fresh frozen plasma, cryoprecipitate, RBCs, and platelets, to correct the patient's coagulation status, may be needed.[78]

Thrombotic Thrombocytopenic Purpura

Thrombotic thrombocytopenic purpura (TTP) is a thrombotic microangiopathy caused by severely reduced activity (<10%) of the von Willebrand factor–cleaving protease *a disintegrin and metalloproteinase with a thrombospondin type 1 motif, member 13* (ADAMTS13). It is characterized by small-vessel platelet-rich thrombi that cause thrombocytopenia, microangiopathic hemolytic anemia, and sometimes organ damage.[81] TTP can be hereditary, due to inherited mutations in *ADAMTS13*, or acquired, due to an autoantibody inhibitor.

Pregnancy is a very strong trigger for acute disease manifestation in patients with hereditary TTP caused by double heterozygous or homozygous mutations of *ADAMTS13*. Without plasma treatment, both the mother and fetus are at risk of dying.[82] The relapse risk during a next pregnancy is almost 100%; however, starting regular plasma transfusion early in pregnancy may prevent acute TTP flareup and lead to a successful outcome.[82] The frequency of plasma transfusion may need to be increased as pregnancy progresses based on the patient's platelet count.

In contrast to hereditary TTP, pregnancy constitutes a mild risk factor for the onset of acute acquired TTP caused by autoantibody-mediated severe ADAMTS13 deficiency. Women having survived acute acquired TTP may not be at very high risk of TTP relapse during an ensuing next pregnancy but seem to have an elevated risk of preeclampsia.[83,84]

Initial and recurrent TTP present most often in the second trimester (55.5%) after 1–2 days of signs/symptoms; postpartum TTP usually occurs following term delivery.[85] Maternal mortality is higher with initial TTP, especially with concurrent preeclampsia. Pregnant women should undergo the same diagnostic testing as nonpregnant adults; however, other diagnostic possibilities may be much more likely and should be considered in these populations.[84]

Monitoring of ADAMTS13 activity and inhibitor titer during pregnancy may help guide management and avoid disease recurrence.[82] Quick diagnosis and initiation of immunosuppression and TPE is needed.[85,86] TPE for TTP is an ASFA Category I indication, meaning that it is a disorder for which apheresis is accepted as the first-line therapy, either as stand-alone therapy or in conjunction with other treatment.[19]

One study of patients with acquired TTP from a large TTP registry found that most pregnancies accompanied with TTP result in normal children.[84] However, a cohort study of acute TTP in pregnancy within the United Kingdom, involving 35 women and nearly 100 pregnancies, reports a 40% fetal loss rate before diagnosis of TTP, almost exclusively in the second trimester, but 100% fetal survival with plasma therapy.[87]

Disseminated Intravascular Coagulation

Pregnancy is associated with physiologic changes of the hemostasis system. To prevent excessive blood loss during labor and after delivery, a procoagulant imbalance is gradually induced by endothelial activation, increased liver synthesis of coagulation factors, and decreased activity of coagulation inhibitors and fibrinolysis.[88] Uncontrolled systemic activation of the hemostatic system can lead to DIC, causing widespread microvascular thrombosis and compromise of the blood supply to different organs and eventually organ failure. The rate of DIC during pregnancy ranges from 0.03% to 0.35% and is associated with significant maternal and fetal morbidity and mortality.[88,89] Obstetric DIC has been associated with pregnancy complications including (1) acute peripartum hemorrhage, (2) placental abruption, (3) preeclampsia/eclampsia/HELLP syndrome, (4) retained stillbirth, (5) septic abortion and intrauterine infection, (6) amniotic fluid embolism, and (7) AFLP.[88,90]

Patients with obstetric DIC may present with severe bleeding (vaginal, intrauterine, intraabdominal) and/or diffuse oozing of blood from skin (at intravenous sites) or mucosa (from a bladder catheter). Some patients may have signs of shock, including tachycardia, hypotension, weak peripheral pulses, altered mental status, cool extremities, narrow pulse pressure (<25 mm Hg), and/or organ dysfunction. Prompt diagnosis and understanding of these rapid and complex coagulation changes is essential and difficult.[91,92]

The International Society for Thrombosis and Hemostasis (ISTH) proposed a DIC scoring system based on coagulation assays including prothrombin time (PT), fibrinogen, and fibrin degradation products.[93] There was good correlation between an abnormal score and DIC in nonpregnant women but not in pregnant women, presumably due to the physiologic changes of the coagulation cascade during gestation.[94] More recently, an Israeli team generated a new DIC score, based on platelet count, fibrinogen concentration, and PT difference[94,95]:

- 1 point for platelet count <100 × 10^9/L, 2 points for <50 × 10^9/L
- 5 points if PT prolonged 0.5- to 1-fold, 12 points if PT prolonged 1.0- to 1.5-fold, 25 points if PT >1.5-fold
- 25 points for fibrinogen <300 mg/dL, 6 points for fibrinogen 300–400 mg/dL, 1 point for fibrinogen 400–450 mg/dL, 0 point if fibrinogen > 450 mg/dL

A score of ≥26 points has better sensitivity (88% vs. 74%) and specificity (96% vs. 95%) for the diagnosis of DIC in pregnant patients compared with the ISTH score system.[94]

The basic principles of obstetric DIC treatment include the following: management of the underlying condition that predisposes to DIC, supportive care with blood components and related measures, regular clinical and laboratory surveillance, and seeking assistance from the relevant specialists at the earliest.[91] The thresholds for transfusing blood components are mainly those recommended by harmonized guidance from the ISTH[96–98]:

- Platelet count <50 × 10^9/L, but if ongoing hemorrhage is occurring, a higher threshold of 75 × 10^9/L may be a starting point
- Fibrinogen <150 mg/dL
- PT and aPTT more than 1.5 times the control

Fetal and Neonatal Alloimmune Thrombocytopenia

Fetal and neonatal alloimmune thrombocytopenia (FNAIT) occurs when a maternal IgG antibody directed against a paternal platelet antigen crosses the placenta and binds to fetal platelets promoting clearance of the antibody-coated platelets, resulting in fetal and/or neonatal thrombocytopenia. FNAIT occurs in 1 in 1000 births and often affects the first pregnancy. Most of the antibodies identified are directed to human platelet antigen (HPA)-1a, but antibodies to other HPA antigens, ABO antigens, and glycoprotein IV (CD36) have also been reported.[99–101]

Two plausible mechanisms have been proposed to explain the occurrence of maternal alloimmunization in FNAIT. One mechanism involves maternal exposure to HPA on fetal platelets due to fetomaternal bleeding related to obstetric complications, trauma, or delivery. The other mechanism is maternal exposure to integrin β3 on placental syncytiotrophoblast cells during pregnancy.[100]

FNAIT can occur early in gestation and is often more severe in fetuses with an older affected sibling who had an antenatal intracranial hemorrhage (ICH). If a previous sibling has had an ICH, the chances that the next affected sibling will have an ICH is at least 80 or 90% unless treatment is administered.[102] Also, if a previous sibling has had an ICH, the platelet count of the next affected fetus is generally lower than that of neonates who did not have a previous affected sibling with ICH.[102]

The mother of a fetus with FNAIT is usually asymptomatic with a normal platelet count. Screening all pregnant women to identify those who are at risk of FNAIT is controversial because of cost, and the optimal management of these women remains unknown. The obstetrician should be suspicious for FNAIT if the pregnant patient has a history of delivering a newborn with thrombocytopenia or known diagnosis of FNAIT. If not previously performed, both the mother and the implicated father should be typed for platelet antigens and the mother should be screened for alloantibodies.[4] Maternal antiplatelet antibody titers correlate poorly with the severity of disease. Noninvasive testing to determine fetal HPA-1a genotype using maternal plasma as the source of fetal DNA has been described.[15]

The primary goal in the treatment of FNAIT is to prevent ICH, especially in utero ICH.[103] Recent ACOG bulletin recommends management of patients with FNAIT based on the presence or absence of an ICH in their previous affected pregnancy and the gestational age of manifestation. Attempts to increase the fetal platelet count and to avoid ICH are required for high-risk patients (fetal platelet counts by umbilical cord blood sampling at 20 weeks of gestation less than $20 \times 10^9/L$ or a sibling with a perinatal ICH), including maternal treatment with IVIG, with or without steroids, and fetal platelet transfusions. This is in contrast to standard-risk patients, those whose previous child had thrombocytopenia without ICH, where IVIG or prednisone therapy is beneficial with no significant advantage of one over the other. It is also recommended to perform a cesarean delivery at 37–38 weeks, without performing amniocentesis for fetal lung maturity.[103]

Serial cordocentesis has been used to monitor fetal platelet count and response to therapy in pregnancies complicated by FNAIT, but this approach has largely been abandoned because of the significant procedure-related risks. However, if fetal blood sampling and in utero platelet transfusion are necessary, they should be performed by an experienced operator. The sampling needle should be of small diameter, 22-gauge, and the procedure should be performed in an operating room in the event that emergent cesarean delivery is needed.[104]

Platelet transfusion should be given to infants with active bleeding or evidence of bleeding (e.g., oozing from the umbilical cord, or the presence of petechiae, large ecchymoses, or cephalohematoma) or to asymptomatic patients with severe thrombocytopenia (platelet count $<50 \times 10^9/L$).[105] The platelets for transfusion may be obtained from an appropriately typed donor who is negative for the implicated platelet antigen or from the mother. If maternal platelets are used, they must be washed before transfusion to remove the offending antibody.[4] If platelet transfusion is needed emergently, there may be no time to acquire antigen-negative platelets. In this case, platelet transfusion from the general inventory, i.e., random donors, is an appropriate management strategy.[106]

MANAGEMENT OF POSTPARTUM HEMORRHAGE

The potential for massive hemorrhage after delivery is high because in late pregnancy uterine artery blood flow is 500–700 mL/min and accounts for about 15% of cardiac output. Normally, with contraction of the myometrium and the release of hemostatic factors, such as tissue factor and type-1 plasminogen activator inhibitors, upon placental separation, hemostasis occurs and bleeding stops. Postpartum hemorrhage (PPH) occurs when there is a disturbance in one or both of these mechanisms.[107]

PPH remains the leading cause of maternal morbidity and mortality worldwide, especially in low-income countries, with an estimated 140,000 women dying annually from this complication, almost 1 every 4 min.[108,109] PPH is commonly defined as blood loss of more than 500 mL after vaginal birth or more than 1000 mL after cesarean delivery within 24 h after birth.[107] Most recently, an international expert panel defined PPH as "active bleeding >1000 mL within the 24 h following birth that continues despite the use of initial measures, including first-line uterotonic agents and uterine massage."[108]

PPH can be divided into minor (500–1000 mL) or major hemorrhage (>1000 mL), with further subdivisions of major hemorrhage as moderate (1001–2000 mL) or severe (>2000 mL).[110] PPH is also classified as primary or secondary: primary PPH occurs within

24 h after delivery, whereas secondary PPH occurs 24 h to 12 weeks after delivery. Most deaths resulting from PPH occur during the 24 h after delivery.[111]

The causes of PPH can be classified into four main groups: (1) uterine atony; (2) placental problems, including retained placenta and abnormal placental implantation; (3) genital tract trauma; and (4) systemic medical disorders (including inherited and acquired coagulation defects).[109] Uterine atony is the major cause of PPH, accounting for up to 80% of cases of primary PPH. Among all causes of PPH, placenta accreta had the highest hysterectomy rate.[112] Women with risk factors for PPH should be identified and counseled before labor. Routine prophylactic use of uterotonic drugs, such as oxytocin, should be considered. Box 11.3 summarizes risk factors associated with PPH.

Management of PPH varies depending on the cause and severity of bleeding and delivery methods. Control of uterine atony is essential in the treatment of PPH. If the patient's hemodynamics do not improve with 2–3 L of crystalloid administration and there is ongoing active PPH, administration of blood components including RBCs, fresh frozen plasma, fibrinogen concentrate (or cryoprecipitate), and platelets may be necessary, and usually begins with RBCs.[107,110] Aggressive use of plasma replacement is also important to reverse dilutional coagulopathy. Coagulation factor concentrates may also be needed. For patients with massive hemorrhage, RBCs, fresh frozen plasma, and platelets are best administered according to an established massive transfusion protocol.[107] Other potentially effective hemostatic agents include tranexamic acid (TXA) and recombinant activated factor VII (rFVIIa).

TXA is an antifibrinolytic that reduces bleeding by inhibiting the enzymatic breakdown of fibrinogen and fibrin by plasmin. TXA has had resurgence in recent years for the management of massive hemorrhage. In the recent WOMAN (World Maternal Antifibrinolytic) trial, the use of TXA in the management of PPH reduced death due to bleeding with no adverse effects.[113] The authors also recommended that TXA be given as soon as possible after bleeding onset.[113]

rFVIIa has been identified as a global hemostatic agent with potential benefit in the management of severe PPH refractory to standard treatment.[114] By transiently reducing blood loss and providing time for more effective replacement therapy, rFVIIa may be lifesaving, especially in an unstable patient requiring transfer to a center in which more surgical expertise and selective arterial embolization are available.[115] It is important to note that administration of RBCs, fresh frozen plasma, fibrinogen concentrate (or cryoprecipitate), and platelets as well as the control of uterine atony are essential

in the treatment of PPH. rFVIIa cannot work optimally if there is a shortage of the basic components of the coagulation cascade such as fibrinogen. Randomized controlled studies are needed to clearly define the value of rFVIIa in PPH management.[115]

BOX 11.3
Risk Factors Associated With PPH

CATEGORY AND RISK FACTOR
Sociodemographic
  Asian ethnicity
  Hispanic ethnicity
  Age ≥ 30 years
Obstetric
  Prolonged Stage 3 labor
  Preeclampsia
  Retained placenta
  Known placenta previa
  Previous PPH
  Suspected or proven placental abruption
  Multiple gestation
  Fetal macrosomia
  HELLP syndrome
  Polyhydramnios
  Oxytocin exposure
  Induction of labor
  Prolonged labor
Surgical
  Emergency cesarean delivery
  Elective cesarean delivery
  Forceps delivery
  Vacuum delivery
  Episiotomy
  Perineal suture
Systemic or medical
  Antepartum hemorrhage
  VWD
  Anemia (<9 g/dL)
  Pyrexia in labor
  Obesity (BMI > 35)
  Cardiac disease

BMI, body mass index; *HELLP*, hemolysis, elevated liver enzymes, low platelets; *PPH*, postpartum hemorrhage; *VWD*, von Willebrand disease.

From Abdul-Kadir R, McLintock C, Ducloy AS, et al. Evaluation and management of postpartum hemorrhage: consensus from an international expert panel. *Transfusion.* 2014;54(7):1756–1768; with permission.

TABLE 11.3
Recommendations for the Prophylactic Treatment of Women With Inherited Bleeding Disorders

Disorder	Management
von Willebrand Disease	
• Type 1	TXA, DDAVP
• Type 2	TXA, VWF concentrates, DDAVP in responders
• Type 3	TXA, VWF concentrates
Afibrinogenemia and hypofibrinogenemia	Fibrinogen concentrate, cryoprecipitate or FFP,[a] and volume status
Dysfibrinogenemia	At risk of both postpartum thrombosis and hemorrhage, therefore require individualized management based on fibrinogen level and personal and family history of bleeding and thrombosis; this also includes individualized postpartum thromboprophylaxis
Coagulation Factor Deficiencies	
• FII	PCCs to maintain FII level >20%–30%
• FV	FFP to increase FV level to >15%–25%
• FV plus FVIII	FV >15%–25%; combination of DDAVP or FVIII concentrate and FFP to increase FVIII >50%
• FVII	rFVIIa or nonactivated plasma-derived FVII concentrate (15–30 μg/kg) for women with FVII level of <10%–20%; hemostatic level for uterine bleeding *or* surgery may be higher
• FX	Replacement therapy during labor and delivery (FX concentrate or PCC as available) if FX levels <10%–20%. If FX >10%–20% and no significant bleeding history, a conservative approach may be appropriate.
• FXI	Prophylactic treatment with TXA should be considered up to 2 weeks after delivery. For those with bleeding phenotype or severe deficiency, give FXI concentrate if available, or FFP *Avoid* concomitant use of TXA and FXI concentrate due to increased thrombogenicity
• FXIII[b]	FXIII concentrate replacement therapy throughout pregnancy in those with FXIII subunit A deficiency; a level of >10%–20% should be considered
Carriers of Hemophilia	
• FVIII carrier	TXA, DDAVP, FVIII replacement
• Factor IX carrier	TXA, FIX replacement

[a]Choice of product may depend on availability.
[b]The incidence of PPH in women with FXIII deficiency is unknown.
DDAVP, desmopressin; *FFP*, fresh frozen plasma; *FII*, factor II; *FV*, factor V; *FVII*, factor VII; *FVIII*, factor VIII; *FX*, factor X; *FXI*, factor XI; *FXIII*, factor XIII; *PCC*, prothrombin complex concentrate; *rFVIIa*, recombinant activated factor VII; *TXA*, tranexamic acid; *VWF*, von Willebrand factor.
Adapted from Abdul-Kadir R, McLintock C, Ducloy AS, et al. Evaluation and management of postpartum hemorrhage: consensus from an international expert panel. *Transfusion*. 2014;54(7):1756–1768 and Peyvandi F, Menegatti M, Siboni SM. Post-partum hemorrhage in women with rare bleeding disorders. *Thromb Res*. 2011;127(suppl 3):S116–S119; with permission.

For women with inherited platelet function disorders, if mild, such as platelet secretion and activation defects, prophylactic administration of TXA is generally sufficient. For moderate bleeding risk cases, if there is no risk of fluid retention, desmopressin (DDAVP) can be added to TXA during the immediate postpartum period. Platelet transfusion with or without rFVIIa may be needed in cases of hemorrhage. For women with severe platelet function disorders, such as Glanzmann thrombasthenia and Bernard-Soulier syndrome, TXA and rFVIIa can be used in cases of uncomplicated vaginal delivery. Platelet transfusion at a dose targeted to achieve a hemostatic response is recommended in cases of operative delivery.[108,116] Women with inherited bleeding disorders may be at increased risk of developing PPH, therefore Table 11.3 outlines the recommended prophylactic hemostatic coverage for these conditions.[108,116]

REFERENCES

1. Bowman JM, Pollock JM, Penston LE. Fetomaternal transplacental hemorrhage during pregnancy and after delivery. *Vox Sang.* 1986;51(2):117–121.
2. Sebring ES, Polesky HF. Fetomaternal hemorrhage: incidence, risk factors, time of occurrence, and clinical effects. *Transfusion.* 1990;30(4):344–357.
3. Bowman JM. The prevention of Rh immunization. *Transfus Med Rev.* 1988;2(3):129–150.
4. Kennedy MS, Delaney M, Scrape S. Perinatal issues in transfusion practice. In: Fung MK, Grossman BJ, Hillyer CD, Westhoff CM, eds. *Technical Manual.* 18th ed. Bethesda, MD: AABB; 2014:561–570.
5. van der Schoot CE, Tax GH, Rijnders RJ, de Haas M, Christiaens GC. Prenatal typing of Rh and Kell blood group system antigens: the edge of a watershed. *Transfus Med Rev.* 2003;17(1):31–44.
6. Markham KB, Rossi KQ, Nagaraja HN, O'Shaughnessy RW. Hemolytic disease of the fetus and newborn due to multiple maternal antibodies. *Am J Obstet Gynecol.* 2015;213(1):68. e61–65.
7. Filbey D, Hanson U, Wesstrom G. The prevalence of red cell antibodies in pregnancy correlated to the outcome of the newborn: a 12 year study in central Sweden. *Acta Obstet Gynecol Scand.* 1995;74(9):687–692.
8. Spong CY, Porter AE, Queenan JT. Management of isoimmunization in the presence of multiple maternal antibodies. *Am J Obstet Gynecol.* 2001;185(2):481–484.
9. Kennedy MS. Hemolytic disease of the fetus and newborn (HDFN). In: Harmening DM, ed. *Modern Blood Banking & Transfusion Practices.* 6th ed. Philadelphia, PA: F. A. Davis Company; 2012:427–438.
10. de Haas M, Thurik FF, Koelewijn JM, van der Schoot CE. Haemolytic disease of the fetus and newborn. *Vox Sang.* 2015;109(2):99–113.
11. Dennery PA, Seidman DS, Stevenson DK. Neonatal hyperbilirubinemia. *N Engl J Med.* 2001;344(8):581–590.
12. Management of Alloimmunization During Pregnancy. ACOG practice bulletin No. 75. American College of Obstetricians and Gynecologists. *Obstet Gynecol.* 2006;108:457–464.
13. Vaughan JI, Manning M, Warwick RM, Letsky EA, Murray NA, Roberts IA. Inhibition of erythroid progenitor cells by anti-Kell antibodies in fetal alloimmune anemia. *N Engl J Med.* 1998;338(12):798–803.
14. Fasano RM. Hemolytic disease of the fetus and newborn in the molecular era. *Semin Fetal Neonatal Med.* 2016;21(1):28–34.
15. Avent ND. Prenatal testing for hemolytic disease of the newborn and fetal neonatal alloimmune thrombocytopenia - current status. *Expert Rev Hematol.* 2014;7(6):741–745.
16. Mari G, Deter RL, Carpenter RL, et al. Noninvasive diagnosis by Doppler ultrasonography of fetal anemia due to maternal red-cell alloimmunization. Collaborative group for Doppler assessment of the blood velocity in anemic fetuses. *N Engl J Med.* 2000;342(1):9–14.
17. Moise Jr KJ, Argoti PS. Management and prevention of red cell alloimmunization in pregnancy: a systematic review. *Obstet Gynecol.* 2012;120(5):1132–1139.
18. Hendrickson JE, Delaney M. Hemolytic disease of the fetus and newborn: modern practice and future investigations. *Transfus Med Rev.* 2016;30(4):159–164.
19. Schwartz J, Padmanabhan A, Aqui N, et al. Guidelines on the use of therapeutic apheresis in clinical practice-evidence-based approach from the writing committee of the American Society for apheresis: the seventh special issue. *J Clin Apher.* 2016;31(3):149–162.
20. Delaney M, Wikman A, van de Watering L, et al. Blood group antigen matching influence on gestational outcomes (AMIGO) study. *Transfusion.* 2017;57(3):525–532.
21. Bowman JM. Controversies in Rh prophylaxis. Who needs Rh immune globulin and when should it be given? *Am J Obstet Gynecol.* 1985;151(3):289–294.
22. Prevention of Rh D Alloimmunization. ACOG practice bulletin No. 4. American College of Obstetricians and Gynecologists. *Obstet Gynecol.* 1999;123.
23. Sandler SG, Flegel WA, Westhoff CM, et al. It's time to phase in RHD genotyping for patients with a serologic weak D phenotype. College of American Pathologists Transfusion Medicine Resource Committee Work Group. *Transfusion.* 2015;55(3):680–689.
24. Schonewille H, Prinsen-Zander KJ, Reijnart M, et al. Extended matched intrauterine transfusions reduce maternal Duffy, Kidd, and S antibody formation. *Transfusion.* 2015;55(12):2912–2919; Quiz 2911.
25. Kim YA, Makar RS. Detection of fetomaternal hemorrhage. *Am J Hematol.* 2012;87(4):417–423.
26. Caruccio L, Wise S. Fundamentals of immunology. In: Harmening DM, ed. *Modern Blood Banking & Transfusion Practices.* 6th ed. Philadelphia, PA: F. A. Davis Company; 2012:45–76.
27. Harmening DM, Rodberg K, Green REB. Autoimmune hemolytic anemias. In: Harmening DM, ed. *Modern Blood Banking & Transfuison Practices.* 6th ed. Philadelphia, PA: F. A. Davis Company; 2012:439–473.
28. Hoppe B, Stibbe W, Bielefeld A, Pruss A, Salama A. Increased RBC autoantibody production in pregnancy. *Transfusion.* 2001;41(12):1559–1561.
29. Sokol RJ, Hewitt S, Stamps BK. Erythrocyte autoantibodies, autoimmune haemolysis and pregnancy. *Vox Sang.* 1982;43(4):169–176.
30. Piatek CI, El-Hemaidi I, Feinstein DI, Liebman HA, Akhtari M. Management of immune-mediated cytopenias in pregnancy. *Autoimmun Rev.* 2015;14(9):806–811.
31. Dhingra S, Wiener JJ, Jackson H. Management of cold agglutinin immune hemolytic anemia in pregnancy. *Obstet Gynecol.* 2007;110(2 Pt 2):485–486.
32. Oteng-Ntim E, Meeks D, Seed PT, et al. Adverse maternal and perinatal outcomes in pregnant women with sickle cell disease: systematic review and meta-analysis. *Blood.* 2015;125(21):3316–3325.

33. Hemoglobinopathies in Pregnancy. ACOG practice bulletin No. 78. American College of Obstetricians and Gynecologists. *Obstet Gynecol.* 2007;109:229–237.

34. Sun PM, Wilburn W, Raynor BD, Jamieson D. Sickle cell disease in pregnancy: twenty years of experience at Grady Memorial Hospital, Atlanta, Georgia. *Am J Obstet Gynecol.* 2001;184(6):1127–1130.

35. Powars DR, Sandhu M, Niland-Weiss J, Johnson C, Bruce S, Manning PR. Pregnancy in sickle cell disease. *Obstet Gynecol.* 1986;67(2):217–228.

36. Koshy M, Burd L, Wallace D, Moawad A, Baron J. Prophylactic red-cell transfusions in pregnant patients with sickle cell disease. A randomized cooperative study. *N Engl J Med.* 1988;319(22):1447–1452.

37. Anemia in Pregnancy. ACOG practice bulletin No. 95. American College of Obstetricians and Gynecologists. *Obstet Gynecol.* 2008;112:201–207.

38. Malinowski AK, Shehata N, D'Souza R, et al. Prophylactic transfusion for pregnant women with sickle cell disease: a systematic review and meta-analysis. *Blood.* 2015;126(21):2424–2435; Quiz 2437.

39. Boga C, Ozdogu H. Pregnancy and sickle cell disease: a review of the current literature. *Crit Rev Oncol Hematol.* 2016;98:364–374.

40. Asma S, Kozanoglu I, Tarim E, et al. Prophylactic red blood cell exchange may be beneficial in the management of sickle cell disease in pregnancy. *Transfusion.* 2015;55(1):36–44.

41. Howard J. Sickle cell disease: when and how to transfuse. *Hematol Am Soc Hematol Educ Program.* 2016; 2016(1):625–631.

42. Oteng-Ntim E, Ayensah B, Knight M, Howard J. Pregnancy outcome in patients with sickle cell disease in the UK–a national cohort study comparing sickle cell anaemia (HbSS) with HbSC disease. *Br J Haematol.* 2015;169(1):129–137.

43. Benites BD, Benevides TC, Valente IS, Marques Jr JF, Gilli SC, Saad ST. The effects of exchange transfusion for prevention of complications during pregnancy of sickle hemoglobin C disease patients. *Transfusion.* 2016;56(1):119–124.

44. Okusanya BO, Oladapo OT. Prophylactic versus selective blood transfusion for sickle cell disease in pregnancy. *Cochrane Database Syst Rev.* 2016;12:CD010378.

45. Naik RP, Lanzkron S. Baby on board: what you need to know about pregnancy in the hemoglobinopathies. *Hematol Am Soc Hematol Educ Program.* 2012;2012: 208–214.

46. Origa R, Piga A, Quarta G, et al. Pregnancy and beta-thalassemia: an Italian multicenter experience. *Haematologica.* 2010;95(3):376–381.

47. Nassar AH, Naja M, Cesaretti C, Eprassi B, Cappellini MD, Taher A. Pregnancy outcome in patients with beta-thalassemia intermedia at two tertiary care centers, in Beirut and Milan. *Haematologica.* 2008;93(10): 1586–1587.

48. Vichinsky EP, Luban NL, Wright E, et al. Prospective RBC phenotype matching in a stroke-prevention trial in sickle cell anemia: a multicenter transfusion trial. *Transfusion.* 2001;41(9):1086–1092.

49. Singer ST, Wu V, Mignacca R, Kuypers FA, Morel P, Vichinsky EP. Alloimmunization and erythrocyte auto-immunization in transfusion-dependent thalassemia patients of predominantly Asian descent. *Blood.* 2000; 96(10):3369–3373.

50. Narchi H, Ekuma-Nkama E. Maternal sickle cell anemia and neonatal isoimmunization. *Int J Gynaecol Obstet.* 1998;62(2):129–134.

51. Castro O, Sandler SG, Houston-Yu P, Rana S. Predicting the effect of transfusing only phenotype-matched RBCs to patients with sickle cell disease: theoretical and practical implications. *Transfusion.* 2002;42(6): 684–690.

52. Stavrou E, McCrae KR. Immune thrombocytopenia in pregnancy. *Hematol Oncol Clin North Am.* 2009; 23(6):1299–1316.

53. Terrell DR, Beebe LA, Vesely SK, Neas BR, Segal JB, George JN. The incidence of immune thrombocytopenic purpura in children and adults: a critical review of published reports. *Am J Hematol.* 2010;85(3):174–180.

54. Gill KK, Kelton JG. Management of idiopathic thrombocytopenic purpura in pregnancy. *Semin Hematol.* 2000;37(3):275–289.

55. Webert KE, Mittal R, Sigouin C, Heddle NM, Kelton JG. A retrospective 11-year analysis of obstetric patients with idiopathic thrombocytopenic purpura. *Blood.* 2003; 102(13):4306–4311.

56. Fujita A, Sakai R, Matsuura S, et al. A retrospective analysis of obstetric patients with idiopathic thrombocytopenic purpura: a single center study. *Int J Hematol.* 2010;92(3):463–467.

57. Sukenik-Halevy R, Ellis MH, Fejgin MD. Management of immune thrombocytopenic purpura in pregnancy. *Obstet Gynecol Surv.* 2008;63(3):182–188.

58. Neunert C, Lim W, Crowther M, Cohen A, Solberg Jr L, Crowther MA. The American Society of Hematology 2011 evidence-based practice guideline for immune thrombocytopenia. *Blood.* 2011;117(16):4190–4207.

59. Rodeghiero F. First-line therapies for immune thrombocytopenic purpura: re-evaluating the need to treat. *Eur J Haematol Suppl.* 2008;(69):19–26.

60. Kaufman RM, Djulbegovic B, Gernsheimer T, et al. Platelet transfusion: a clinical practice guideline from the AABB. *Ann Intern Med.* 2015;162(3):205–213.

61. Sun D, Shehata N, Ye XY, et al. Corticosteroids compared with intravenous immunoglobulin for the treatment of immune thrombocytopenia in pregnancy. *Blood.* 2016;128(10):1329–1335.

62. Weinstein L. Syndrome of hemolysis, elevated liver enzymes, and low platelet count: a severe consequence of hypertension in pregnancy. *Am J Obstet Gynecol.* 1982;142(2):159–167.

63. Haram K, Svendsen E, Abildgaard U. The HELLP syndrome: clinical issues and management. A Review. *BMC Pregnancy Childbirth.* 2009;9:8.

64. Aloizos S, Seretis C, Liakos N, et al. HELLP syndrome: understanding and management of a pregnancy-specific disease. *J Obstet Gynaecol J Inst Obstet Gynaecol.* 2013;33(4):331–337.

65. Audibert F, Friedman SA, Frangieh AY, Sibai BM. Clinical utility of strict diagnostic criteria for the HELLP (hemolysis, elevated liver enzymes, and low platelets) syndrome. *Am J Obstet Gynecol.* 1996;175(2):460–464.

66. Sibai BM, Ramadan MK, Usta I, Salama M, Mercer BM, Friedman SA. Maternal morbidity and mortality in 442 pregnancies with hemolysis, elevated liver enzymes, and low platelets (HELLP syndrome). *Am J Obstet Gynecol.* 1993;169(4):1000–1006.

67. Sibai BM. Diagnosis, controversies, and management of the syndrome of hemolysis, elevated liver enzymes, and low platelet count. *Obstet Gynecol.* 2004;103(5 Pt 1): 981–991.

68. Abildgaard U, Heimdal K. Pathogenesis of the syndrome of hemolysis, elevated liver enzymes, and low platelet count (HELLP): a review. *Eur J Obstet Gynecol Reprod Biol.* 2013;166(2):117–123.

69. Catanzarite VA, Steinberg SM, Mosley CA, Landers CF, Cousins LM, Schneider JM. Severe preeclampsia with fulminant and extreme elevation of aspartate aminotransferase and lactate dehydrogenase levels: high risk for maternal death. *Am J Perinatol.* 1995;12(5):310–313.

70. Julius CJ, Dunn ZL, Blazina JF. HELLP syndrome: laboratory parameters and clinical course in four patients treated with plasma exchange. *J Clin Apher.* 1994;9(4): 228–235.

71. Martin Jr JN, Rose CH, Briery CM. Understanding and managing HELLP syndrome: the integral role of aggressive glucocorticoids for mother and child. *Am J Obstet Gynecol.* 2006;195(4):914–934.

72. Martin Jr JN, Rinehart BK, May WL, Magann EF, Terrone DA, Blake PG. The spectrum of severe preeclampsia: comparative analysis by HELLP (hemolysis, elevated liver enzyme levels, and low platelet count) syndrome classification. *Am J Obstet Gynecol.* 1999;180(6 Pt 1): 1373–1384.

73. Roberts WE, Perry Jr KG, Woods JB, Files JC, Blake PG, Martin Jr JN. The intrapartum platelet count in patients with HELLP (hemolysis, elevated liver enzymes, and low platelets) syndrome: is it predictive of later hemorrhagic complications? *Am J Obstet Gynecol.* 1994;171(3):799–804.

74. Socollov D, Ilea C, Lupascu IA, et al. Maternal-fetal prognosis in HELLP syndrome in a level 3 maternal-fetal care centre. *Clin Exp Obstet Gynecol.* 2016;43(3):374–378.

75. Asicioglu O, Gungorduk K, Yildirim G, Aslan H, Gunay T. Maternal and perinatal outcomes of eclampsia with and without HELLP syndrome in a teaching hospital in western Turkey. *J Obstet Gynaecol J Inst Obstet Gynaecol.* 2014;34(4):326–331.

76. Riely CA. Liver disease in the pregnant patient. American College of Gastroenterology. *Am J Gastroenterol.* 1999;94(7):1728–1732.

77. Knight M, Nelson-Piercy C, Kurinczuk JJ, Spark P, Brocklehurst P. A prospective national study of acute fatty liver of pregnancy in the UK. *Gut.* 2008;57(7):951–956.

78. Liu J, Ghaziani TT, Wolf JL. Acute fatty liver disease of pregnancy: updates in pathogenesis, diagnosis, and management. *Am J Gastroenterol.* 2017;112.

79. Minakami H, Morikawa M, Yamada T, Yamada T, Akaishi R, Nishida R. Differentiation of acute fatty liver of pregnancy from syndrome of hemolysis, elevated liver enzymes and low platelet counts. *J Obstet Gynaecol Res.* 2014;40(3):641–649.

80. Nelson DB, Yost NP, Cunningham FG. Hemostatic dysfunction with acute fatty liver of pregnancy. *Obstet Gynecol.* 2014;124(1):40–46.

81. Battinelli EM. TTP and pregnancy. *Blood.* 2014;123(11): 1624–1625.

82. von Auer C, von Krogh AS, Kremer Hovinga JA, Lammle B. Current insights into thrombotic microangiopathies: thrombotic thrombocytopenic purpura and pregnancy. *Thromb Res.* 2015;135(suppl 1):S30–S33.

83. Vesely SK. Life after acquired thrombotic thrombocytopenic purpura: morbidity, mortality, and risks during pregnancy. *J Thromb Haemost.* 2015;13(suppl 1):S216–S222.

84. Jiang Y, McIntosh JJ, Reese JA, et al. Pregnancy outcomes following recovery from acquired thrombotic thrombocytopenic purpura. *Blood.* 2014;123(11):1674–1680.

85. Martin Jr JN, Bailey AP, Rehberg JF, Owens MT, Keiser SD, May WL. Thrombotic thrombocytopenic purpura in 166 pregnancies: 1955-2006. *Am J Obstet Gynecol.* 2008;199(2):98–104.

86. Scully M. Thrombotic thrombocytopenic purpura and atypical hemolytic uremic syndrome microangiopathy in pregnancy. *Semin Thromb Hemost.* 2016;42(7):774–779.

87. Scully M, Thomas M, Underwood M, et al. Thrombotic thrombocytopenic purpura and pregnancy: presentation, management, and subsequent pregnancy outcomes. *Blood.* 2014;124(2):211–219.

88. Erez O, Mastrolia SA, Thachil J. Disseminated intravascular coagulation in pregnancy: insights in pathophysiology, diagnosis and management. *Am J Obstet Gynecol.* 2015;213(4):452–463.

89. Szecsi PB, Jorgensen M, Klajnbard A, Andersen MR, Colov NP, Stender S. Haemostatic reference intervals in pregnancy. *Thromb Haemost.* 2010;103(4):718–727.

90. Richey ME, Gilstrap 3rd LC, Ramin SM. Management of disseminated intravascular coagulopathy. *Clin Obstet Gynecol.* 1995;38(3):514–520.

91. Erez O. Disseminated intravascular coagulation in pregnancy - clinical phenotypes and diagnostic scores. *Thromb Res.* 2017;151(suppl 1):S56–s60.

92. Lurie S, Feinstein M, Mamet Y. Disseminated intravascular coagulopathy in pregnancy: thorough comprehension of etiology and management reduces obstetricians' stress. *Arch Gynecol Obstet.* 2000;263(3):126–130.

93. Taylor Jr FB, Toh CH, Hoots WK, Wada H, Levi M. Towards definition, clinical and laboratory criteria, and a scoring system for disseminated intravascular coagulation. *Thromb Haemost.* 2001;86(5):1327–1330.
94. Erez O, Novack L, Beer-Weisel R, et al. DIC score in pregnant women–a population based modification of the International Society on Thrombosis and Hemostasis score. *PLoS One.* 2014;9(4):e93240.
95. Jonard M, Ducloy-Bouthors AS, Fourrier F. Comparison of two diagnostic scores of disseminated intravascular coagulation in pregnant women admitted to the ICU. *PLoS One.* 2016;11(11):e0166471.
96. Iba T. Harmonized guidance for disseminated intravascular coagulation from the International Society on Thrombosis and Haemostasis and the current status of anticoagulant therapy in Japan. *J Thromb Haemost.* 2013;11(11):2076–2078.
97. Wada H, Thachil J, Di Nisio M, et al. Guidance for diagnosis and treatment of DIC from harmonization of the recommendations from three guidelines. *J Thromb Haemost.* 2013. http://dx.doi.org/10.1111/jth.12155.
98. Wada H, Thachil J, Di Nisio M, Kurosawa S, Gando S, Toh CH. Harmonized guidance for disseminated intravascular coagulation from the International Society on Thrombosis and Haemostasis and the current status of anticoagulant therapy in Japan: a rebuttal. *J Thromb Haemost.* 2013;11(11):2078–2079.
99. Bussel JB, Berkowitz RL, Lynch L, et al. Antenatal management of alloimmune thrombocytopenia with intravenous gamma-globulin: a randomized trial of the addition of low-dose steroid to intravenous gamma-globulin. *Am J Obstet Gynecol.* 1996;174(5):1414–1423.
100. Curtis BR. Recent progress in understanding the pathogenesis of fetal and neonatal alloimmune thrombocytopenia. *Br J Haematol.* 2015;171(5):671–682.
101. Peterson JA, McFarland JG, Curtis BR, Aster RH. Neonatal alloimmune thrombocytopenia: pathogenesis, diagnosis and management. *Br J Haematol.* 2013;161(1):3–14.
102. Bussel JB, Zabusky MR, Berkowitz RL, McFarland JG. Fetal alloimmune thrombocytopenia. *N Engl J Med.* 1997;337(1):22–26.
103. Thrombocytopenia in Pregnancy. ACOG practice bulletin No. 166. American College of obstetricians and gynecologists. *Obstet Gynecol.* 2016;128(3):e43–e53.
104. Lakkaraja M, Berkowitz RL, Vinograd CA, et al. Omission of fetal sampling in treatment of subsequent pregnancies in fetal-neonatal alloimmune thrombocytopenia. *Am J Obstet Gynecol.* 2016;215(4):471. e471–479.
105. Chakravorty S, Roberts I. How I manage neonatal thrombocytopenia. *Br J Haematol.* 2012;156(2):155–162.
106. Kiefel V, Bassler D, Kroll H, et al. Antigen-positive platelet transfusion in neonatal alloimmune thrombocytopenia (NAIT). *Blood.* 2006;107(9):3761–3763.
107. WHO. *WHO Recommendations for the Prevention and Treatment of Postpartum Hemorrhage;* 2012. http://apps.who.int/iris/bitstream/10665/75411/1/9789241548502_eng.pdf?ua=1.
108. Abdul-Kadir R, McLintock C, Ducloy AS, et al. Evaluation and management of postpartum hemorrhage: consensus from an international expert panel. *Transfusion.* 2014;54(7):1756–1768.
109. Oyelese Y, Ananth CV. Postpartum hemorrhage: epidemiology, risk factors, and causes. *Clin Obstet Gynecol.* 2010;53(1):147–156.
110. Prevention, Management of Postpartum Haemorrhage: Green-top guideline No. 52. *BJOG Int J Obstet Gynaecol.* 2017;124(5):e106–e149.
111. Klufio CA, Amoa AB, Kariwiga G. Primary postpartum haemorrhage: causes, aetiological risk factors, prevention and management. *Papua New Guin Med J.* 1995;38(2):133–149.
112. Green L, Knight M, Seeney FM, et al. The epidemiology and outcomes of women with postpartum haemorrhage requiring massive transfusion with eight or more units of red cells: a national cross-sectional study. *BJOG Int J Obstet Gynaecol.* 2016;123(13):2164–2170.
113. Effect of early tranexamic acid administration on mortality, hysterectomy, and other morbidities in women with post-partum haemorrhage (WOMAN): an international, randomised, double-blind, placebo-controlled trial. *Lancet (London, Engl).* 2017;389(10084):2105–2116.
114. Lavigne-Lissalde G, Aya AG, Mercier FJ, et al. Recombinant human FVIIa for reducing the need for invasive second-line therapies in severe refractory postpartum hemorrhage: a multicenter, randomized, open controlled trial. *J Thromb Haemost.* 2015;13(4):520–529.
115. Ahonen J. The role of recombinant activated factor VII in obstetric hemorrhage. *Curr Opin Anaesthesiol.* 2012;25(3):309–314.
116. Peyvandi F, Menegatti M, Siboni SM. Post-partum hemorrhage in women with rare bleeding disorders. *Thromb Res.* 2011;127(suppl 3):S116–S119.

CHAPTER 12

Transfusion Approaches in the Transplanted Patient

LJILJANA V. VASOVIC, MD • ROBERT A. DESIMONE, MD • RUCHIKA GOEL, MD, MPH

BACKGROUND

Transplantation is one of the most intriguing and challenging advances of modern medicine with a rapidly expanding scope of application. Blood transfusion support is critical in transplant patient recovery.[1] A careful consideration needs to be given to balancing the benefits and risks of transfusions in transplant populations owing to their complex management. Patient blood management (PBM) programs have had a major impact on transfusion practices in all subspecialties, including hematology and oncology, but nuances specific for transplant recipients remain to be standardized.

A bone marrow transplant (BMT) program requires dedicated and knowledgeable personnel, as well as administrative support, and a close working relationship with their institution's blood bank (BB) to streamline the procurement of required blood components to support transplant patients.

For patients with advanced stages of hematologic malignancies such as acute myeloid leukemia and acute lymphoblastic leukemia, an allogeneic hematopoietic stem cell transplant (HSCT) is often the only therapeutic option that offers either potential for cure or prolongation of lifespan.[2] Hematopoietic progenitor cell (HPC) transplants have resulted in survival rates greater than 90% for some hematologic malignancies.[3] According to the National Marrow Donor Program, approximately 20,000 patients in the United States receive either autologous transplants, or, if needed, allogeneic HSCT each year from a matched related donor (MRD) or matched unrelated donors (MUD).[4–6] However, this is dependent on an optimal or best available graft source selected between bone marrow, mobilized peripheral-blood stem cells, or umbilical cord blood based on the degree of matching and stem cell dose required.[7–9]

COMPLEX IMMUNE SYSTEM INTERACTIONS IN TRANSPLANT PATIENTS

Exposure to cells foreign to a transplant recipient leads to immune system activation or suppression brought about by tumor cells, transplant, transfusion, pregnancy, and infectious microorganisms. The interaction of two distinct allogeneic immune systems following transplant, that of the donor and that of the recipient, leads to a major immune system imbalance. A recipient's immune system is presented with a plethora of new antigens (Ag) after a transplant. Human leukocyte antigens (HLAs) belong to major histocompatibility complexes and are a major player in graft rejection, graft-versus-host disease (GVHD), and a graft-versus-tumor effect.[10,11] HLAs are of primary clinical significance because the HLA mismatch represents one of the major barriers to a successful HSCT. Anti-HLA antibodies (Ab) in conjunction with cellular immune responses can cause either acute or chronic transplant rejection, and donor specific antibody reactivity can directly influence transplant outcome.[12] However, immunization rates are dependent not only on the immunogenicity of a specific Ag but also on donor-recipient HLA differences and the relative immunocompromised state of the recipient secondary to chemotherapy. HLA matching often determines the degree of reactivity; however, with current immunosuppressive therapy even haploidentical transplants are feasible.[13] In some cases, transplant can be even more complicated with multiple transplant donors of unrelated stem cells such as cord transplant in which cells from each cord vie for dominance (double cord) or in the setting of a combination of cord transplant and haploidentical hematopoietic progenitor cell transplant (HPCT) (Haplo-Cord).[14] Minor histocompatibility antigens contribute to the complexity of the immune interactions, including human erythrocyte antigen (HEA), and human platelet antigens (HPAs) are among those well described in the literature. Another important challenge to the host's immune system comes from the allogeneic transfusion support itself so that transfused blood has been described as a form of a "liquid transplant."[15] Blood transfusion can immunize recipients to allogeneic HEA, HLA, and HPA. Clinically, significant alloantibodies against HEA, HLA, and platelets (PLTs) can be detected well before the actual transplant. Pregnancy-related alloimmunization is a major source of pretransplant anti-HLA and anti-HEA antibodies. Interestingly, pregnancy also can be a source of tolerance based on long-term fetomaternal microchimerism and generation of protective antitumor immunity. Characterization of graft-recipient interactions based on acquired immunologic hyporesponsiveness to noninherited maternal antigens[16] or inherited paternal antigens can be considered for improving transplant outcome.[17,18] ABO Ag have wide tissue expression, most notably expressed on the endothelium and soluble plasma proteins, including vWF.[19,20] Other HEAs have divergent patterns of tissue distribution.[21,22] Rh Ag are restricted to red blood cells (RBCs); however, Lewis (Le), Duffy (Fy) have both epithelial and endothelial expression.[23] In regard to PLT transfusions, both anti-HLA and anti-HPA alloimmunization can contribute to poor posttransplant PLT recovery as well as to unsuccessful response to PLT transfusions, i.e., PLT transfusion refractoriness. Separately, a noteworthy body of literature on transfusion-related immunomodulation especially in the setting of solid organ transplants (SOTs) may lead to a greater dependency on stronger immunosuppression protocols.[24,25] ABO-incompatible neonatal heart transplant has been successfully achieved if performed before the production of anti-donor A/B.[26,27] This is because children more readily accept ABO-incompatible organs because of the potential to induce donor-specific tolerance.[28,29] Immunization occurring post transplant can be caused by the graft itself. Transfusion in the posttransplant period can stimulate residual cells of a recipient's immune system, mature donor derived "passenger" lymphocytes or de novo produced naïve lymphocytes after engraftment. At present, this is more commonly observed because of the use of reduced-intensity conditioning. In addition, graft-derived passenger lymphocytes of donor origin are sources of alloimmunization against recipient-mismatched antigens. Donor registries do not routinely perform extended RBC phenotyping of potential donors. As a result, it is indeed challenging to provide blood components fully antigen matched or even compatible to both the recipient and the donor beyond basic ABO/Rh matching. At times, it can be difficult to distinguish alloimmunization because of the graft or posttransplant transfusions, and in these cases, chimerism analyses can be extended to RBC Ag in specific situations.[30,31] In light of these immune interactions, treatment with immunosuppressive medications must carefully balance a recipient's underlying disease state, transplant match, and potential for infections.

ABO Incompatibility in Stem Cell Transplant

ABO-incompatible stem cell transplants are feasible because hematopoietic stem cells, early pluripotent stem cells, and early committed HPCs do not express ABO antigens. HLA and ABO antigens are expressed on different genes and have independent inheritance. In this type of transplants, because HLA matching supersedes ABO matching, approximately 20%–40% of allogeneic transplants are ABO incompatible, which demands special requirements for blood matching in this population.[32,33] To minimize transplant-related complications, a combination of immunosuppression, anticipatory adverse effect management that includes transfusion support, and ultimately long-term tolerance is key to transplant success. In view of the immunization challenges described previously, the basic doctrine of matching in transplants is to minimize as much as possible the effect of the mismatch based on the following hierarchy: HLA > ABO > HEA in the immunized recipient.

In allogeneic transplant, relationships between the donor and recipient ABO fall into four categories:
1. ABO identical transplant
2. ABO major incompatible transplant
3. ABO compatible, e.g., minor incompatible transplant
4. ABO bidirectional incompatible transplant

ABO identical transplants have the same consideration regarding transfusion as any other oncology patient. ABO-compatible transplants are characterized by the recipient's anti-A or anti-B isohemagglutinins reacting against the corresponding donor ABO Ag. This minor incompatibility is directed against the recipient RBC and ABO antigens expressed throughout (solid organ) and plasma-soluble substances. Please refer to Fig. 12.1 for ABO major and minor compatibility combinations and an illustration of isohemagglutinin immunoreactivity direction.

On the other hand, major ABO-incompatible transplants are characterized by the presence of A or B or both Ag on donor RBCs and in the case of SOTs on the endothelium, which can be recognized by a recipient's isohemagglutinins. Furthermore, there are several considerations that are unique to ABO and other HEA-mismatched antigens in allogeneic transplants that need to be taken into account. These may include the relationship between the timing of cellular therapy product (CTP) infusion and prompt postinfusion test result interpretation in the management of immune-mediated hemolysis.[34,35]

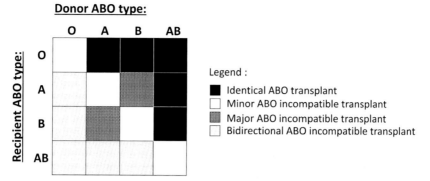

FIG. 12.1 ABO compatibility relationships in transplant.

Clinical Consequences Associated With Red Blood Cell Antigen-Mismatched Allogeneic Hematopoietic Progenitor Cell Transplant

Hemolysis can be encountered at the time of hematopoietic stem cell infusion as an acute reaction or at a later time as a chronic presentation of varying length ranging from few days to months (see Fig. 12.2).[33,36]

Acute hemolytic reaction due to major ABO incompatibility

CTP can contain significant amounts of donor RBCs and plasma. Mostly, the HPC source determines the volume of contaminating RBC in the stem cell product. The total volume of bone marrow (BM) products is generally large, 1–1.5 liters (L); they usually have a high hematocrit (20%–30%) and large amount of isohemagglutinins and thus have a significant risk of immediate immune-mediated hemolysis. Since the mid 1980s, transplants have been increasingly conducted with mobilized HPCs collected by apheresis (HPC-A) from peripheral blood. Compared with HPC from marrow (HPC-M), HPC-A products contain a much smaller RBC volume (20–40 mL) and smaller plasma volume (150–300 mL), minimizing the risk of immediate immune-mediated hemolysis. Similarly, after standard RBC and plasma reduction, the total volume of the cord blood product is about 20 mL, which results in minimal to no risk of acute hemolysis.

In contrast, for major ABO incompatibility, if the RBC content of the BM product is determined to be above the tolerable limit (20–40 mL for adult recipients), red cell reduction may be necessary. For pediatric recipients, RBC reduction is done if the estimated RBC volume is found to be more than 0.4 mL/kg of the recipient's weight. RBC depletion may also be done on an ABO-identical or autologous bone marrow product before cryopreservation if large amounts of RBCs are present. The reason for this is to minimize significant hemolysis secondary to product processing; however, this is part of standard laboratory practice (see Chapter 14).[23] If hemolysis does occur, treatment includes hydration, acidification, and postponement of the remainder of the infusion. RBC or plasma exchange can potentially be done in severe cases following the blood type selection outlined in transplant patients' guidelines given later in the discussion.

Delayed engraftment/pure red cell aplasia

Very high recipient isohemagglutinin titers in major ABO-incompatible transplants can cause chronic hemolysis of donor RBCs, leading to delayed engraftment and in severe cases development of pure red cell aplasia (PRCA).[37,38] Red cell lineage engraftment can be defined as the number of days until the reticulocyte count is $\geq 25 \times 10^9/L$.[39] The patient is transfusion dependent until a recipient's isohemagglutinin titer declines sufficiently to allow engraftment of newly emerging donor reticulocytes, and this may take up to 3–4 months. Time to red cell engraftment is further prolonged if nonmyeloablative regimens or reduced-intensity conditioning is used. In the BB, direct antiglobulin test (DAT) positivity with isohemagglutinin in eluate tested on A and/or B expressing reagent cells precedes full engraftment. As RBC engraftment proceeds, DAT becomes negative, and with sustained RBC production transfusion needs gradually decrease.

Various therapeutic modalities have been used for the treatment of prolonged PRCA, which include high-dose corticosteroids and rituximab.[40,41] Efficacy of therapeutic plasma exchange (TPE) for PRCA treatment has been established, but it is currently reserved only for severe cases.[42] An additional option is the use

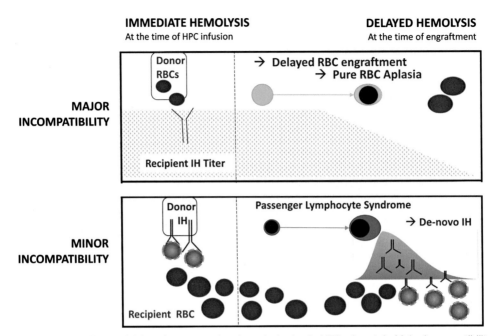

FIG. 12.2 Immediate and delayed posttransplant hemolysis due to HEA mismatch. Major incompatibility, e.g., A to O can lead to immediate hemolysis at the time of infusion or delayed engraftment. Minor incompatibility, e.g., O to A, whereby the recipient is transfused O RBC in anticipation of transplant to minimize potential of immediate or delayed hemolysis. Bidirectional incompatibility, e.g., A to B can cause both complications. *HEA*, human erythrocyte antigen; *IH*, isohemagglutinin; *RBC*, red blood cell.

of immunoadsorption for the removal of residual persistent isohemagglutinins in refractory cases; however, these processes are not currently approved for use in the United States.[43–45] Factors that complicate the diagnosis of PRCA are the determination of stem cell dose appropriateness, extent of disease, and chemotherapy conditioning regimen effect on BM niche, as well as concurrent iron deficiency and presence of microangiopathic hemolytic anemia (MAHA) processes.

Acute hemolytic reaction due to minor ABO incompatibility
If isohemagglutinin titers in an HPC collection product exceed 1:256, acute infusion-related hemolysis attributable to ABO incompatibility may be seen. For donors with known high plasma isohemagglutinin titers, to reduce risk of minor incompatibility, HPC products are plasma reduced. This type of HPC plasma reduction is performed routinely and is part of cryopreservation protocols. This is analogous to RBC depletion in major incompatible transplants.

Passenger lymphocyte syndrome
In minor-incompatible HSCT, about 5–15 days post transplant, the presence of donor lymphocytes can lead to the generation of significant titers of anti-A and/or anti-B against residual recipient RBCs. This phenomenon, called "passenger lymphocyte syndrome" (PLS), can result in recipients experiencing acute, immune-mediated hemolysis.[46] Fortunately, in most cases, hemolysis is not severe and eventually subsides with clearance of recipient RBCs.[37] If hemolysis is severe, automated red cell exchange (RCE) might be needed to remove recipient RBCs and replace with donor-compatible RBCs. Prophylactic RCE can be performed in recipients at high risk of PLS. Treatment with anti-CD20 Ab (rituximab) is also available for persistent cases.[47] Isohemagglutinins derived from passenger lymphocytes frequently do not persist for long, presenting only as posttransplant ABO discrepancy.[36]

OTHER CAUSES OF POSTTRANSPLANT HEMOLYSIS
In some cases, autoimmune hemolytic anemia (AIHA), DAT-negative IgA AIHA, and thrombotic microangiopathy have to be considered in the differential diagnosis of posttransplant hemolysis. Cases have been reported in both HPCT and SOTs. Nonimmune causes of hemolysis also need to be in the differential diagnosis of a

hemolysis workup. Cryopreservation can lead to hemolysis owing to osmotic shock after cryopreservation injury. This is dependent on the RBC volume, especially after BMT, which may necessitate washing of the product before administration.

Other Consequences of Transplant Mismatch Pertinent to Transplant Outcomes

ABO incompatibility has been extensively investigated in allogeneic bone marrow transplant, and its impact does not preclude successful transplant outcome. However, ABO incompatibility has been shown to be an independent adverse risk factor for GVHD and lowers the disease-free and overall survival rates. Increased risks with major, minor, and bidirectional incompatibility have been reported over time. Isohemagglutinin titers change after ABO-incompatible allogeneic stem cell transplant and become less consequential as time progresses after transplant. Also, improved overall clinical management and transfusion support contribute to successful outcomes.[48]

Graft-Versus-Host Disease Has Higher Risk in ABO Minor Incompatible Transplant

GVHD is a common complication of allogeneic CTPs containing mature lymphocytes against minor histocompatibility genes. There is a higher risk in minor ABO incompatibility mediated by isohemagglutinin reacting to ABO Ag on the recipient endothelium leading to cell activation. Another possibility is the formation of immune complexes between isohemagglutinins and soluble ABO antigens contributing to amplification of a bystander effect.[49] Importantly, donor lymphocytes express A, B, H (ABO antigen family) in addition to Le[a] and Le[b] Ag depending on the ABH secretor status of the donor, which might result in removal of GVHD reactive lymphocytes.[50]

Cellular Therapy Product Manipulations to Prevent Acute Hemolysis Postinfusion

The direction of ABO incompatibility and strength of isohemagglutinin titers may require product processing to avoid infusion that can be associated with hemolysis. For major ABO-incompatible transplants, RBC reduction, and for minor ABO-incompatible HPCT, volume reduction, or both for bidirectional ABO-incompatible HPCT are standard laboratory procedures before cryopreservation (see Table 12.1).

CD34 selected cellular therapy product

Recipients of CD34-selected HPCs, which are devoid of plasma and passenger lymphocytes, are not at risk of developing acute or delayed hemolytic reactions.

TABLE 12.1
Standard Cellular Therapy Product Modifications Based on ABO Incompatibility and Isohemagglutinin (IH) Titer

ABO Mismatched Transplant	IH Titer	Cellular Therapy Product Processing
Major	Recipient IH Anti-donor titer: ≥32	RBC depletion: if RBC content is >20 mL or >0.4 mL/kg
Minor	Donor IH Anti-recipient RBC titer: ≥1:256	Plasma depletion of graft

RBC, red blood cell.

TRANSFUSION STRATEGIES FOR TRANSPLANT PATIENTS

Human Erythrocyte Antigen–Compatible Blood Product Selection for Transfusion

Special consideration is given to provision of safe and appropriate components in the transplant setting. Measures regarding prevention of communicable diseases and other potential adverse effects of transfusion are vigilantly enforced in transplant recipients because they encompass a vulnerable population prone to infections, thrombosis, and bleeding.[51,52] General requirements such as irradiation, leukoreduction, and cytomegalovirus-negative transfusion of cellular blood components are generally accepted by the transplant medical community. However, regarding the selection of ABO, Rh(D), and other HEA-matched units for transfusion support remains without clear guidance, and there is no unequivocal evidence obtained by randomized clinical trials suggesting the best strategy to follow.[53] Therefore decisions are left to the individual BB, transfusion medicine physicians, and transplant center to establish when, what, and why to transfuse. Existing protocols for component selection are based on several published transfusion guideline strategies supported by experience of individual transplant centers and literature review.

BB tests to be performed in the setting of transplant should include at a minimum: ABO front and back type (paying close attention to reaction strength and isohemagglutinin titer), antibody screen/antibody identification, DAT, and eluate testing if indicated. Once testing is performed, there should be an evaluation by clinicians with assistance from transfusion medicine physicians to establish the need of transfusion and to resolve instances in which less than optimal blood component units may need to be washed, or if ABO-incompatible PLTs need to be transfused owing inventory limitations. Decision to transfuse incompatible PLTs must take into account acceptable risks, specifically possibility of bleeding versus remote risk due to infusion of incompatible plasma. This situation is especially difficult if PLT refractoriness is a concern.

ABO-Compatible Blood Transfusion Selection

Transfusion requirements can be significant after HPCT, may be associated with transplant-related morbidity, and can affect long-term survival outcome. To provide transfusion support to a recipient, the transplant procedure is subdivided into three phases:

- Phase I: Pretransplant conditioning.
- Phase II: Peritransplant. Dynamic chimera: both recipient and donor RBCs and isohemagglutinins are detectable. Mixed-field ABO testing, positive DAT.
- Phase III: Post donor RBC engraftment, loss of recipient RBC and isohemagglutinins, negative DAT.

Pretransplant or phase I

Blood component support and transfusion indications are similar to any hematologic malignancy. Irradiated, leukoreduced, CMV-safe or CMV-negative components are provided. Special needs should be communicated to the BB so that information is recorded in the laboratory information system (LIS). Additional information to be included is avoidance of donations from family members of RBC, PLT, or granulocytes to prevent alloimmunization against minor histocompatibility and private antigens, thereby increasing risk of graft rejection.

Peritransplant or phase II

RBCs and plasma must be ABO compatible to both the recipient and the donor(s) in phase II (see Box 12.1, Fig. 12.3).

Major ABO-incompatible transplant. These transplants include type O recipient with donor of type A, B, or AB; AB donor to type A or type B recipient; type A donor to type B recipient; or type B donor to type A recipient.

Complications. During stem cell infusion severe hemolysis can occur; as a result, RBC depletion must be done during processing of product (HPC-M containing large RBC volume). As mentioned before, HPC-A products usually have less than 20–30 mL of RBC and usually do not cause severe hemolysis. If a recipient has

very high anti-A or anti-B titers, TPE can be considered before HPC product infusion. In this type of transplant, posttransplant RBC transfusion requirement may be high.

Blood transfusion. During phase II, a recipient's anti A or anti B continues to circulate in the recipient's blood (half-life 3 weeks) and DAT is positive. During this phase, transfused RBC should be of recipient type until DAT is negative. However, plasma components must be of donor type to prevent delayed engraftment of donor cells. However, if the recipient's anti-A or anti-B titer is high, there can be delayed RBC engraftment, and in very rare cases PRCA can develop.

An interesting and nearly forgotten method of in vivo adsorption of recipient isohemagglutinins is a low-cost technique performed in Europe to circumvent immediate and delayed hemolysis after ABO-incompatible stem cell transplant. In this approach, if a recipient's isohemagglutinin titer is <1:32, ABO-incompatible RBCs (matching donor type in major ABO-incompatible HPCT) are slowly transfused, monitoring the recipient's vital signs at an intensive care unit. The antibodies would bind to RBC, leading to a decrease in the antibody titer. Isohemagglutinin titers were controlled after each ABO-incompatible transfusion, and in the case of O/A recipient/donor blood group transplant, one or two units of A2 and A1 RBCs were sufficient. Additional benefit was that ABO-incompatible transfusion strategy also obviated the need for RBC reduction, improving the quality of an unmanipulated graft.[54]

Minor ABO-incompatible transplant. This can occur, for example, if the recipient is type A and the donor is type O, among other combinations.

Complications. The HPC product should undergo plasma depletion during processing to avoid hemolysis of incompatible circulating recipient RBCs.

Blood transfusion. Red cells must be of the donor's type. PLTs and plasma must be of the recipient's type and continue in phase III and indefinitely. The reason is to protect the endothelium from damage, as they express ABO antigens.

Bidirectional ABO-incompatible transplant. This can occur, for example, if the recipient is type A and the donor is type B, or vice versa.

Complications. HPC bone marrow product may require both RBC depletion and plasma depletion to minimize hemolysis.

Blood transfusion. It is recommended to use type O RBCs and type AB plasma and platelets indefinitely post-transplant.

BOX 12.1
Practical Considerations for Transfusion Component Selection in Transplant Recipients

Provide all blood components compatible to both the recipient and the donor(s) whenever possible.

RBC SELECTION
1. RBCs must be ABO compatible to both the recipient and the donor(s) in phase II; see Figs. 12.3 and 12.4.
   - For minor ABO-incompatible transplants: RBC transfusions must always be of donor type.
   - For major and bidirectional ABO-incompatible transplants: Donor type RBCs should be provided in phase III after RBC engraftment, isohemagglutinins are undetectable, and DAT becomes negative.
   - Change ABO type to donor blood type if recipient's isohemagglutinins are not detectable in two consecutive blood samples, DAT is negative, and no RBC transfusions for at least 90 days.
   - For AB-identical transplant, the second choice for RBC is A, followed by B RBC, and lastly followed by O RBC.
   - Complex ABO matching for double transplant might be required.
2. Rh-negative RBC should be provided if either the recipient or the donor is Rh negative to prevent anti-D alloimmunization until the blood type is changed.
3. Extended phenotypically matched RBC, compatible to both the recipient and the donor may be provided when unexpected alloantibodies are present.

PLASMA SELECTION
1. Plasma should be ABO compatible to both the recipient and the donor(s) in all phases indefinitely.
   - The second choice for plasma is always AB, except for an O-identical transplant in which type A is the second choice owing to inventory management.

PLATELET SELECTION
1. Platelets contain large amounts of plasma and should be ABO compatible to both the recipient and the

donor given availability, or follow plasma compatibility/second choice as outlined in Fig. 12.4.
   - Platelets resuspended in platelet additive solution have a reduced volume of incompatible plasma, and are an alternative at many institutions to washing of ABO-incompatible platelets.
   - Low-titer A-type platelets or A2-platelets may be acceptable choices in the absence of AB platelets.
   - *Major transplant incompatibility*: Donor-compatible platelets are preferred as a second choice to avoid isohemagglutinins directed against donor RBCs leading to delayed RBC engraftment.
   - *Minor transplant incompatibility*: Recipient-compatible platelets are the preferred second choice to avoid hemolysis of residual recipient RBCs and formation of ABO isohemagglutinins-Ag immune complexes, and to protect the recipient's endothelium.
   - *Bidirectional transplant incompatibility*: Donor-compatible platelets are the preferred second choice.
2. Rh-negative platelet products should be provided if either the recipient or the donor is Rh negative.
   - Rh immunoglobulin IM or IV administration may be provided following Rh-positive platelet transfusions if both the recipient and the donor are Rh negative and/or after engraftment and Rh change to Rh negative (donor type).
3. If required, HLA-matched or crossmatched platelets take precedence over ABO selection.
   - Washed platelets as per Fig. 12.4. Matching takes into account ABO expression on platelets.
4. For practical reasons, many centers may select incompatible platelets close to their expiration date even if younger matched/identical platelets are available. Increased risks of thrombosis and negative transplant outcome when using incompatible platelet transfusion have not been widely studied and might require larger studies.

DAT, direct antiglobulin test; *HLA*, human leukocyte antigen; *IM*, intramuscular; *IV*, intravenous; *RBC*, red blood cells.

Postengraftment or phase III

Once engraftment has occurred, special needs can be changed to transfuse donor type RBCs for any ABO-incompatible transplant.

Major ABO-incompatible transplant: PLTs and plasma should be of donor type.

Minor ABO-incompatible and bidirectional incompatible transplant: PLTs and plasma should be of recipient type.

Post-engraftment of donor RBCs, disappearance of recipient RBCs and isohemagglutinins, and confirmation that the DAT is negative, one can change the recipient's ABO blood type to the donor blood type, as long as the recipient has been transfusion-independent for at least 90 days (Fig. 12.4).

In phase III, when recipient RBCs and isohemagglutinins become undetectable, donor RBCs have

ABO Type Selection for RBC Transfusion		
	Phase II: Peri-Transplant Recipient IH detectable / DAT+	Phase III: Post engraftment ABO type switched to donors
Major ABO Incompatible Transplant	RECIPIENT TYPE RBC	DONOR TYPE RBC
Minor ABO Incompatible Transplant	DONOR TYPE RBC	DONOR TYPE RBC
Bidirectional Transplant	O RBC	DONOR TYPE RBC

ABO Type Selection for Plasma (Platelet) Transfusion		
	Phase II: Peri-Transplant Recipient IH detectable / DAT+	Phase III: Post engraftment ABO type switched to donors
Major ABO Incompatible Transplant	DONOR TYPE PLASMA	DONOR TYPE PLASMA
Minor ABO Incompatible Transplant	RECIPIENT TYPE PLASMA	DONOR TYPE PLASMA
Bidirectional Transplant	AB Plasma	AB Plasma

FIG. 12.3 Strategy for provision of blood components in ABO-mismatched HPCT. *DAT*, direct antiglobulin test; *HPCT*, hematopoietic progenitor cell transplant; *IH*, isohemagglutinin; *RBC*, red blood cell. (Adapted from Murphy MF, Stanworth SJ. Haematological disease. In: Murphy MF, Pamphilon DH, eds. *Practical Transfusion Medicine*. 3rd ed. Hoboken: Wiley-Blackwell Publishers; 2009; with permission.)

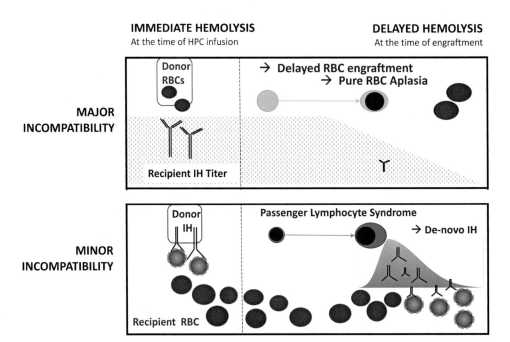

FIG. 12.4 Transfusion components ABO type selection for ABO-mismatched transplant recipients.

engrafted, and DAT becomes negative, then donor type RBCs should be provided.

For minor ABO-incompatible transplants, RBC transfusions should be of the recipient type.

ABO-Compatible Blood Components Provision for Patients With Multiple Transplants

In the case of multiple transplants such as double cord and Haplo-Cord, all components should be compatible to both the donors and the recipient. Plasma and PLTs should be selected to protect cord cells in the case of Haplo-Cord. These transplants have similar RBC and PLT recovery as adult MRD/MUD transplants. In Haplo-Cord transplants, ABO and RhD incompatibility and acute GVHD are the major determinants of erythroid recovery. Acute GVHD is a major determinant of PLT recovery.[55]

Beyond ABO, HEA: RhD, K, Fy, Jk Matching

Transfusions that are matched for ABO type represent the first example of "precision medicine."[53] Non-ABO RBC alloantibodies have been reported as causes of posttransplant hemolysis following allogeneic hematopoietic stem cell transplant. A number of published reports have described clinically significant RBC Ag, such as Rh, Kell, Duffy, and Kidd system, mismatch leading to acute major and minor hemolysis, as well as delayed RBC engraftment, PRCA, and PLS.[56,57] HEA antigens are also expressed in other tissues and may act as minor histocompatibility antigens in solid organ transplants, e.g., renal allograft rejection. The most common example is RhD alloimmunization. Rh-negative RBCs should be provided if either the recipient or the donor is Rh negative to prevent generation of anti-D until the blood type can be changed. Extended phenotypically matched RBCs, compatible to both the recipient and the donor, may be provided when unexpected alloantibodies are present.

Pretransplant Genotyping

The molecular basis of HEA has been established for more than 300 antigens grouped into 34 antigenic group systems by the International Society of Blood Transfusion. Molecular gene polymorphisms responsible for the different blood-group antigens have been identified.[58] A single mutation in the DNA sequence, i.e., single-nucleotide polymorphism, has led to the development of several blood groups by molecular- and protein-based testing systems.

The RBC phenotype can be reliably predicted from genotype results. Interestingly, genotyping is more challenging for ABO and Rh systems. This is because genes encoding ABO transferases, enzymes involved in carbohydrate antigen modification, and Rh system Ag are associated with a large number of insertions and deletions and hybrid gene formation.

Methodologies for genotyping, such as multiplex systems, can be optimized for the simultaneous detection of multiple HLA, HEA, and HPA antigens to coordinate transplant and transfusion management. In this regard, RBC genotyping may be implemented in the future for routine pretransplant testing of transplant recipients and donors.[59] Multiplex genotyping systems for the simultaneous detection of RBC, HPA, and molecular HLA may allow the screening of individuals and large populations of donors. This practice can be coimplemented along with informatics systems to compare transplant patients' antigen profiles with available antigen-negative and/or rare blood-typed donors. This practice shows promise for improving the efficiency, reliability, and extent of RBC-matching in transplant-recipient populations.[60]

GENERAL CONSIDERATIONS FOR BLOOD COMPONENT TRANSFUSIONS FOR HEMATOPOIETIC PROGENITOR CELL TRANSPLANT

Certain modifications are necessary for transplant recipients. This involves leukoreduction, CMV-safe/CMV-negative status, and irradiation of cellular components.[61] Depending on a transplant center's needs, these special requirements may need to be implemented as a universal policy or entered under "special needs" in the BB LIS.[62]

Irradiated Components

Transfusion-associated graft-versus-host disease (TA-GVHD), a rare but extremely serious adverse effect that occurs after transfusion in immunocompromised patients, is associated with a mortality rate of >90%.[63] TA-GVHD often presents with nonspecific clinical symptoms similar to underlying transplant complications, such as fever, skin rash, diarrhea, and pancytopenia. Recognition and proper diagnosis may be delayed, thereby delaying treatment and contributing to high mortality. Furthermore, TA-GVHD has been reported in SOT recipients.[64] Irradiation of all cellular components for transfusion has been recommended as a standard modification for HPC transplant recipients. Universal irradiation has been adopted as a pragmatic approach in large medical centers with a significant at-risk recipient population. Leukoreduction does not prevent TA-GVHD (see later discussion).

Granulocyte components have a high content of lymphocytes and must be irradiated. Donor leukocyte infusions in certain posttransplant protocols are also irradiated to prevent GVHD.[65] However, HPC products must not be irradiated or leukoreduced. HLA-matched and partially matched PLTs have especially high risk of TA-GVHD owing to possible matched donor homozygosity. It is important to note that TA-GVHD might be difficult to distinguish from transplant-related acute and chronic GVHD. DNA short tandem repeat analysis can be performed to distinguish these processes by detecting the presence of multiple donor cells in affected recipients.[66,67]

Leukoreduced Components
Leukoreduction of RBC and PLT units is a standard procedure provided in all phases of transplant. Leukoreduction is important in reducing febrile nonhemolytic transfusion reactions, decreasing the rate of alloimmunization to HLA antigens, and reducing viral transmission risk. Currently, many centers perform universal leukoreduction as a standard procedure.

CMV-Negative Blood Products
CMV infection is a significant comorbidity in allogeneic transplants. It can affect almost any organ and result in pneumonia, gastrointestinal ulcers, or retinitis. Without prophylaxis, approximately 80% of CMV-seropositive patients develop CMV infection after allogeneic HCT.[68,69] Leukoreduced components are considered "CMV safe." These components are considered equally effective to CMV-negative components in preventing CMV transmission secondary to transfusion. "CMV-negative" components are usually reserved for cases in which both the recipient and the donor are CMV negative. However, safety of these components has been challenged because of the possibility that donor is in the window period of an active infection.

Pathogen Reduction
Infectious complications remain the most serious consequence of transfusion; CMV, Epstein–Barr virus (EBV), parvovirus, hepatitis B and C virus, and human immunodeficiency virus may have a more severe course in transplant patients who are immunosuppressed.[70-72] The pathogen residual risk of infectivity of blood components in immunocompromised transplant recipients might be substantial. In addition, there remains a risk of infectious agents, including Babesia, Zika, EBV, and many others, for which testing is still not performed or available, which could be mitigated with pathogen-reduction strategies. Pathogen-reduced RBCs are not yet available and are currently under investigation in clinical trials. Pathogen-reduced PLTs are now increasingly available. In regard to plasma, use of a solvent detergent to treat pooled plasma leading to destruction of enveloped viruses adds another layer of safety in immunocompromised recipients.

PATIENT BLOOD MANAGEMENT
PBM plays an essential role in optimizing the transfusion needs of a transplant service. PLT and RBC transfusion support is prescribed by institutional PBM guidelines following the three pillars of PBM:
1. optimization of hemostasis;
2. minimization of blood loss; and
3. elimination of unnecessary transfusions.

Red Blood Cell Transfusion
HPCT recipients have substantial transfusion needs until RBC engraftment occurs. Cord transplant recipients have especially prolonged time periods to RBC transfusion independence and have the slowest engraftment. Delayed engraftment in cord and double cord HPCT is a frequent phenomenon. As an effort toward minimizing transfusion needs, blood losses should be minimized. This could be achieved by minimizing phlebotomy and minimizing blood loss through potential bleeding sites (e.g., chronic gastrointestinal bleed, ulcers, genitourinary bleed, and menstrual losses in women). All necessary tooth extractions should be done before the transplant. Current guidelines in pediatric BMT recommend the use of combined hormonal contraceptive pills for menstrual suppression.[73] Nontransfusion alternatives for treating iron deficiency need to be used when possible. Lastly, for any hemorrhagic complication following diagnostic biopsies and interventions, optimization of hemostasis status to minimize perioperative transfusions should be done.

RBC transfusion guidelines
Most institutions still maintain posttransplant hemoglobin >8 g/dL and hematocrit ≥24% or higher in cases of symptomatic management of anemia or acute bleed. However, there is growing clinical evidence suggesting that successful implementation of health system-wide PBM program initiatives for transplant programs results in substantial reduction in blood component use and costs without increased morbidity or mortality in patients receiving intensive chemotherapy for HSCT.[74]

Platelet Transfusion

PLT transfusion guidelines: Prophylactic PLT transfusions have generally adopted a threshold of 10×10^9/L. When thrombocytopenia is associated with fever, sepsis, or splenomegaly, a threshold of 20×10^9/L may be appropriate. In an actively bleeding patient or if an invasive procedure is planned, a threshold of $>50 \times 10^9$/L is recommended, although individual services, such as neurology and ophthalmology, might establish a higher threshold of 100×10^9/L.[75]

PLTs express ABO antigens and only HLA class I antigens on their surface. They do not express Rh or HLA class II antigens. PLT components contain large amounts of plasma and thus should be ABO compatible to both the recipient and the donor, given availability, as outlined in Box 12.1 and Platelet first choice in Fig. 12.4. In some settings, washed PLTs compatible with both the donor and the recipient have been proposed.[76,77] Patients refractory to PLT transfusion should first be provided with "front type" ABO-compatible PLT as outlined in Fig. 12.4 D. Washed blood components (all). Platelet additive solution (PAS) PLTs have a reduced volume of incompatible plasma and are currently the preferred alternative to washed PLTs at many institutions, as washing results in poor PLT function or losses.[78] PLT units with low anti-A/anti-B titers are preferred to type O PLTs, as they are known to have higher anti-A and anti-B titers. PLTs from A2 can be screened as an alternative to AB PLTs.[79] However, if required, HLA matching or crossmatched PLTs take precedence over ABO selection for the purpose of treating PLT refractoriness.[80]

Rh-negative recipients should be given PLTs from Rh-negative donors to prevent Rh alloimmunization by remaining RBCs in a PLT unit. Rh immune globulin should be given when Rh-positive PLTs are transfused to Rh-negative recipients in phase I and II. The same applies in phase III after engraftment has occurred in a previously Rh-positive patient now typing as Rh negative.

The expected PLT count after transfusion of a unit is $>30,000$ PLT/μL. When the count fails to increment on more than one occasion (1 h post transfusion), the patients are considered PLT refractory and are further classified as either immune or nonimmune in nature. HSCT patients are particularly prone to be PLT refractory given their high transfusion burden.

Common causes of PLT refractoriness include both immune-mediated and non-immune-mediated processes. If immune mediated, anti-HLA antibodies, anti-A/anti-B antibodies, and anti-PLT specific antibodies (i.e., anti-HPA-1) may be responsible. Etiologies of non-immune-mediated refractoriness include bleeding, fever, sepsis, disseminated intravascular coagulation, splenomegaly, and medications, to name a few.

To determine if a patient is refractory and to classify the type, two consecutive PLT-corrected count increments (CCIs) at 1 and 24 h post ABO-matched PLT transfusions are needed. A baseline count is taken before transfusion and the postcount is obtained between 10 min and 1 h after the completion of the PLT transfusion. If a patient is given a PLT drip (slow infusion), the precount should be taken immediately before starting the next transfusion (after prior unit is completed). If both CCIs are <7500 PLT/μL, the patient is considered refractory. Immune-mediated causes have poor 1 and 24 h CCI. In contrast, non-immune-mediated causes usually have an adequate 1-h CCI but a poor 24-h CCI.

HLA-matched PLTs should be provided early to avoid further anti-HLA alloimmunization and to prevent expansion of anti-HLA Ab specificity as proposed in Fig. 12.5. If the patient is not responding to HLA-matched and/or crossmatched PLTs, and screening is positive for PLT-specific antibodies, a PLT antibody identification panel (i.e., anti-HPA-1a) should be considered. In this scenario, other treatment options such as PLT drip should be discussed with the clinical team. PLT transfusion support is further complicated when there is a combination of immune-mediated and non-immune-mediated mechanisms mediating poor responses to PLT transfusions.[81] However, this is beyond the scope of this chapter.

Granulocyte Transfusion

Granulocyte transfusions have not been proven effective and should be reserved only for neutropenic patients with severe invasive infections not responding to maximal antibiotic therapy when there is a reasonable opportunity of marrow recovery. Granulocyte ABO matching follows the RBC scheme explained earlier. Granulocyte transfusions must be irradiated and naturally cannot be leukoreduced! It is important to remember that granulocyte transfusions are supposed to be used only as bridge therapy in patients in whom cure is otherwise anticipated, and by no means as a life-prolonging measure in otherwise treatment-refractory patients. Granulocyte-colony stimulating factor can be coadministered to the patient if engraftment has not occurred.

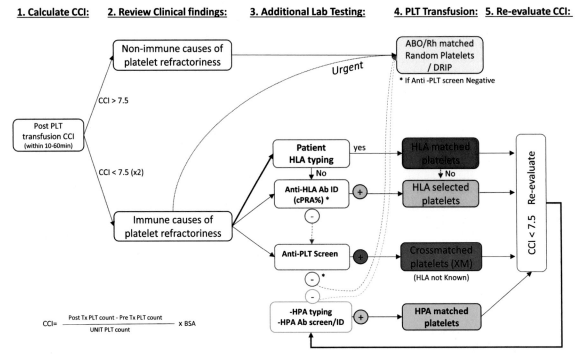

FIG. 12.5 Refractory platelet transfusion workup and management algorithm. *BSA*, Body surface area; *CCI*, corrected count increments; *cPRA*, Calculated Panel Reactive Antibodies; *HLA*, human leukocyte antigens; *HPA*, human platelet antigens; *PLT*, platelet; *Tx*, Transfusion.

SPECIAL CONSIDERATIONS FOR HEMATOPOIETIC PROGENITOR CELL TRANSPLANT

Autologous Transplant

As in any patient with a hematologic malignancy, ABO-identical or ABO-compatible RBC, PLT, and plasma components selected for autologous transplant recipients should be irradiated, leukoreduced, and CMV safe. Any additional special needs should be communicated to the BB so that information is entered in the BB LIS.

Pediatric Transplant

Although the overarching principles regarding transfusion support of pediatric HSCT recipients are similar to those for adults, indications for transplant, stem cell source, and donor selection may be different in children. For example, children with inherited diseases (such as sickle cell disease [SCD] or thalassemia major) may be more likely to be treated with HSCT than adults. Furthermore, high-dose chemotherapy with autologous stem cell rescue is more often used to treat some childhood malignancies (including advanced stage

neuroblastoma) and better tolerated than in adults. Moreover, cord blood may be used more frequently for transplant to treat some diseases in pediatric recipients. HPCs obtained from cords (HPC-C) usually provide a sufficient dose for a child, but not for an adult, because of a child's smaller size.[82]

Transplant in Patients with Sickle Cell Disease

Patients with SCD with significant morbidity and mortality might benefit from HPCT. Identification of a completely HLA-matched sibling donor is a major challenge in patients with SCD. Importantly, hemolytic anemia and vasoocclusive episodes can be seen after stem cell product infusion. Symptoms can include painful crisis, splenic sequestration, and multiorgan failure. Patients with SCD should generally be scheduled for RBC exchange before major ABO-incompatible transplant with a goal of <30%–45% hemoglobin S. They should receive RBCs that are ABO compatible with the donor ABO type so that when donor cells engraft, there will be reduced hemolysis of the residual RBCs in the recipient. In this situation, if the recipient is Rh positive and the donor is Rh negative it may be prudent to perform the RCE with Rh-negative units and continue with Rh-negative RBC transfusions to avoid significant hemolysis when anti-D is produced after engraftment of donor cells.

Red cell phenotyping of the stem cell donor is recommended to prevent alloimmunization in the recipient against donated cells to guide both donor selection and product processing. If possible, stem cell donors who are negative for cognate red cell antigens against which recipients have red cell alloantibodies should be considered.[83] This is particularly important for reduced-intensity or nonmyeloablative conditioning regimens, which can induce long-term mixed chimerism.[84] If antigen-positive donors are used, RBC reduction of the stem cell product is recommended even in the absence of ABO incompatibility to avoid a transfusion reaction during stem cell infusion.

Acquired Thrombotic Thrombocytopenic Purpura/Venoocclusive Disease

MAHA/thrombotic thrombocytopenic purpura (TTP) is rarely seen in transplant recipients, usually has poor prognosis, and does not respond well to usual treatments such as TPE. Venoocclusive disease (VOD) with or without multiorgan dysfunction post HSCT can be influenced by PLT transfusion containing ABO-incompatible plasma and is a major limiting factor of high-dose chemotherapy in children.[85] Posttransplant TTP and VOD should be always considered in the differential diagnosis of anemia and thrombocytopenia in the posttransplant period, as they require specialized management.

Iron Overload

Transfusion dependency before and during transplant should be minimized to prevent hemosiderosis-related adverse effects. Patients with thalassemia major, SCD, or myelodysplastic syndrome who have received multiple lifetime RBC transfusions and show evidence of hepatic iron overload often have poor transplant outcomes.

DONORS: TRANSFUSION SUPPORT FOR ALLOGENEIC HEMATOPOIETIC PROGENITOR CELL FROM MARROW DONORS DURING COLLECTION

BM donors can lose 1–2 L or more of blood during marrow harvesting. It is prudent to flag the donor in the BB laboratory LIS to receive irradiated, leukoreduced, CMV-safe/CMV-negative blood components in the uncommon event that they require transfusion. An option for autologous blood donation before marrow harvest can be discussed with a donor.

SOLID ORGAN TRANSPLANT

ABO-Incompatibility in Solid Organ Transplant

The most important transplant antigen system to be considered in solid organ transplant is the ABO blood group system. ABO compatibility rules are cornerstones of matching SOT recipients and donors.[63] ABO antigens are widely expressed on endothelial and epithelial cells and in soluble form in plasma. They are responsible for hyperacute or acute graft rejection. They also stimulate chronic graft rejection that occurs concomitantly with HLA antigen expression on epithelial cells. Crossing the ABO barrier in solid organ transplant is done only in emergency transplants or when there is significant organ shortage.[28,37,86] Early experiences of crossing the ABO barriers in renal transplant were disappointing. In the 1970s, clinical trials started with transplants of renal grafts of subgroup A2 into blood group O recipients. A2 subgroup individuals express a reduced amount of A-antigens compared with subgroup A1. Transplants of A2 kidneys to non-A-recipients have been successful owing to lower A2 antigen tissue expression and pretreatment with standard immunosuppression.[86] Existing data confirm that ABO-incompatible renal transplants without splenectomy is feasible using rituximab induction as long as the isohemagglutinin titers are <16 before transplant.[87] These patients benefit from continued monitoring of titers.

Special Considerations for Blood Component Transfusion in Solid Organ Transplant

Unlike stem cell transplants, blood components only need to be leukoreduced and no irradiation is needed in solid organ transplant.

Liver transplant

Commonly, candidates for liver transplant have profound coagulation defects. Massive transfusion protocols to improve efficiency of blood component delivery must ensure proper ratios of RBC:Plasma:PLT to improve outcomes. Excessive bleeding is usually managed with plasma administration, cryoprecipitate, and fibrinogen concentrates.[88] Real-time viscoelastic monitoring with rotational thromboelastometry and thromboelastography have been proved to be valuable methods for optimizing blood component selection during and after liver transplant.[89,90]

REFERENCES

1. Nisbet-Brown E. Transfusion support of the transplant patient. *Can Fam Physician.* 1988;34:2503–2508.
2. Bortin MM, Bach FH, van Bekkum DW, Good RA, van Rood JJ. 25th anniversary of the first successful allogeneic bone marrow transplants. *Bone Marrow Transplant.* 1994;14(2):211–212.
3. Bishop MR, Logan BR, Gandham S, et al. Long-term outcomes of adults with acute lymphoblastic leukemia after autologous or unrelated donor bone marrow transplantation: a comparative analysis by the National Marrow Donor Program and Center for International Blood and Marrow Transplant Research. *Bone Marrow Transplant.* 2008;41(7):635–642.
4. Hollenbach JA, Saperstein A, Albrecht M, et al. Race, ethnicity and ancestry in unrelated transplant matching for the national Marrow Donor Program: a comparison of multiple forms of self-identification with genetics. *PLoS One.* 2015;10(8):e0135960.
5. Shaw BE, Logan BR, Kiefer DM, et al. Analysis of the effect of race, socioeconomic status, and center size on unrelated national Marrow Donor Program donor outcomes: donor toxicities are more common at low-volume bone marrow collection centers. *Biol Blood Marrow Transplant.* 2015;21(10):1830–1838.
6. van Besien K, Shore T, Cushing M. Peripheral-blood versus bone marrow stem cells. *N Engl J Med.* 2013;368(3):287–288.
7. Burns LJ, Logan BR, Chitphakdithai P, et al. Recovery of unrelated donors of peripheral blood stem cells versus recovery of unrelated donors of bone marrow: a prespecified analysis from the phase III blood and marrow transplant clinical trials network protocol 0201. *Biol Blood Marrow Transplant.* 2016;22(6):1108–1116.
8. Anasetti C, Logan BR, Lee SJ, et al. Peripheral-blood stem cells versus bone marrow from unrelated donors. *N Engl J Med.* 2012;367(16):1487–1496.
9. Ballen KK, Koreth J, Chen YB, Dey BR, Spitzer TR. Selection of optimal alternative graft source: mismatched unrelated donor, umbilical cord blood, or haploidentical transplant. *Blood.* 2012;119(9):1972–1980.
10. Richter KV. Histocompatibility and bone marrow transplantation (BMT). *Folia Haematol Int Mag Klin Morphol Blutforsch.* 1989;116(3–4):445–450.
11. Choi SW, Levine JE, Ferrara JL. Pathogenesis and management of graft-versus-host disease. *Immunol Allergy Clin North Am.* 2010;30(1):75–101.
12. Hsu KC, Keever-Taylor CA, Wilton A, et al. Improved outcome in HLA-identical sibling hematopoietic stem-cell transplantation for acute myelogenous leukemia predicted by KIR and HLA genotypes. *Blood.* 2005;105(12):4878–4884.
13. Ciceri F, Labopin M, Aversa F, et al. A survey of fully haploidentical hematopoietic stem cell transplantation in adults with high-risk acute leukemia: a risk factor analysis of outcomes for patients in remission at transplantation. *Blood.* 2008;112(9):3574–3581.
14. Liu H, Rich ES, Godley L, et al. Reduced-intensity conditioning with combined haploidentical and cord blood transplantation results in rapid engraftment, low GVHD, and durable remissions. *Blood.* 2011;118(24):6438–6445.
15. Thomas D, Thomson J, Ridler B. *All Blood Counts: A Manual for Blood Conservation and Patient Blood Management.* TFM Publishing Limited; 2016.
16. Claas FH, Gijbels Y, Van der Velden-de Munck J, van Rood JJ. Induction of B cell unresponsiveness to noninherited maternal HLA antigens during fetal life. *Science.* 1988;241(4874):1815–1817.
17. van Rood JJ, Loberiza Jr FR, Zhang MJ, et al. Effect of tolerance to noninherited maternal antigens on the occurrence of graft-versus-host disease after bone marrow transplantation from a parent or an HLA-haploidentical sibling. *Blood.* 2002;99(5):1572–1577.
18. Van der Zanden HG, Van Rood JJ, Oudshoorn M, et al. Noninherited maternal antigens identify acceptable HLA mismatches: benefit to patients and cost-effectiveness for cord blood banks. *Biol Blood Marrow Transplant.* 2014;20(11):1791–1795.
19. Matsui T, Shimoyama T, Matsumoto M, et al. ABO blood group antigens on human plasma von Willebrand factor after ABO-mismatched bone marrow transplantation. *Blood.* 1999;94(8):2895–2900.
20. Nydegger UE, Tevaearai H, Berdat P, et al. Histo-blood group antigens as allo- and autoantigens. *Ann N Y Acad Sci.* 2005;1050:40–51.
21. Storry JR, Castilho L, Daniels G, et al. International Society of Blood Transfusion Working Party on red cell immunogenetics and blood group terminology: cancun report (2012). *Vox Sang.* 2014;107(1):90–96.
22. Van Rood JJ. Tissue typing and organ transplantation. *Lancet.* 1969;1(7606):1142–1146.
23. Rowley SD, Donato ML, Bhattacharyya P. Red blood cell-incompatible allogeneic hematopoietic progenitor cell transplantation. *Bone Marrow Transplant.* 2011;46(9):1167–1185.
24. Kanda J, Ichinohe T, Matsuo K, et al. Impact of ABO mismatching on the outcomes of allogeneic related and unrelated blood and marrow stem cell transplantations for hematologic malignancies: IPD-based meta-analysis of cohort studies. *Transfusion.* 2009;49(4):624–635.
25. Roelen DL, van Rood JJ, Brand A, Claas FH. Immunomodulation by blood transfusions. *Vox Sang.* 2000;78(suppl 2):273–275.
26. Robertson A, Issitt R, Crook R, et al. A novel method for ABO-incompatible heart transplantation. *J Heart Lung Transplant.* 2017;(17).
27. Urschel S, Larsen IM, Kirk R, et al. ABO-incompatible heart transplantation in early childhood: an international multicenter study of clinical experiences and limits. *J Heart Lung Transplant.* 2013;32(3):285–292.
28. Triulzi DJ, Nalesnik MA. Microchimerism, GVHD, and tolerance in solid organ transplantation. *Transfusion.* 2001;41(3):419–426.

29. de Vries-van der Zwan A, van der Pol MA, Besseling AC, de Waal LP, Boog CJ. Stem cell transfusion as a new method for the induction of tolerance in organ transplantation. *Transplant Proc.* 1997;29(1–2):1209–1210.

30. Liu F, Li G, Mao X, Hu L. ABO chimerism determined by real-time polymerase chain reaction analysis after ABO-incompatible haematopoietic stem cell transplantation. *Blood Transfus.* 2013;11(1):43–52.

31. Worel N, Bojic A, Binder M, et al. Catastrophic graft-versus-host disease after lung transplantation proven by PCR-based chimerism analysis. *Transpl Int.* 2008;21(11):1098–1101.

32. Blacklock HA, Katz F, Michalevicz R, et al. A and B blood group antigen expression on mixed colony cells and erythroid precursors: relevance for human allogeneic bone marrow transplantation. *Br J Haematol.* 1984;58(2):267–276.

33. Janatpour KA, Kalmin ND, Jensen HM, Holland PV. Clinical outcomes of ABO-incompatible RBC transfusions. *Am J Clin Pathol.* 2008;129(2):276–281.

34. Flegel WA. Pathogenesis and mechanisms of antibody-mediated hemolysis. *Transfusion.* 2015;55(suppl 2):S47–S58.

35. Zubair A, Benjamin RJ. Transfusion medicine illustrated. Erythrophagocytosis after an ABO-mismatched stem cell transplant. *Transfusion.* 2001;41(12):1463.

36. Raimondi R, Soli M, Lamparelli T, et al. ABO-incompatible bone marrow transplantation: a GITMO survey of current practice in Italy and comparison with the literature. *Bone Marrow Transplant.* 2004;34(4):321–329.

37. Yazer MH, Triulzi DJ. Immune hemolysis following ABO-mismatched stem cell or solid organ transplantation. *Curr Opin Hematol.* 2007;14(6):664–670.

38. Kanda Y, Tanosaki R, Nakai K, et al. Impact of stem cell source and conditioning regimen on erythrocyte recovery kinetics after allogeneic haematopoietic stem cell transplantation from an ABO-incompatible donor. *Br J Haematol.* 2002;118(1):128–131.

39. van Besien K, Nichols CR, Tricot G, et al. Characteristics of engraftment after repeated autologous bone marrow transplantation. *Exp Hematol.* 1990;18(7):785–788.

40. Sharma SK, Kumar S, Agrawal N, Mishra P, Seth T, Mahapatra M. Oral high dose dexamethasone for pure red cell aplasia following ABO-mismatched allogeneic peripheral blood stem cell transplantation: a case report. *Indian J Hematol Blood Transfus.* 2015;31(2):317–318.

41. Kopinska A, Helbig G, Frankiewicz A, Grygoruk-Wisniowska I, Kyrcz-Krzemien S. Rituximab is highly effective for pure red cell aplasia and post-transplant lymphoproliferative disorder after unrelated hematopoietic stem cell transplantation. *Contemp Oncol (Pozn, Pol).* 2012;16(3):215–217.

42. Stussi G, Halter J, Bucheli E, et al. Prevention of pure red cell aplasia after major or bidirectional ABO blood group incompatible hematopoietic stem cell transplantation by pretransplant reduction of host anti-donor isoagglutinins. *Haematologica.* 2009;94(2):239–248.

43. Park SH, Lee MH, Lee SH, et al. The outcomes of hypertransfusion in major ABO incompatible allogeneic stem cell transplantation. *J Korean Med Sci.* 2004;19(1):79–82.

44. Rabitsch W, Knobl P, Prinz E, et al. Prolonged red cell aplasia after major ABO-incompatible allogeneic hematopoietic stem cell transplantation: removal of persisting isohemagglutinins with Ig-Therasorb immunoadsorption. *Bone Marrow Transplant.* 2003;32(10):1015–1019.

45. Rabitsch W, Knobl P, Greinix H, et al. Removal of persisting isohaemagglutinins with Ig-Therasorb immunoadsorption after major ABO-incompatible non-myeloablative allogeneic haematopoietic stem cell transplantation. *Nephrol Dial Transplant.* 2003;18(11):2405–2408.

46. Jacobs LB, Shirey RS, Ness PM. Hemolysis due to the simultaneous occurrence of passenger lymphocyte syndrome and a delayed hemolytic transfusion reaction in a liver transplant patient. *Arch Pathol Lab Med.* 1996;120(7):684–686.

47. Tsujimura K, Ishida H, Tanabe K. Is efficacy of the Anti-Cd20 antibody rituximab preventing hemolysis due to passenger lymphocyte syndrome? *Ther Apher Dial.* 2017;21(1):22–25.

48. Canaani J, Savani BN, Labopin M, et al. ABO incompatibility in mismatched unrelated donor allogeneic hematopoietic cell transplantation for acute myeloid leukemia: a report from the acute leukemia working party of the EBMT. *Am J Hematol.* 2017;92(8):789–796.

49. Stussi G, Muntwyler J, Passweg JR, et al. Consequences of ABO incompatibility in allogeneic hematopoietic stem cell transplantation. *Bone Marrow Transplant.* 2002;30(2):87–93.

50. Dunstan RA. Status of major red cell blood group antigens on neutrophils, lymphocytes and monocytes. *Br J Haematol.* 1986;62(2):301–309.

51. Dahl D, Hahn A, Koenecke C, et al. Prolonged isolated red blood cell transfusion requirement after allogeneic blood stem cell transplantation: identification of patients at risk. *Transfusion.* 2010;50(3):649–655.

52. Greener D, Henrichs KF, Liesveld JL, et al. Improved outcomes in acute myeloid leukemia patients treated with washed transfusions. *Am J Hematol.* 2017;92(1):E8–E9.

53. Klein HG, Flegel WA, Natanson C. Red blood cell transfusion: precision vs imprecision medicine. *JAMA.* 2015;314(15):1557–1558.

54. Moog R. In vivo adsorption of isoagglutinins with incompatible red blood cell transfusion in stem cell transplant recipients. *Transfus Med Hemother.* 2016;43(4):307.

55. Gergis U, Al-Mulla NA, Javier S, et al. Hematopoietic recovery after in-vivo T-cell depleted allogeneic stem cell transplant - effects of ABO incompatibility, rhesus incompatibility and acute Gvhd. *Blood.* 2016;128(22):5745.

56. Franchini M, Gandini G, Aprili G. Non-ABO red blood cell alloantibodies following allogeneic hematopoietic stem cell transplantation. *Bone Marrow Transplant.* 2004;33(12):1169–1172.

57. Mijovic A. Alloimmunization to RhD antigen in RhD-incompatible haemopoietic cell transplants with non-myeloablative conditioning. *Vox Sang.* 2002;83(4):358–362.

58. Westhoff CM. The potential of blood group genotyping for transfusion medicine practice. *Immunohematology.* 2008;24(4):190–195.

59. Hillyer CD, Shaz BH, Winkler AM, Reid M. Integrating molecular technologies for red blood cell typing and compatibility testing into blood centers and transfusion services. *Transfus Med Rev.* 2008;22(2):117–132.

60. Fasano RM, Sullivan HC, Bray RA, et al. Genotyping applications for transplantation and transfusion management: the emory experience. *Arch Pathol Lab Med.* 2017;141(3):329–340.

61. Hillyer CD, Snydman DR, Berkman EM. The risk of cytomegalovirus infection in solid organ and bone marrow transplant recipients: transfusion of blood products. *Transfusion.* 1990;30(7):659–666.

62. Tormey CA, Snyder E. Transfusion support for the oncology patient. In: Simon TL, Snyder EL, Stowell CP, et al., eds. *Rossi's Principles of Transfusion Medicine.* 4th ed. Bethesda, MD: AABB; 2009:482–497.

63. Shimoda T. On postoperative erythroderma. *Geka.* 1955;17:487–492.

64. Wisecarver JL, Cattral MS, Langnas AN, et al. Transfusion-induced graft-versus-host disease after liver transplantation. Documentation using polymerase chain reaction with HLA-DR sequence-specific primers. *Transplantation.* 1994;58(3):269–271.

65. Porter DL. Donor leukocyte infusions in acute myelogenous leukemia. *Leukemia.* 2003;17(6):1035–1037.

66. Liesveld JL, Rothberg PG. Mixed chimerism in SCT: conflict or peaceful coexistence? *Bone Marrow Transplant.* 2008;42(5):297–310.

67. Khan F, Agarwal A, Agrawal S. Significance of chimerism in hematopoietic stem cell transplantation: new variations on an old theme. *Bone Marrow Transplant.* 2004;34(1):1–12.

68. Ljungman P, Hakki M, Boeckh M. Cytomegalovirus in hematopoietic stem cell transplant recipients. *Hematol Oncol Clin North Am.* 2011;25(1):151–169.

69. Tomblyn M, Chiller T, Einsele H, et al. Guidelines for preventing infectious complications among hematopoietic cell transplantation recipients: a global perspective. *Biol Blood Marrow Transplant.* 2009;15(10):1143–1238.

70. Cancelas JA, Dumont LJ, Rugg N, et al. Stored red blood cell viability is maintained after treatment with a second-generation S-303 pathogen inactivation process. *Transfusion.* 2011;51(11):2367–2376.

71. Cushing M, Shaz B. Transfusion-transmitted babesiosis: achieving successful mitigation while balancing cost and donor loss. *Transfusion.* 2012;52(7):1404–1407.

72. Simon MS, Leff JA, Pandya A, et al. Cost-effectiveness of blood donor screening for *Babesia microti* in endemic regions of the United States. *Transfusion.* 2014;54(3 Pt 2):889–899.

73. Adegite EA, Goyal RK, Murray PJ, Marshal M, Sucato GS. The management of menstrual suppression and uterine bleeding: a survey of current practices in the Pediatric Blood and Marrow Transplant Consortium. *Pediatr Blood Cancer.* 2012;59(3):553–557.

74. Leahy MF, Trentino KM, May C, Swain SG, Chuah H, Farmer SL. Blood use in patients receiving intensive chemotherapy for acute leukemia or hematopoietic stem cell transplantation: the impact of a health system-wide patient blood management program. *Transfusion.* 2017;57.

75. Kaufman RM, Djulbegovic B, Gernsheimer T, et al. Platelet transfusion: a clinical practice guideline from the AABB. *Ann Intern Med.* 2015;162(3):205–213.

76. Schmidt AE, Refaai MA, Blumberg N. Platelet transfusion and thrombosis: more questions than answers. *Semin Thromb Hemost.* 2016;42(2):118–124.

77. Henrichs KF, Howk N, Masel DS, et al. Providing ABO-identical platelets and cryoprecipitate to (almost) all patients: approach, logistics, and associated decreases in transfusion reaction and red blood cell alloimmunization incidence. *Transfusion.* 2012;52(3):635–640.

78. Dunbar NM, Katus MC, Freeman CM, Szczepiorkowski ZM. Easier said than done: ABO compatibility and D matching in apheresis platelet transfusions. *Transfusion.* 2015;55(8):1882–1888.

79. Cid J, Harm SK, Yazer MH. Platelet transfusion – the art and science of compromise. *Transfus Med Hemother.* 2013;40(3):160–171.

80. Heal JM, Blumberg N, Masel D. An evaluation of cross-matching, HLA, and ABO matching for platelet transfusions to refractory patients. *Blood.* 1987;70(1):23–30.

81. Dai WJ, Zhang RR, Yang XC, Yuan YF. Efficacy of standard dose rituximab for refractory idiopathic thrombocytopenic purpura in children. *Eur Rev Med Pharmacol Sci.* 2015;19(13):2379–2383.

82. Goel R, Cushing MM, Tobian AA. Pediatric patient blood management programs: not just transfusing little adults. *Transfus Med Rev.* 2016;30(4):235–241.

83. Canals C, Muniz-Diaz E, Martinez C, et al. Impact of ABO incompatibility on allogeneic peripheral blood progenitor cell transplantation after reduced intensity conditioning. *Transfusion.* 2004;44(11):1603–1611.

84. Mijovic A, Abdallah A, Pearce L, Tobal K, Mufti GJ. Effects on erythropoiesis of alemtuzumab-containing reduced intensity and standard conditioning regimens. *Br J Haematol.* 2008;142(3):444–452.

85. Lapierre V, Mahe C, Auperin A, et al. Platelet transfusion containing ABO-incompatible plasma and hepatic veno-occlusive disease after hematopoietic transplantation in young children. *Transplantation.* 2005;80(3):314–319.

86. Rydberg L. ABO-incompatibility in solid organ transplantation. *Transfus Med.* 2001;11(4):325–342.

87. Muramatsu M, Gonzalez HD, Cacciola R, Aikawa A, Yaqoob MM, Puliatti C. ABO incompatible renal transplants: good or bad? *World J Transplant.* 2014;4(1):18–29.

88. Franchini M, Lippi G. Fibrinogen replacement therapy: a critical review of the literature. *Blood Transfus.* 2012;10(1):23–27.

89. Blasi A, Beltran J, Pereira A, et al. An assessment of thromboelastometry to monitor blood coagulation and guide transfusion support in liver transplantation. *Transfusion.* 2012;52(9):1989–1998.

90. Zubair AC, Torp K, Eichbaum Q. How we provide blood transfusion support in two large US liver transplant programs. *Transfusion.* 2016;56(8):1938–1943.

CHAPTER 13

Hematopoietic Stem Cell Collections and Cellular Therapies

LJILJANA V. VASOVIC, MD • RONIT REICH-SLOTKY, PHD, MSC • RUCHIKA GOEL, MD, MPH

HEMATOPOIETIC PROGENITOR CELL TRANSPLANTATION

Hematopoietic progenitor cell transplant (HPCT) is a therapeutic procedure that enables bone marrow (BM) reconstitution after chemotherapy and radiation and increases the chance of cure for hematologic malignancies relative to standard chemotherapy alone. Stem cells (SCs) and progenitor cells are defined by their ability to self-renew and differentiate to form all lineages of blood cells. Hematopoietic stem cells (HSCs) and hematopoietic progenitor cells (HPCs) have the capacity to reconstitute hematopoiesis in aplastic or ablated BM. Small populations of HPCs that express CD34 provide multilineage hematopoietic engraftment of myeloid, erythroid megakaryocytic, and immune lineages.[1]

Historically, BM was the primary HPC graft source during early transplant field development. It provided large amounts of measured and unmeasured SCs, more differentiated HPCs, and mesenchymal feeder cells. With the development of excellent mobilization regimens, namely, granulocyte colony-stimulating factor (G-CSF), HPCs were mobilized to circulation and successfully harvested by large-volume apheresis. As a result, peripheral blood stem cells (PBSCs) became the preferred graft source because of procurement of higher doses and convenience of collection, easy access through peripheral or central lines without operating room procedures, fewer side effects for donors, and lower costs. They were initially named PBSCs, but their name was changed to HPC-apheresis (HPC-A) following efforts to internationally standardize nomenclature.[2]

HPC-A are considered to have an equivalent engraftment potential compared with BM-derived SCs (HPC-M). Umbilical cord HPCs are being used more frequently, especially in pediatric settings. However, if a full human leukocyte antigen (HLA) match is not available, HPC-Cord (HPC-C) are used owing to lesser propensity for development of graft-versus-host disease (GVHD).

HPCs can be collected from a patient, stored, and reinfused back to the patient when indicated as an autologous HPCT. Autologous HPCs are usually obtained from patients in remission, post chemotherapy, and cryopreserved for long-term storage. Fresh autologous infusion is rarely done in current practice. Allogeneic infusion of HPCs from another individual constitutes allogeneic HPCT.

Annual numbers of transplant recipients in the United States and worldwide are steadily increasing as illustrated by data from the Center for International Blood and Marrow Transplant Research (CIBMTR) (Fig. 13.1).[3] More than 50,000 transplants are performed annually worldwide. Indications for HPCT are predominantly because of hematologic malignancies and, to a lesser extent, nonmalignant hematologic disorders (Fig. 13.2). HPCT is also accepted for therapy of solid tumors, mostly in pediatric patients. Moreover, there are increasing numbers of controlled clinical trials providing evidence that HPCTs increase overall survival (OS) and relapse-free survival.[4,5]

Autologous transplants account for more than 50% of all HPCT. The most common indications for an autologous HPCT are multiple myeloma and lymphoma. In multiple myeloma, patients' 3-year, 5-year, and overall survival trends have steadily improved in the last few decades owing to increased numbers of autologous transplants and enhanced posttransplant maintenance therapy. Likewise, what is considered as an acceptable age limit for HPCTs has steadily increased over the years and is currently over 70 years. Patients older than 60 years account for more than 50% of autologous HPCT recipients.

The number of allogeneic HPCT recipients exceeds 8000 per year in the United States. Hematologic

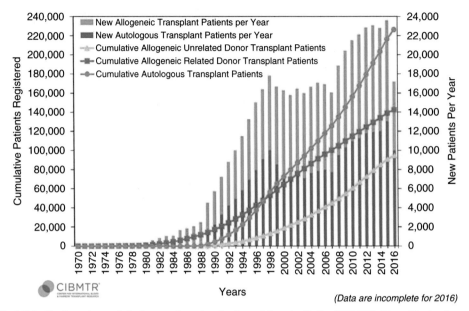

FIG. 13.1 Continued growth in the number of patients registered with the CIBMTR. (From Center for International Blood & Marrow Transplant Research (CIBMTR). *2016 Annual Report*. Available at: https://www. cibmtr.org/ReferenceCenter/Newsletters/Documents/2016%20CIBMTR%20Annual%20Report%20final.pdf; with permission.)

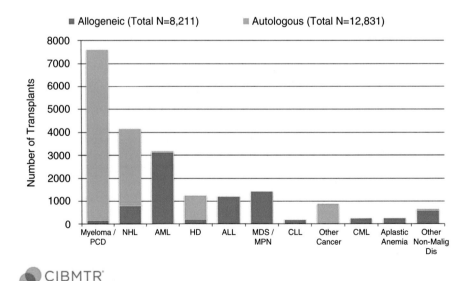

FIG. 13.2 The most common indications for hematopoietic cell transplantation in the United States, 2014. *ALL*, acute lymphoid leukemia; *AML*, acute myeloid leukemia; *CLL*, chronic lymphoid leukemia; *CML*, chronic myeloid leukemia; *HD*, Hodgkin Lymphoma; *NHL*, non-Hodgkin Lymphoma; *MDS*, myelodysplastic syndrome; *MPN*, myeloproliferative neoplasms; *PCD*, plasma cell disorder. (From D'Souza A, Zhu X. *Current Uses and Outcomes of Hematopoietic Cell Transplantation (HCT): CIBMTR Summary Slides*; 2016. Available at: https://www.cibmtr.org/ReferenceCenter/SlidesReports/SummarySlides/pages/index.aspx# DownloadSummarySlides; with permission.)

malignancies, such as acute leukemia and myelo-proliferative/myelodysplastic disorders, are the most common indications for allogeneic transplants. More than 70% of allogeneic HPCTs are performed as treatment of acute myeloid leukemia (AML), acute lymphoid leukemia, and myelodysplastic/myelo-proliferative neoplasms. Aplastic anemia, sickle cell disease, thalassemia, and other nonmalignant and nonhematologic indications, such as metabolic diseases, are also increasingly being treated with allogeneic HPCT. The number of allogeneic HPCTs for lymphomas, chronic lymphoid leukemia, and chronic myeloid leukemia (CML) has declined because of advances in diagnostic techniques and chemotherapeutic regimens, including imatinib mesylate. In this regard, CML was once the most common indication for allogeneic HPCT.

Historical Perspective

The first insight on blood-forming SCs dates back to observations of individuals exposed to lethal doses of radiation in the 1940s. Experimental models in 1950s confirmed transplantability of BM-derived SCs. Drs. Medawar and Burnet received the 1960 Nobel Prize for the discovery of acquired immunologic tolerance. Drs. Snell, Dausset, and Benacerraf received the 1980 Nobel Prize for their discoveries of the major histocompatibility complex (MHC) that regulate immunologic reactions.[6]

In the subsequent years, this led to the characterization of hematopoietic and stromal SC differentiation. However, initial success of the first BM transplant in 1958 of five workers irradiated during a nuclear accident ended with graft rejection.[7-9] The first successful human BM transplant between identical twins was performed by Dr. E. Donnall Thomas for which he received the 1990 Nobel Prize in Medicine for his work on transplantation.[10,11] The first successful human allogeneic HPCT, an HLA-matched marrow from a sibling to a patient with X-linked Severe Combined Immunodeficiency (SCID) to correct the immune deficiency was performed in 1968 by Gatti et al.[12] John Kersey performed the first successful BM transplant to cure lymphoma.[13] In utero, HSC transplant has been mostly performed and reported as a treatment for genetic hematologic diseases.[14] Enrichment of donor marrow with CD34+ cells was necessary to minimize infusion volume.[15-19] Clinical transplant for hematologic malignancies, other tumors, and nonmalignant indications followed, expanding the field even further.[20,21]

DONOR SELECTION, EVALUATION, AND MANAGEMENT

Consent to Donate

Consent to donate must be obtained before collection after risks and benefits are discussed with the potential donor. Because there is no immediate benefit to the allogeneic donor, it might be necessary to include donor advocates in this process, especially for young pediatric donors and teenagers donating for their siblings. Counseling can be provided to deal with fear of needles, bone pain due to G-CSF mobilization, apprehension of graft adequacy, and responsibility for transplant failure. More challenging ethical legal issues can occur when one donor is available for two siblings in need or in instances when parents conceive a child to be a donor for a sick relative in need of transplant.

Autologous Donors

Autologous HPCs are collected from the patient and stored in a cryopreserved state while the patient is treated with high-dose chemotherapy with or without radiotherapy to eradicate malignant cells.[22] Autologous HPCT will repopulate a patient's marrow during a period of engraftment lasting a few weeks. Autologous transplants have less risk of infection because of faster immune function recovery.

Engraftment failure is rare because of virtual absence of rejections. When it does occur, engraftment failure may be attributed to cell damage during any step from product collection to product distribution or severe viral infection post transplant. There is an increased risk of disease relapse and related mortality in high-grade disease due to autologous graft contamination with malignant cells. Nonmyeloablative autologous HPCT has been explored for treatment of novel and gene transfer therapies.[23] Autologous collections are frequently performed on patients with a history of chronic underlying diseases, such us congestive heart failure or lung, liver, renal, or psychologic disease. Therefore, medical clearance, including cardiology clearance, might be required before apheresis collection. A central line is usually needed owing to poor peripheral access. Precollection transfusion needs should be evaluated, and transfusions should be scheduled before collection. Pediatric patients, particularly low-weight patients, have been successfully collected with apheresis systems by utilizing blood primes.[24,24a]

Allogenic Donors

Finding an optimal donor match for allogeneic HPCT is a formidable task. HLA allele mismatches reduce the probability of posttransplant OS. The initial donor search usually starts by evaluating matched related donors (MRDs), such as siblings and family members. On the other hand, finding a suitable matched unrelated donor (MUD) can be very difficult and involves substantial effort by the transplant service and at times by centers across the world. As a result, identifying the best match and organizing the donor's HPC collection might be a lengthy procedure and for emergent cases a less optimal match might be acceptable.

HLA matching between donor and recipient is the most important factor for transplant outcome. Current standards require high-resolution molecular typing for MUD matching. HLA class I: HLA-A, HLA-B, HLA-C and class II: HLA-DRB1, HLA-DQB1, and HLA-DP1 are currently used for a 12 of 12 allele HLA match. An identical twin would have an identical HLA gene profile, minor histocompatibility antigens, and ABO antigens and would be termed a syngeneic transplant donor. Siblings have a 25% chance of being HLA-identical or mismatched and a 50% chance of being haploidentical. Parents and children are at least haploidentical, although specific ethnic populations demonstrate homozygosity, thereby increasing the chance of a match. Related donors can be initially screened using low-resolution HLA typing because of linked gene inheritance. MRDs have an additional advantage of potentially sharing minor MHC antigens that are not routinely evaluated. With a larger donor pool it becomes easier to find a suitable match, although provision of adequately HLA-matched SCs to patients of all ethnic groups is not always possible because of the limited number of registered donors.[25]

Cord Donors

Umbilical cord blood is a proven source of HPCs for transplant. Cord blood for transplant, collected from the umbilical cord and placenta after the baby is delivered, is screened for infectious diseases, HLA typed, and cryopreserved until needed. To collect cord blood, a detailed health history is obtained from the mother before collection, with special reference to genetic disorders and malignancies to prevent transmission of genetic diseases that may be present but not evident at the time of birth.

Eligibility Determination

As stated previously, suitable donors that are HLA matched have to be evaluated for eligibility.[26] The primary safety concern is communicable infectious disease transmission. Cellular therapy products (CTPs)

should be quarantined until completion of donor eligibility determination. All donors of human cells, tissue, and cellular and tissue-based products (HCT/Ps) must be screened and tested for relevant communicable disease agents or diseases (RCDADs) as required in § 1271.85(a) using US Food and Drug Administration (FDA)-licensed, approved, or cleared screening tests as described in Section V (§ 1271.80(c)) performed in a CLIA-approved laboratory, unless subject to an exemption in § 1271.90(a).[27,28] Within 30 days before collection, HPCT donors should be tested for human immunodeficiency virus type 1 and type 2, hepatitis B virus, hepatitis C virus, human T-lymphotropic virus (HTLV) types 1 and 2, cytomegalovirus (CMV), and *Treponema pallidum*. In addition, donors of viable, leukocyte-rich HCT/Ps are tested within 7 days before or after collection for HTLV types 1 and 2 and CMV.[29,30] With global travel, fast infectious disease spread has become a reason for major concern. Graft exchange between international organizations has led to new concern for Zika virus (ZikV) transmission. As a consequence, FDA amended its eligibility determination guidance in 2015 to include ZikV. In addition, allogeneic donors are also tested for Epstein-Barr virus as per Foundation for the Accreditation of Cellular Therapy requirement.[31-33]

National Marrow Donor Program

National Marrow Donor Program (NMDP), initially established as the National Bone Marrow Donor Registry in 1986, is an organization that facilitates MUD volunteer hematopoietic cell donors and umbilical cord blood units in the United States through the Be The Match Registry.[34] Suitable donors who are HLA typed and matched, and their willingness to donate, have to be evaluated for eligibility. National and international Bone Marrow Transplant (BMT) registries have continued to grow and volunteer donors are actively recruited to increase ethnic representation of as many groups as possible. To the success of the initiative, an important milestone occurred when the 11 millionth HPCT donor was registered in 2012.[3]

The World Marrow Donor Association

The World Marrow Donor Association was established in 1988 to address and facilitate resolution of issues arising when donors and recipients do not reside in the same country. This association has proposed recommendations and requirements for standardizing practices throughout the world.[24] These recommendations include established guidelines for international collection, transportation of marrow,

TABLE 13.1	
Organizations Promoting Advancement of Cellular Therapies	
Organization	**Web Page**
AABB	www.aabbcct.org
America's Blood Centers (ABC)	www.americasblood.org
American Association of Tissue Banks (AATB)	www.aatb.org
American Red Cross (ARC)	www.redcross.org
American Society for Apheresis (ASFA)	www.apheresis.org
American Society for Blood and Marrow Transplantation (ASBMT)	www.asbmt.org
ClinicalTrial.gov US National Institutes of Health	https://clinicaltrials.gov
College of American Pathologists (CAP)	www.cap.org
Cord Blood Association (CBA)	www.cb-association.org
EuroStemCell	http://www.eurostemcell.org
Food and Drug Administration (FDA)	https://www.accessdata.fda.gov
Foundation for the Accreditation of Cellular Therapy (FACT)	www.factwebsite.org
ICCBBA	www.iccbba.org
International Blood and Marrow Transplant Research (CIBMTR)	https://www.cibmtr.org
International NetCord Foundation	www.netcord.org
International Society for Cellular Therapy (ISCT)	www.celltherapysociety.org
JACIE Accreditation Office	www.jacie.org
National Marrow Donor Program (NMDP)	www.nmdp.org
World Health Organization (WHO) Transplantation	http://www.who.int/transplantation
Worldwide Network for Blood & Marrow Transplantation (WBMT)	http://www.wbmt.org

and financial and insurance-related issues. Long international travel requires expedited clearance and transportation of CTP across borders without delays. Participating couriers must guarantee that the product is not tampered with and not irradiated at the borders and airports. Complete documentation of donor eligibility and product characteristics must accompany the CTP. Efforts to harmonize international laws and requirements for enabling better CTP exchange are promoted by numerous organizations for advancement of cellular therapies (Table 13.1).[35]

CELLULAR THERAPY PRODUCT COLLECTION PROCEDURES
HPC-Marrow Collection
HPC-Marrow (HPC-M) is obtained from the posterior iliac crests by multipass aspirations, collecting 500–2000 mL of BM (usually less than 20 mL/kg of

donor weight according to NMDP guidelines). Adequacy of collection yield may be monitored by intraprocedure total nucleated cell (TNC) counts or a goal of 10–15 mL/kg of recipient weight. There has been some evidence of decreased incidence and severity of GVHD owing to the lower amount of contaminating lymphoid cells.[36] In the case that the donor needs to receive a blood transfusion because of procedural blood loss, red blood cells (RBCs) must be irradiated to prevent third-party GVHD because transfused blood donor lymphocytes become incorporated in the HPC-M product. Alternatively, BM donors can be offered the opportunity to donate an autologous unit in case transfusion is needed. Patients with AML, myelodysplastic syndrome (MDS), and non-Hodgkin lymphoma have been reported to have similar outcomes with either BM or PBSC transplants with reduced-intensity conditioning during unrelated donor transplant.[37]

HPC-Apheresis Collection
Donor mobilization
The apheresis procedure is conducted as per transplant program policy.[38,39] Typically four total blood volumes are processed but in some cases less if a high CD34 yield is expected based on the high number of circulating CD34+ cells in a blood sample drawn immediately before apheresis. For apheresis donations, use of pediatric donors is restricted to donors who are older than 14 years and weigh more than 50 kg.

Allogeneic HPC-A donors are usually mobilized with G-CSF.[40] Occasionally, donors difficult to mobilize, such as elderly donors or those with undiagnosed BM disease, cannot achieve adequate dose collection after two consecutive days of large-volume apheresis. Among autologous donors, those frequently deemed "poor mobilizers" can be secondary to extent of disease,[41] treatment-related marrow fibrosis, and advanced age. These patients may need additional days of mobilization or mobilization with chemotherapy. If there is a failure to mobilize and collect an adequate dose, Mozobil, a CXCR-4 antagonist, is an alternative mobilizing agent that can be added to the G-CSF regimen. If these approaches are not feasible, HPC-M collection is an option.

HPCs collected by apheresis usually contain a high number of mononuclear cells, variable amounts of granulocytes, and a small amount of RBCs (2%–5% hematocrit).[42] Large numbers of mature lymphocytes in HPC-A products carry a higher risk of GVHD than HPC-M and HPC-C products. Products with <20 mL of RBCs are well tolerated without evidence of acute hemolytic reactions in major ABO-incompatible transplants. HPC-A products may induce acute hemolysis of recipient RBCs in minor ABO-incompatible transplants if the donor isohemagglutinin titer is high (>1: 256) and infused plasma volume is more than 200 mL. Consequently, donor mature memory B lymphocytes producing anti-A and anti-B can cause delayed hemolysis in minor ABO-incompatible recipients because of the "passenger lymphocyte syndrome" (PLS) (for additional description see chapter titled Transfusion Approaches in the Transplanted Patient).[43]

Optimization of the collection process and the quality of collected products are assured by having a competent staff. Experienced senior personnel should perform training and competency assessment of collection procedures. High-quality initial training of apheresis staff requires performing multiple procedures until competency is achieved.[44] The key elements of competency assessment include direct observation comparing performance to written standard operating procedures

(SOP), written examination, and evaluation of product quality. Staff retraining should be performed at scheduled intervals or as needed.[45]

Cord (HPC-C) Collection
Cord blood can be collected in utero or after the baby is delivered. There are two types of cord blood banks, public and private. In public banks, cord blood units are stored free of charge for general population use. The larger number of units in the public bank allows for a diverse HLA representation, so that different ethnic populations can potentially benefit. On the other hand, private cord blood banks allow for cord blood units to be stored for an annual fee for the use of specific individuals or family members. Each HPC-C unit is required by the FDA to have a minimum TNC count of at least 5×10^8 and a minimum viable CD34+ count of 1.25×10^6 in a volume of approximately 25 mL with an expiration date of up to 15 years.

First related cord blood transplant was performed in France on a child with Fanconi anemia with successful engraftment.[21] After a successful unrelated cord blood transplant in 1993, several thousand transplants have been completed for various diseases such as malignant and nonmalignant hematologic disorders and congenital metabolic disorders, mostly in children and to a lesser extent in adults from related and unrelated donors with fairly good results.[37] HPC-C transplant success rates are higher in children than in adults.[38] This is because the lower number of HPCs present in an HPC-C unit may be insufficient to populate a larger adult marrow. In the past several years, double HPC-C transplants are being done in adults to provide adequate number of SCs for successful engraftment. Infusion reactions can occur anytime during the process and may even continue for several hours after its completion. If a second HPC-C unit needs to be infused on the same day, it should be delayed until the reactions of the previous unit have resolved.

When HLA-MRDs are not available to provide BM or HPC-A for a patient, it can take several months to identify an unrelated compatible donor. In that situation, it may be easier to obtain compatible HPC-C units from a public cord blood bank, as they are readily available. Although HLA matching is very important in allogeneic BM transplants, with HPC-C transplants, minor HLA mismatch can still result in successful engraftment. Furthermore, there is a lower incidence of GVHD with HPC-C transplants than in HPC-M or HPC-A transplants, and even when it occurs it tends to be less severe. Overall, there is delayed granulocyte and platelet (PLT) recovery compared with other HPCT. There is also delayed immune reconstitution that can lead to increased incidence of viral infections.

Various methods are being developed to enhance the efficacy of HPC-C transplants. Expansion strategies to increase the yield of CD34$^+$ cells, increasing the homing to and nurturing of cells within the hematopoietic microenvironment, and directly injecting the HPC-C unit into the BM are all in experimental stage.[46]

Children with genetic diseases cannot use autologous cord blood cells, as the same disease can recur after transplant. Also, children with leukemia cannot get autologous cord blood, as they may have leukemic mutations. When the Stem Cell Therapeutic and Research Act of 2005 was enacted into law by the US federal government, the C.W. Bill Young Cell Transplantation Program was created. Through this program in 2006 NMDP was awarded the function of the country's Cord Blood Coordinating Center. Through various cord blood banks, NMDP recruits expectant parents for umbilical cord blood donations with the goal of having ethnic diversity.[25,47]

CELLULAR THERAPY PRODUCT PROCESSING

Standard Labeling—Cellular Therapy Products

Standards for the terminology and labeling of CTPs *are based on International Society of Blood Transfusion (ISBT) 128.*[48] *The Global Information Standard for Medical Products of Human Origin* published the ISBT 128 Standard Labeling of Cellular Therapy Products document available at the ICCBBA site.[49] This document is intended to help facilities and software developers design appropriate ISBT 128 labels for CTPs recognized worldwide. Biohazard labeling is performed according to regulatory requirements.[29]

Graft Characterization

Product characterization should include steps to ensure product identity, measure applicable cell dose, confirm sterility, and assess RBC volume for incompatible allogeneic donors. Confirmation of product identity is achieved by tracing the product from the donor to the recipient. This is usually achieved by requiring two qualified personnel to identify and confirm that the product corresponds to a specific donor at all disposition steps. In addition, ABO/Rh and HLA confirmatory testing is performed on all allogeneic products or donors. Measurement of TNC count of

CTPs, using a hematology analyzer, provides a quick way to assess product content but does not specifically identify cells of interest (i.e., hematopoietic progenitor cells, T-cells). TNC viability can be assessed by a trypan blue exclusion assay. Flow cytometry is used to specifically identify the cells of interest and determine their viability. Cellular markers typically used for progenitor cells and T cells are CD34 and CD3, respectively. The 7-aminoactinomycin (AAD) flow cytometric stain is used to determine specific cell viability. Another test, the colony-forming unit assay is a very valuable potency test for HPC assessment, despite poor interlaboratory reproducibility.[50] A long turnaround time (TAT) for the assay, including a 2-week incubation, prompted a number of researchers to look for alternative tests with a shorter TAT depending on HPC metabolic activity, but these have not achieved clinical use.[51] Frozen aliquot samples should be stored for future genetic testing and further microbial testing if needed.

In cases of minor and major ABO incompatibility between graft recipient and donor, the product has to be assessed for RBC content and plasma for donor antibodies, respectively. If necessary, RBC reduction or plasma reduction methods are used, as applicable. Per FDA standards, sterility testing with bacterial and fungal cultures must be performed at a minimum at the end of processing and before product infusion to the recipient. Many laboratories test products before and after processing. Sterility culture usually requires 7–14 days incubation before final results are available. However, these results may not be available before infusion, especially for fresh product infusions.

Enumeration of Hematopoietic Stem Cells

The dose and quality of stem cell products are determined by viable CD34-positive HPC enumeration. Analysis and quantitation of CD34$^+$ cells are performed in accordance with the International Society for Hematotherapy and Graft Engineering (ISHAGE) guidelines. The ISHAGE protocol is based on a sequential gating strategy of HPCs stained with CD45- and CD34-labeled antibodies and 7-7AAD exclusion viability dye.[52] HPC dose is reported as the number of CD34$^+$ cells/kg of recipient weight. The dose of CD34$^+$ cells is a predictor of long-term survival.[53]

Management of Positive Microbial Cultures

CTPs with positive cultures must be quarantined, appropriately labeled, and stored in a designated area. Follow-up of the donor must occur in case of a positive culture because of the potential for bacteremia or sepsis. The recipient's physician should be informed of the donor's positive cultures and should obtain consent from the patient before product infusion. The recipient should receive appropriate medical monitoring and preventive antibiotic treatment and follow-up. Positive microbial cultures are a type of biological product deviation. The clinical program is accountable to provide reports of positive microbial cultures to the applicable regulatory agencies, such as FDA, if the product is administered to a patient. Alternatively, if possible, another collection can be scheduled.

Volume Reduction

ABO incompatibility (ABOi) between the blood types of the donor and the transplant recipient could result in similar types of adverse reactions as seen in blood transfusions because HPC products contain variable amounts of donor RBCs and plasma. In minor ABO-incompatible HPC transplant, the patient may experience acute and/or delayed hemolysis because of the presence of isohemagglutinin in the donor plasma. In this case, reducing the amount of donor plasma in the product helps to remove potential antibodies against the recipient's ABO antigen. This is achieved by product centrifugation, extraction of plasma, and replacement with isotonic solution. Reducing product volume before cryopreservation can also help to reduce the amount of dimethyl sulfoxide (DMSO) used for cryopreservation, thus decreasing its potential toxicity upon infusion.

Red Blood Cell Reduction for Marrow

A major ABO incompatibility implies that the recipient has circulating isohemagglutinin antibodies against the donor's RBCs, which can cause acute RBC hemolysis, delayed red cell engraftment, and even red cell aplasia. RBC reduction can significantly reduce the RBC volume in the HPC product and reduce the likelihood of acute hemolysis at the time of infusion. Owing to the relatively large total volume of BM products (0.5–1.5 L) and high hematocrit content (typically 25%–45%), RBC reduction should be performed on BM products with major ABO incompatibilities. RBC reduction is also recommended for all cryopreserved BM products because of RBC hemolysis during cryopreservation that can cause adverse reactions. Reduction can be achieved either manually, by centrifugation, or by sedimentation with hydroxyethyl starch. Alternatively, automated cell washing devices can be used. There are no specific regulations

regarding RBC volume allowed in an HPC product, and many laboratories use self-determined thresholds. A threshold of ≤0.4 mL/kg RBC volume is commonly used. For bidirectional mismatch, a combination of procedures and techniques used in major and minor mismatched transplants may be considered. Fresh collections before cryopreservation can be T-cell depleted using the Miltenyi Clinimacs depletion device. The target is to obtain a product containing less than 1×10^4 CD3$^+$ cells per kg of recipient body weight and approximately 3×10^6/kg CD34$^+$ cells. The CD34 selection procedure is to be performed in the stem cell laboratory of the transplant center.

Cryopreservation of Cellular Therapy Product

Cryopreservation of CTPs allows for collection and storage of products for later use. CTP cryopreservation is an essential practice for autologous transplants, since the patient is collected prior to conditioning regiment and transplant subsequently, often at the later time. CTP cryopreservation is also helpful to manage allogeneic collections, especially to assure the adequate dose is obtained. HPC-C units, which are collected immediately following birth, must be cryopreserved. Other allogeneic products are typically infused fresh, but in cases of limited donor availability or when there is a need to further optimize the patient's condition before transplant, cryopreservation can be a powerful tool. Owing to the limited lifespan of fresh products and to minimize the risk of microbial contamination, cryopreservation should be done in a timely manner shortly after collection. The main advantage of cryopreservation is that it provides assurance that adequate product is available before patient conditioning, optimizing the management of high-dose myeloablative chemotherapy treatment protocol. It also reduces the risk of inadequate collection dose, contamination, and accidental loss of product when a patient is already conditioned for transplant.

Successful cryopreservation based on cell type and product composition using a variety of different protocols, cryoprotectants, cell concentrations, and freezing temperatures is based on rigorous validation. The most commonly used cryoprotectant is DMSO at a final concentration of 5%–10%. DMSO is a highly lipid soluble, rapid cell membrane permeable substance that prevents intracellular ice formation. A nonpermeating cryoprotectant such as Hetastarch can also be used in combination with DMSO and a high concentration of autologous plasma/AB plasma or albumin (>10%). The basic principle of successful cryopreservation is a slow freeze time. Requirements vary with different cell types and as a general guide CTP should be cooled at a rate of 1–3 °C per minute. Although cryopreserved products have been proved to be viable even after 20 years of storage time, expiration time is based on standard validated protocols, currently up to 5–10 years.

Ultra Low-Temperature Storage of Cellular Therapy Product

CTP can be successfully cryopreserved for long periods provided a temperature of less than –155 °C is continuously maintained.[54] Storage temperature is continuously monitored and alarms must go off before fluctuating out of range, providing ample time for immediate corrective action. Variation in validated cryopreservation protocols can include either dump freezing or through controlled rate freezing at –80 °C for as long as 2 years with subsequent transfer to liquid nitrogen (LN). Ultralow temperatures can be maintained by immersion in LN, vapor phase nitrogen, or specialized ultralow electric freezers. Owing to reports of CTP cross-contamination by viral pathogens through immersion in the LN medium, vapor phase LN is the recommended storage modality. Low LN level alarms should be in place. Insulated LN freezers can maintain ultralow temperatures in case of emergencies, even for up to 10–14 days. For mechanical freezers, adequate backup should be provided in case of malfunction.

Safety Considerations (Liquid Nitrogen)

Proper training of personnel, which includes use of personal protective attire, goggles, full-face visors, and thermally insulated gloves, will minimize risk of frostbite, burns, and other adverse incidents. The hazard of asphyxiation due to nitrogen vapor displacement of atmospheric oxygen has to be kept in mind. This is critical because oxygen depletion can be a rapid cause of loss of consciousness without warning. LN freezers should be placed in well-ventilated areas to minimize this risk and be subject to planned preventative maintenance. Large-volume stores should have low oxygen alarm systems.

Inventory Control

Inventory systems designed and validated for accurate record keeping and inventory control should at least record date and time, placement of CTPs into freezers, storage location, rack/position, and retrieval by responsible qualified personnel performing all steps. CTPs must be linked to all quality control (QC) documents, continuous temperature records, alarms caused by out-of-range freezer temperatures, and other associated events.

Thawing

Methods to thaw cryopreserved CTPs for transplant should minimize cell loss, maintain cell viability, and prevent introduction of microbial contamination. Thawing should be done rapidly to avoid the possibility of recrystallization of any small intracellular ice nucleation. If needed, steps should be taken to reduce DMSO concentration. There are three common thawing and processing methods and they include direct thaw without manipulation, thaw with dilution and wash, and dilution without wash.

The direct thaw is the most common method used for cryopreserved peripheral blood CTPs administered to adult patients. It is usually performed in the CTP laboratory or at the patient's bedside to reduce cells exposure time to DMSO. The cryopreserved product bag is typically delivered in a validated container to the infusion site, placed in an additional overwrap and submerged in a 37 °C water bath for 3–6 min or until ice crystals dissolve and is infused. This is a simple method that can be done by trained technologists or a trained nurse at the bedside. In addition, it results in little cell loss, especially if the empty bag is flushed with additional saline. Alternatively, dry baths can be validated to minimize risk of microbial contamination.

The thaw and wash methods designed by Rubinstein et al.[55] address the potential risk to cell viability immediately after thaw, and need to remove toxic elements, such as DMSO, to reduce additional risk of long-term cell damage and potential adverse infusion reactions. It is mostly used for HPC-C products and pediatric transplants. After thawing the product in a 37 °C water bath, it is reconstituted with equal volume of an isotonic solution containing a protein source such as human serum albumin or colloids such as dextran 40. The product is then centrifuged, most of the DMSO and hemolyzed cells are removed, and cells are resuspended in the same solution. Unlike bedside thaw, this process is done in a controlled laboratory environment, allowing sampling for prospective testing such as viability and potency. This method is proven to maintain cell viability for 4 h post thaw and result in lower rates of adverse reactions. The procedure does carry some disadvantages, including potential cell loss and increased risk of bag breakage that can cause introduction of microbial contamination.

To overcome the risk of cell loss, some programs use an alternative method that does not include the centrifugation step. This method is used mostly for HPC-C. It provides a simpler approach and takes advantage of the fact that most adults and larger pediatric patients can tolerate small volumes of DMSO with no significant adverse reactions. The toxicity of DMSO to cells is bypassed by diluting the thawed unit with a solution similar to the one used for the wash procedure but without the additional centrifugation step. The method was reported to result in tolerable infusion reactions and high rates of sustainable engraftment. Like the wash procedure, the reconstitution steps are performed in the laboratory to allow sampling for testing, and the progenitor cell viability and potency is comparable with that of the thaw and wash procedure.

Infusion of Cellular Therapy Product

The infusion part of CTP is as important as product collection and processing. Because in most cases products are given after chemotherapy and radiation treatments that severely deplete or eradicate progenitor cells in the BM, it is essential to provide the patient with a product containing viable and potent cells to achieve a successful transplant. Allogeneic products are usually given fresh, and most transplant centers infuse them within 48–72h of collection.[56,57] Autologous products are usually cryopreserved and are infused fast to reduce potential cell damage caused by DMSO exposure.[58,59]

To ensure that the recipient is ready, the infusion time is confirmed with the patient's physician or designee on the day of transplant. Before infusion, the patient can be premedicated with acetaminophen, diphenhydramine, and hydrocortisone. The laboratory personnel deliver the fresh or cryopreserved product to the infusion site. Allogeneic transplants are always performed in the inpatient setting, but autologous infusion can sometimes be performed in an outpatient setting depending on each individual case.

It is important to confirm that the patient is receiving the correct product as prescribed by the transplant physician. Before the product is released for transplant the laboratory medical director or designee should review the processing records and confirm that the product meets release criteria. Minimal release criteria include the applicable cell dose (i.e., progenitor cells, T cells), product sterility, and ABO/Rh verification (required for allogeneic products). In cases of minor or major ABO/Rh incompatibility, release criteria also include product antibody titer and RBC content, respectively.

The identity and integrity of the product on disposition between the laboratory personnel and infusion nurse is confirmed. The clinical team usually follows additional blood product infusion guidelines to confirm the product. Products are infused

through nontunneled single-, double-, or triple-lumen peripherally inserted central catheters or tunneled catheters (double and triple lumen Broviac/Hickman). A 170- to 260-μm blood filter can be used to help prevent any clots in the product from reaching the patient.[2,60,61] If more than one product bag is required, the bags are infused sequentially. In cases where products from multiple donors are infused, most standards require that there be at least 1h between infusions to allow for proper investigation of infusion reactions should they occur. The patient should be monitored by the clinical team during and after infusion for any signs of mild or severe adverse events and treated accordingly.

Adverse Reactions

Infusion of CTPs have been associated with a variety of immunologic and nonimmunologic reactions, including DMSO toxicity, acute and delayed hemolytic reactions, febrile nonhemolytic reactions, allergic reactions, transfusion-related acute lung injury (TRALI), circulatory overload, hypothermia, septic infusion reactions, fat emboli, alloimmunization to antigens, GVHD, and transmission of infectious agents. Many of these reactions are not specific to CTPs but are more broadly seen with transfusions. Here, we review the reactions most commonly associated with CTP infusions.

DMSO Toxicity

DMSO is a rapidly penetrating molecule that increases cells tolerance to osmotic stress induced by cryopreservation. DMSO was originally used as an antiinflammatory reagent but was later found to cause an array of side effects when administered to patients.[62–65] DMSO toxicity in HPC product infusions was shown to affect multiple organs, including respiratory, cardiovascular, gastrointestinal, hepatic, and renal systems.[66,67] DMSO is also associated with intravascular hemolysis.[64] Side effects related to infusion of thawed products are usually mild to moderate, most commonly nausea, vomiting, hypertension, or allergic reactions.[68] Severe side effects are rare but cardiovascular, neurologic, and respiratory side effects have been reported, with some of them being severe or fatal.[69] The rate of side effects was shown to correlate with higher DMSO volume.[70,71] Current recommendation is to infuse less than 1mL DMSO/kg recipient weight.

Acute Hemolytic Reactions

Acute hemolytic reactions can be observed in the setting of major or minor ABO blood group incompatibility or in the setting of other blood group incompatibilities. They may occur immediately or up to 24 h following infusion. Signs and symptoms are nonspecific and include chills, fever, headache, lower back pain, facial flushing, chest pain, labored respirations, and tachycardia. Patients must be managed symptomatically, with measures taken to correct blood pressure and coagulopathy. In addition, practitioners must promote and maintain adequate urine flow to prevent renal damage. Cellular processing techniques before infusion, such as RBC reduction in the case of major ABO incompatibility and plasma reduction in the case of minor ABO incompatibility, help to mitigate these reactions.

Febrile Nonhemolytic Reactions

Febrile nonhemolytic reactions may reflect the action of cytokines either in the product or generated by recipient antibodies against donor white blood cells. Signs and symptoms include chills and a temperature rise of 1°C or more during or within 2 h of product administration. Treatment and prevention is with antipyretics. The main feared differential is an acute hemolytic reaction.

Allergic Reactions

Allergic reactions are thought to be caused by the presence of atopic substances interacting with antibodies present in the donor or recipient plasma. In rare cases, anaphylaxis may occur. Anaphylaxis has been reported in patients with hereditary IgA or haptoglobin deficiency caused by IgA-specific or haptoglobin-specific antibodies of the IgG and/or IgE subclasses. In regards to CTPs, allergic reactions to hydroxyethyl starch or DMSO may also occur in sensitized patients. Signs and symptoms include urticaria, pruritus, bronchospasm, hypotension, severe dyspnea, facial/glottal/laryngeal edema, nausea, vomiting, diaphoresis, or dizziness. For mild cases antihistamines are effective, but in more serious cases patients may require fluids, epinephrine, or steroids. Antihistamines are useful for prevention in mild cases, and washing of products can help prevent symptoms in patients with more severe reactions.

Transfusion-Related Acute Lung Injury

TRALI occurs owing to an acute increase in permeability of the pulmonary microcirculation resulting in massive fluid and protein leakage into alveolar spaces and the interstitium. Anti-HLA and anti-human neutrophil antigen antibodies in the donor or recipient have been implicated. In HLA-matched products TRALI is rare. Symptoms include acute respiratory distress within 6 h of administration, hypoxemia, and bilateral pulmonary infiltrates. Treatment is largely supportive. Plasma-reduction or washing can help to mitigate the risk of TRALI.

Alloimmunization

Alloimmunization to antigens on RBCs, white blood cells, PLTs, or plasma proteins may occur after infusion of CTPs. Alloimmunization is usually asymptomatic but may contribute to accelerated removal of cellular elements, contributing to graft failure, transfusion refractoriness, and red cell aplasia.

Graft-Versus-Host Disease (GVHD)

GVHD is an extremely serious condition complicating allogeneic CTPs. GVHD is the result of viable donor T lymphocytes reacting against recipient tissue antigens. Signs and symptoms are variable in their organ involvement and severity and are sometimes fatal. First-line therapy includes posttransplant immunosuppression and extracorporeal photopheresis,[72] which have been shown to be effective as a second-line therapy as well.[73]

POSTTRANSPLANT ASSESSMENT

If successful, transplants result in the production of normal blood reconstitution and possibly cure of the underlying disorder. To hasten the recovery of SCs a drug called filgrastim (G-CSF) is administered daily from Day +1 (first day following transplant) until blood counts have completely recovered. All subjects regardless of disease histology receive filgrastim (G-CSF) 5 μg/kg (rounded to 300 or 480 μg, depending on the patient's weight) subcutaneously daily from Day 1 until absolute neutrophil count (ANC) >5 × 10⁹/L. Earlier discontinuation, more prolonged administration, or reinitiation may be required for different clinical reasons.

The posttransplant period is associated with high morbidity and transplant-related mortality. Major complications are associated with delayed neutrophil and PLT engraftment and graft rejection, GVHD, disease relapse, and secondary malignancy. Despite a controlled environment and prophylactic antibiotics, which include antiviral and antifungal regimens, bacterial sepsis, mucositis, and viral and other infections are frequently observed. Graft-versus-tumor effect or graft-versus-leukemia effect are observed as part of the GVHD.[74] Patients with allogeneic transplant and chronic GVHD may have a lower risk of cancer relapse.

Engraftment

After transplant, the patient is monitored closely for engraftment by evaluating ANC, PLT, and reticulocyte count (Retic):

- Neutrophil engraftment is defined as the first day of three consecutive days with ANC $\geq 0.5 \times 10^9$/L.
- PLT engraftment is defined as a PLT count $\geq 20 \times 10^9$/L without PLT transfusion support in previous 3 or 7 days.
- Red cell lineage engraftment is the number of days until the Retic has surpassed $\geq 25 \times 10^9$/L.[75]

A delay in time to engraftment may put the patient at risk for infection, bleeding, and other complications. The delayed engraftment standard for each product type has been defined.[76] Different patient categories might have different criteria that should be established based on the diagnosis, conditioning regimen, transplant modification, and use of supporting growth factors.

An example of delayed engraftment based on graft source:

- HPC-M: ANC $\geq 0.5 \times 10^9$/L within 42 days post transplant and PLT $\geq 20,000 \times 10^9$/L within 60 days post transplant.
- HPC-A: ANC $\geq 0.5 \times 10^9$/L within 28 days post transplant and PLT $\geq 20,000 \times 10^9$/L within 60 days post transplant.
- HPC-C: ANC $\geq 0.5 \times 10^9$/L within 42 days post transplant and PLT $\geq 20,000 \times 10^9$/L within 100 days post transplant.[77]

Transfusion Dependence

Transfusion dependence is an obvious but less well-defined criterion of poor engraftment.[78,79] From the transfusion medicine standpoint, the number of days from the last RBC or PLT transfusion is not routinely used because the transfusion threshold varies and transfusion can be due to interventions.[80] Change in blood type in the case of ABO/Rh-mismatched transplants, no matter how prolonged the phase with mixed-field typing, Direct Antiglobulin Test (DAT) positivity, and transfusion with O blood, makes this approach less amenable for monitoring and standardization. The blood bank does not report the ABO/Rh change until the patient becomes transfusion independent for at least 3 months (for additional description see chapter titled Transfusion Approaches in the Transplanted Patient).

QUALITY ASSURANCE AND QUALITY CONTROL

A reliable quality assurance (QA) plan includes measurements and monitoring tools to ensure that all the steps that affect product quality are performed as expected and meet regulatory requirements. Regulatory agencies and accreditation organizations require collection and processing facilities to have a quality program (i.e., FDA, JACIE, CAP, AABB, NMDP, and FACT).[81]

The QA program should ensure that there is consistency in the methods, material, and equipment and that all personnel involved in processing are appropriately trained. The QA plan should include a detailed quality management plan, appropriate monitoring tools to ensure that all activities are executed as defined in the laboratory procedures, effective ways to communicate with informed personnel, and templates to reduce error and process improvement.

Process QC should include measurements to monitor all activities during all processing steps that can affect the final product and can result in compromised performance. In the United States, QC measurements are mandated by federal agencies (i.e., FDA, CMS, CLIA), state health departments, and voluntary accreditation organizations (AABB, CAP, FACT). A QC program should include steps to define necessary QC measurements, review and approval procedures, appropriate acceptability criteria, and appropriate corrective action steps.

The quality program includes provisions for training, qualification, and competency assessment of all employees. SOP must be established for all critical procedures.[82] Product reviews and audits must be performed regularly. Complaint reviews need to be documented, and deviations, errors, and accidents thoroughly documented, evaluated, and investigated using root cause analyses with complete corrective action and follow-up documentation.

Review of records must be completed before distribution and includes tracking records linking donor and recipient identifiers, review of donor-eligibility determination, and collection, processing, and storage records. A verification and attestation is made that release criteria have been met and the determination is made that HPC is available for distribution.

QA investigation of positive microbial cultures: cause, documentation and labeling, product release including approvals, and notification of other facilities involved in the manufacture of the product are required. Recipient outcome review must include any evidence of infection related to the infusion of the contaminated product and additional information of treatment of the recipient. An investigation into the source of the product contamination, such as donor bacteremia or environmental exposure during product collection or processing in the laboratory, must be conducted.

REGULATORY CONSIDERATIONS

The FDA, the leading regulatory body in the United States issued a final rule that HCT/Ps are regulated as drugs, devices, and/or biological products. Establishments processing/manufacturing HCT/Ps are required to register and list their products with the FDA. Federal law prohibits dispensing HPC CTP without a prescription.

Autologous HPCs are regulated solely under Section 361 of the Public Health Service Act (PHS Act) and regulations in Title 21, Section 1271 of the Code of Federal Regulations (§ 21 CFR 1271) because they consist of human cells or tissues that are intended for implantation, transplant, infusion, or transfer into a human recipient (§ 21 CFR 1271.3(d)) and must meet all criteria in § 21 CFR 1271.10, such as that they are minimally manipulated, intended for homologous use only, not combined with other cells or tissues or another article except as specifically listed, for allogeneic use in a first-degree or second-degree blood relative, or for reproductive use if they have a systemic effect as depending on the metabolic activity of living cells for their primary function. These regulations, also known as "tissue rules," define procedures for registration and listing, donor eligibility determination, current good tissue practice (GTP), and qualification of suppliers of critical materials and services.[27]

HCT/Ps such as HPC-C or unrelated peripheral blood SCs are regulated as drug, device, and/or biological products under Section 351 of the PHS Act and/or The Federal Food, Drug, and Cosmetic Act (FD&C Act), biologics/drug regulations, § 21 CFR 207,210, 211, 600–680, and § 21 CFR 1271 subparts A–D, if they are more than minimally manipulated, combined with another article other than a preservation or storage agent, used in a way that is not homologous to their normal function, or they have a systemic effect and are dependent on the metabolic activity of living cells for their primary function. The investigational new drug requirements are outlined in part 312, and drug manufacturing requirements in parts § 211 and § 212.[28]

Transplant Centers Accreditation

Transplant facilities have to abide by federal, state, and hospital regulations. Different states may have different regulations. Mandatory accreditation by state and voluntary peer-based accreditation are raising the quality of transplants. Across the country, insurance companies require such accreditation to provide reimbursement. Computed tomography processing laboratory accreditations are available from AABB and CAP. AABB also provides accreditation for collection facilities and has deemed status with FDA. FACT is approved as an accrediting organization by the United States Health Resources Services and Administration for the C.W. Bill Young Cord Blood Transplantation Program.[31]

OUTCOME DATA MANAGEMENT

Posttransplant recipient follow-up includes outcome analysis. This analysis includes timely engraftment and day 100 and day 365 mortality and is reported to NMDP/CIBMTR.[83] CIBMTR collects transplant data and outcomes in a large observational database. CIBMTR focuses on hematopoietic cell transplantation research together with NMDP and provides summary statistics (Figs. 13.1–13.3).[84]

CLINICAL RESEARCH

Increasing the number of interventional and observational studies involving standard HPCs used in novel protocols, in combination with drugs and devices, for new indications, or new investigational CTP are currently offered to physicians and patients.[85] All clinical research must be conducted under an investigational new drug label and have institutional review board approval. Advanced cell therapies clinical trials are registered with ClinicalTrials.gov. This registry offers searchable database of clinical studies and results conducted around the world. However, even in an investigational setting current Good Manufacturing Practices requirements must be followed.[86]

Novel Cellular Therapy Product

Introduction of novel cell therapies is rapidly growing in the last 2 decades. The number of cellular therapy registered trials is constantly increasing, especially those sponsored by industry. Most of these trials are phase I, phase I/II, and phase II, but the biologics license application of at least one novel CTP already has been approved for the treatment of patients with diffuse large

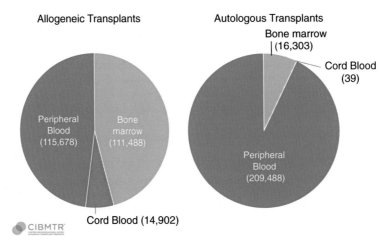

FIG. 13.3 Distribution of patients in the CIBMTR research database by graft source. (From Center for International Blood & Marrow Transplant Research (CIBMTR). *2016 Annual Report*. Available at: https://www.cibmtr.org/ReferenceCenter/Newsletters/Documents/2016%20CIBMTR%20Annual%20Report%20final.pdf; with permission.)

B-cell lymphoma using chimeric antigen receptor T-cell therapy, and more companies are expected to join in the coming year.[87,88] Novel therapies can use existing HSC product sources to target different disease categories, but other cell sources such as mesenchymal SCs, human embryonic SCs, or other pluripotent cells are being increasingly used. To accommodate these new therapies, transplant centers and processing laboratories are required to develop new protocols for receiving, processing, administering, and treating sometimes unpredictable adverse events. In 2017 FACT released its first standard for immunotherapy encouraging transplant centers to establish procedures for treating patients with this new generation of CTPs (Table 13.1).[89]

REFERENCES

1. *EBMT-ESH Handbook on Haematopoietic Stem Cell Transplantation*. 2012.
2. AABB, AAoTB, American Red Cross, American Society for Blood and Marrow, Transplantation ASfA, America's Blood Centers, College of American Pathologists, Cord Blood Association, Foundation for the Accreditation of, Cellular Therapy I, International NetCord Foundation, International Society for Cellular Therapy, JACIE Accreditation Office, Program NMD. *Circular of Information for the Use of Cellular Therapy Products*. Bethesda, MD: AABB; 2016.
3. van Rood JJ, Oudshoorn M. Eleven million donors in bone marrow donors worldwide! Time for reassessment? *Bone Marrow Transplant*. 2008;41(1):1–9.
4. Koreth J, Schlenk R, Kopecky KJ, et al. Allogeneic stem cell transplantation for acute myeloid leukemia in first complete remission: systematic review and meta-analysis of prospective clinical trials. *JAMA*. 2009;301(22):2349–2361.
5. Li D, Wang L, Zhu H, et al. Efficacy of allogeneic hematopoietic stem cell transplantation in intermediate-risk acute myeloid leukemia adult patients in first complete remission: a meta-analysis of prospective studies. *PLoS One*. 2015;10(7):e0132620.
6. Cosimi AB. Nobel prizes in medicine in the field of transplantation. *Transplantation*. 2006;82(12):1558–1562.
7. Mathe G, Schwarzenberg L. Bone marrow transplantation (1958–1978): conditioning and graft-versus-host disease, indications in aplasias and leukemias. *Pathol Biol (Paris)*. 1979;27(6):337–343.
8. Mathe G, Schwarzenberg L, Larrieu MJ. Transfusion and graft of bone marrow in man: technic. *Sangre (Barc)*. 1959;30:784–788.
9. Mathe G, Jammet H, Pendic B, et al. Transfusions and grafts of homologous bone marrow in humans after accidental high dosage irradiation. *Rev Fr Etud Clin Biol*. 1959;4(3):226–238.
10. Aldhous P. Nobel Prize. Transplantation wins again. *Nature*. 1990;347(6293):507.
11. Palca J. Overcoming rejection to win a Nobel Prize. *Science*. 1990;250(4979):378.

12. Gatti RA, Meuwissen HJ, Allen HD, Hong R, Good RA. Immunological reconstitution of sex-linked lymphopenic immunological deficiency. *Lancet.* 1968;2(7583):1366–1369.

13. O'Leary M, Ramsay NK, Nesbit Jr ME, et al. Bone marrow transplantation for non-Hodgkin's lymphoma in children and young adults. A pilot study. *Am J Med.* 1983;74(3): 497–501.

14. Flake AW, Roncarolo MG, Puck JM, et al. Treatment of X-linked severe combined immunodeficiency by in utero transplantation of paternal bone marrow. *N Engl J Med.* 1996;335(24):1806–1810.

15. Almeida-Porada G, Atala A, Porada CD. In utero stem cell transplantation and gene therapy: rationale, history, and recent advances toward clinical application. *Mol Ther Methods Clin Dev.* 2016;5:16020.

16. Loewendorf AI, Csete M, Flake A. Immunological considerations in in utero hematopoetic stem cell transplantation (IUHCT). *Front Pharmacol.* 2014;5:282.

17. Chowdhury N, Asakura A. In utero stem cell transplantation: potential therapeutic application for muscle diseases. *Stem Cells Int.* 2017;2017:3027520.

18. MacKenzie TC, David AL, Flake AW, Almeida-Porada G. Consensus statement from the first international conference for in utero stem cell transplantation and gene therapy. *Front Pharmacol.* 2015;6:15.

19. McClain LE, Flake AW. In utero stem cell transplantation and gene therapy: recent progress and the potential for clinical application. *Best Pract Res Clin Obstet Gynaecol.* 2016;31:88–98.

20. Birkeland SA. The history of transplantation. *Dan Medicinhist Arbog.* 1999:163–185.

21. Kurtzberg JA. History of cord blood banking and transplantation. *Stem Cells Transl Med.* 2017;6(5):1309–1311.

22. Spitzer G, Verma DS, Fisher R, et al. The myeloid progenitor cell-its value in predicting hematopoietic recovery after autologous bone marrow transplantation. *Blood.* 1980;55(2):317–323.

23. Pazarentzos E, Mazarakis ND. Anticancer gene transfer for cancer gene therapy. *Adv Exp Med Biol.* 2014;818: 255–280.

24. Bone marrow transplants using volunteer donors–recommendations and requirements for a standardized practice throughout the world. The Executive Committee of the World Marrow Donor Association. *Bone Marrow Transplant.* 1992;10(3):287–291.

24a. Maitta RW, Vasovic LV, Mohandas K, Music-Aplenc L, Bonzon-Adelson A, Uehlinger J. A safe therapeutic apheresis protocol in paediatric patients weighing 11 to 25 kg. *Vox Sang.* 2014;107(4):375–380.

25. Dew A, Collins D, Artz A, et al. Paucity of HLA-identical unrelated donors for African-Americans with hematologic malignancies: the need for new donor options. *Biol Blood Marrow Transplant.* 2008;14(8):938–941.

26. Food, Drug Administration HHS. Eligibility determination for donors of human cells, tissues, and cellular and tissue-based products. Final rule. *Fed Regist.* 2004;69(101):29785–29834.

27. Human cells, tissues, and cellular and tissue-based products; establishment registration and listing. Food and Drug Administration, HHS. Final rule. *Fed Regist.* 2001;66(13):5447–5469.

28. Food, Drug Administration HHS. Current good tissue practice for human cell, tissue, and cellular and tissue-based product establishments; inspection and enforcement. Final rule. *Fed Regist.* 2004;69(226): 68611–68688.

29. Food, Drug Administration HHS. Human cells, tissues, and cellular and tissue-based products; donor screening and testing, and related labeling. Interim final rule; opportunity for public comment. *Fed Regist.* 2005;70(100):29949–29952.

30. Food, Drug Administration HHS. Revisions to exceptions applicable to certain human cells, tissues, and cellular and tissue-based products. Final rule. *Fed Regist.* 2016;81(120):40512–40518.

31. Warkentin PI. Foundation for the accreditation of cellular T. Voluntary accreditation of cellular therapies: Foundation for the Accreditation of Cellular Therapy (FACT). *Cytotherapy.* 2003;5(4):299–305.

32. American Society for B, Marrow T, American Association of Blood B, et al. ASBMT Position Statement. Joint public policy on legislative and regulatory affairs. *Biol Blood Marrow Transplant.* 2004;10(4):283–284.

33. Anthias C, O'Donnell PV, Kiefer DM, et al. European group for blood and marrow transplantation centers with FACT-JACIE accreditation have significantly better compliance with related donor care standards. *Biol Blood Marrow Transplant.* 2016;22(3):514–519.

34. Standards of the National Marrow Donor Program. NMDP Standards Committee. *Transfusion.* 1993;33(2):172–180.

35. Hurley CK, Foeken L, Horowitz M, et al. Standards, regulations and accreditation for registries involved in the worldwide exchange of hematopoietic stem cell donors and products. *Bone Marrow Transplant.* 2010;45(5):819–824.

36. Choi SW, Levine JE, Ferrara JL. Pathogenesis and management of graft-versus-host disease. *Immunol Allergy Clin North Am.* 2010;30(1):75–101.

37. Eapen M, Logan BR, Horowitz MM, et al. Bone marrow or peripheral blood for reduced-intensity conditioning unrelated donor transplantation. *J Clin Oncol.* 2015;33(4):364–369.

38. Howell C, Douglas K, Cho G, et al. Guideline on the clinical use of apheresis procedures for the treatment of patients and collection of cellular therapy products. British Committee for Standards in Haematology. *Transfus Med.* 2015;25(2):57–78.

39. Schwartz J, Padmanabhan A, Aqui N, et al. Guidelines on the use of therapeutic apheresis in clinical practice-evidence-based approach from the Writing Committee of the American Society for Apheresis: the seventh special issue. *J Clin Apher.* 2016;31(3):149–162.

40. Kessinger A, Sharp JG. The whys and hows of hematopoietic progenitor and stem cell mobilization. *Bone Marrow Transplant.* 2003;31(5):319–329.

41. Sugrue MW, Williams K, Pollock BH, et al. Characterization and outcome of "hard to mobilize" lymphoma patients undergoing autologous stem cell transplantation. *Leuk Lymphoma.* 2000;39(5–6):509–519.

42. Schwartz J, Winters JL, Padmanabhan A, et al. Guidelines on the use of therapeutic apheresis in clinical practice-evidence-based approach from the Writing Committee of the American Society for Apheresis: the sixth special issue. *J Clin Apher.* 2013;28(3):145–284.

43. Jacobs LB, Shirey RS, Ness PM. Hemolysis due to the simultaneous occurrence of passenger lymphocyte syndrome and a delayed hemolytic transfusion reaction in a liver transplant patient. *Arch Pathol Lab Med.* 1996;120(7):684–686.

44. Marques MB. The American Society for Apheresis (ASFA) is pleased to offer a Qualification in Apheresis (QIA) in partnership with The Board of Certification (BOC) of the American Society for Clinical Pathology (ASCP) starting in January of 2016!. *Transfus Apher Sci.* 2016;54(2):319–320.

45. Celluzzi CM, Keever-Taylor C, Aljurf M, et al. Training practices of hematopoietic progenitor cell-apheresis and -cord blood collection staff: analysis of a survey by the Alliance for Harmonisation of Cellular Therapy Accreditation. *Transfusion.* 2014;54(12):3138–3144.

46. Ramirez PA, Wagner JE, Brunstein CG. Going straight to the point: intra-BM injection of hematopoietic progenitors. *Bone Marrow Transplant.* 2010;45(7):1127–1133.

47. Gragert L, Eapen M, Williams E, et al. HLA match likelihoods for hematopoietic stem-cell grafts in the U.S. registry. *N Engl J Med.* 2014;371(4):339–348.

48. Ashford P, Distler P, Gee A, et al. Standards for the terminology and labeling of cellular therapy products. *Transfusion.* 2007;47(7):1319–1327.

49. Koistinen J. ICCBBA (International Council for Commonality in Blood Bank Automation). *Vox Sang.* 2000; 78(suppl 2):307–309.

50. Clarke E. Colony-forming cell assays for determining potency of cellular therapy products. In: Areman EM, Loper K, eds. *Cellular Therapy: Principles, Methods, and Regulations.* Bethesda, MD: AABB; 2009:573–580.

51. Spellman S, Hurley CK, Brady C, et al. Guidelines for the development and validation of new potency assays for the evaluation of umbilical cord blood. *Cytotherapy.* 2011;13(7):848–855.

52. Sutherland DR, Anderson L, Keeney M, Nayar R, Chin-Yee I. The ISHAGE guidelines for CD34+ cell determination by flow cytometry. International Society of Hematotherapy and Graft Engineering. *J Hematother.* 1996;5(3):213–226.

53. Servais S, Porcher R, Xhaard A, et al. Pre-transplant prognostic factors of long-term survival after allogeneic peripheral blood stem cell transplantation with matched related/unrelated donors. *Haematologica.* 2014;99(3):519–526.

54. McCullough J, Haley R, Clay M, Hubel A, Lindgren B, Moroff G. Long-term storage of peripheral blood stem cells frozen and stored with a conventional liquid nitrogen technique compared with cells frozen and stored in a mechanical freezer. *Transfusion.* 2010;50(4):808–819.

55. Rubinstein P, Dobrila L, Rosenfield RE, et al. Processing and cryopreservation of placental/umbilical cord blood for unrelated bone marrow reconstitution. *Proc Natl Acad Sci USA.* 1995;92(22):10119–10122.

56. Frey NV, Lazarus HM, Goldstein SC. Has allogeneic stem cell cryopreservation been given the 'cold shoulder'? An analysis of the pros and cons of using frozen versus fresh stem cell products in allogeneic stem cell transplantation. *Bone Marrow Transplant.* 2006;38(6):399–405.

57. Ghobadi A, Fiala MA, Ramsingh G, et al. Fresh or cryopreserved CD34+-selected mobilized peripheral blood stem and progenitor cells for the treatment of poor graft function after allogeneic hematopoietic cell transplantation. *Biol Blood Marrow Transplant.* 2017;23(7):1072–1077.

58. Rodrigues JP, Paraguassú-Braga FH, Carvalho L, Abdelhay E, Bouzas LF, Porto LC. Evaluation of trehalose and sucrose as cryoprotectants for hematopoietic stem cells of umbilical cord blood. *Cryobiology.* 2008;56(2):144–151.

59. Richard HL. Thawing and infusing cellular therapy products. In: Areman EM LK, ed. *Cellular Therapy: Principles, Methods, and Regulations.* 2nd ed. Bethesda, MD: AABB; 2016:459–467.

60. Totoe G, Lindgren B, Emrick E, Kadidlo D, McKenna D. Postthaw filtration of umbilical cord blood does not affect product quality or likelihood of engraftment. *Transfusion.* 2011;51(10):2257–2258.

61. Berg A, Kao GS. Impact of filtering thawed hematopoietic progenitor cells (HPC) with routine blood filter on CD34+ cell number (abstract). *Transfusion.* 2006;46.

62. Yellowlees P, Greenfield C, McIntyre N. Dimethylsulphoxide-induced toxicity. *Lancet.* 1980;2(8202):1004–1006.

63. Runckel DN, Swanson JR. Effect of dimethyl sulfoxide on serum osmolality. *Clin Chem.* 1980;26(12):1745–1747.

64. Samoszuk M, Reid ME, Toy PT. Intravenous dimethylsulfoxide therapy causes severe hemolysis mimicking a hemolytic transfusion reaction. *Transfusion.* 1983;23(5):405.

65. Davis JM, Rowley SD, Braine HG, Piantadosi S, Santos GW. Clinical toxicity of cryopreserved bone marrow graft infusion. *Blood.* 1990;75(3):781–786.

66. Smith DM, Weisenburger DD, Bierman P, Kessinger A, Vaughan WP, Armitage JO. Acute renal failure associated with autologous bone marrow transplantation. *Bone Marrow Transplant.* 1987;2(2):195–201.

67. Benekli M, Anderson B, Wentling D, Bernstein S, Czuczman M, McCarthy P. Severe respiratory depression after dimethyl-sulphoxide-containing autologous stem cell infusion in a patient with AL amyloidosis. *Bone Marrow Transplant.* 2000;25(12):1299–1301.

68. Dhodapkar M, Goldberg SL, Tefferi A, Gertz MA. Reversible encephalopathy after cryopreserved peripheral blood stem cell infusion. *Am J Hematol.* 1994;45(2):187–188.

69. Zenhausern R, Tobler A, Leoncini L, Hess OM, Ferrari P. Fatal cardiac arrhythmia after infusion of dimethyl sulfoxide-cryopreserved hematopoietic stem cells in a patient with severe primary cardiac amyloidosis and end-stage renal failure. *Ann Hematol.* 2000;79(9):523–526.

70. Rapoport AP, Rowe JM, Packman CH, Ginsberg SJ. Cardiac arrest after autologous marrow infusion. *Bone Marrow Transplant.* 1991;7(5):401–403.

71. Windrum P, Morris TC, Drake MB, Niederwieser D, Ruutu T, Subcommittee ECLWPC. Variation in dimethyl sulfoxide use in stem cell transplantation: a survey of EBMT centres. *Bone Marrow Transplant.* 2005;36(7):601–603.

72. Dunbar NM, Raval JS, Johnson A, et al. Extracorporeal photopheresis practice patterns: an international survey by the ASFA ECP subcommittee. *J Clin Apher.* 2017;32(4):215–223.

73. Shimoda T. On postoperative erythroderma. *Geka.* 1955; 17:487–492.

74. Howrey RP, Martin PL, Driscoll T, et al. Graft-versus-leukemia-induced complete remission following unrelated umbilical cord blood transplantation for acute leukemia. *Bone Marrow Transplant.* 2000;26(11):1251–1254.

75. van Besien K, Nichols CR, Tricot G, et al. Characteristics of engraftment after repeated autologous bone marrow transplantation. *Exp Hematol.* 1990;18(7):785–788.

76. Kanda J, Kaynar L, Kanda Y, et al. Pre-engraftment syndrome after myeloablative dual umbilical cord blood transplantation: risk factors and response to treatment. *Bone Marrow Transplant.* 2013;48(7):926–931.

77. Escolar ML, Poe MD, Provenzale JM, et al. Transplantation of umbilical-cord blood in babies with infantile Krabbe's disease. *N Engl J Med.* 2005;352(20):2069–2081.

78. Worel N, Panzer S, Reesink HW, et al. Transfusion policy in ABO-incompatible allogeneic stem cell transplantation. *Vox Sang.* 2010;98(3 Pt 2):455–467.

79. Solh M, Brunstein C, Morgan S, Weisdorf D. Platelet and red blood cell utilization and transfusion independence in umbilical cord blood and allogeneic peripheral blood hematopoietic cell transplants. *Biol Blood Marrow Transplant.* 2011;17(5):710–716.

80. Cohn CS. Transfusion support issues in hematopoietic stem cell transplantation. *Cancer Control.* 2015;22(1):52–59.

81. Snowden JA, McGrath E, Duarte RF, et al. JACIE accreditation for blood and marrow transplantation: past, present and future directions of an international model for healthcare quality improvement. *Bone Marrow Transplant.* 2017;52(10).

82. Keever-Taylor CA, Slaper-Cortenbach I, Celluzzi C, et al. Training practices of cell processing laboratory staff: analysis of a survey by the Alliance for Harmonization of Cellular Therapy Accreditation. *Cytotherapy.* 2015;17(12):1831–1844.

83. Mariotto AB, Noone AM, Howlader N, et al. Cancer survival: an overview of measures, uses, and interpretation. *J Natl Cancer Inst Monogr.* 2014;2014(49):145–186.

84. D'Souza A, Zhu X. *Current Uses and Outcomes of Hematopoietic Stem Cell Transplantation: 2016 CIBMTR Summary Slides;* 2016.

85. Sanchez R, Silberstein LE, Lindblad RW, Welniak LA, Mondoro TH, Wagner JE. Strategies for more rapid translation of cellular therapies for children: a US perspective. *Pediatrics.* 2013;132(2):351–358.

86. Lindblad RW, Ibenana L, Wagner JE, et al. Cell therapy product administration and safety: data capture and analysis from the Production Assistance for Cellular Therapies (PACT) program. *Transfusion.* 2015;55(3):674–679.

87. Fesnak AD, June CH, Levine BL. Engineered T cells: the promise and challenges of cancer immunotherapy. *Nat Rev Cancer.* 2016;16(9):566–581.

88. Levine BL, Miskin J, Wonnacott K, Keir C. Global manufacturing of CAR T cell therapy. *Mol Ther Methods Clin Dev.* 2017;4:92–101.

89. FACT-JACIE. Immune Effector Cell Standards. http://www.factweb.org/forms/store/ProductFormPublic/first-edition-fact-standards-for-immune-effector-cells-free-download. First edition. 2017.

CHAPTER 14

Therapeutic Apheresis

CHISA YAMADA, MD

INTRODUCTION

Apheresis is a process whereby blood is removed from the subject, continuously separated into component parts, one or more components are removed, and the remainder is then returned to the subject. Since its first application to Waldenström macroglobulinemia in 1960,[1] the applications of therapeutic apheresis have been expanding. The American Society for Apheresis (ASFA) was formed in 1982, and the first guidelines for clinical application of therapeutic apheresis were published in 1986. The guidelines have been revised multiple times, and currently more than 85 diseases have been reviewed with an evidence-based approach for therapeutic apheresis.[2] The ASFA guidelines groups diseases into category I through IV: category I for diseases for which apheresis is accepted as the first-line therapy, category II for diseases for which apheresis is accepted as the second-line therapy, category III for diseases in which the role of apheresis is not established, and category IV for diseases for which apheresis is ineffective. Table 14.1 shows 24 diseases or conditions classified as category I per ASFA guidelines. In this chapter, the clinical applications of common procedures, such as therapeutic plasma exchange (TPE), red cell exchange (RBC Ex), leukocytapheresis, low-density lipoprotein and (LDL) apheresis, and their common diseases applicable for each procedure are explained. In addition, hematopoietic progenitor cell (HPC) collections and extracorporeal photopheresis (ECP) are discussed.

Access

Therapeutic apheresis procedures require lines that allow adequate blood flow from and to the apheresis device (draw and infusion lines). The flow rates are 60–150 mL/min for adults and minimum 10 mL/min for pediatric patients. When patients have adequate veins, peripheral access on both arms may be the best choice using 16- to 18-gauge steel needles as draw lines. However, when their veins collapse during the procedure or they do not have good veins, central lines are required, and tunneled catheters are recommended when patients receive multiple procedures

during a prolonged period to avoid infectious risk. Rigid double-lumen central catheters for apheresis or dialysis are usually used, and they need maintenance with heparin flush at least once a week.

THERAPEUTIC PLASMA EXCHANGE

Procedure

There are three types of techniques used for plasma removal: centrifugation technique, immunoadsorption technique, and double filtration technique. Among these, the main technique currently used for TPE in the United States is centrifugation. The subject's blood is drawn to the apheresis device, which separates the blood into roughly red blood cell (RBC), buffy coat, and plasma layer using centrifugation. Anticoagulant (usually citrate acid or heparin) is added before the blood enters the device, plasma is held by the device, and the RBCs and buffy coat are returned to the subject with replacement fluid. Therefore plasmapheresis using the centrifugation technique is now called plasma exchange. Replacement fluid can be 5% albumin, donor plasma, normal saline, or a combination of these depending on the patient's condition or disease.

TPE is used to remove pathologic proteins in the plasma. The efficacy of removal of the target protein depends on the volume of blood processed by the TPE and the volume of distribution of the protein. In general, one plasma volume exchange removes approximately 60% of protein in plasma. When the offending protein or substance removed has a large volume of distribution, however, the rebound is high and the overall efficacy of the procedure can be much lower. One plasma volume exchange per procedure is a common protocol, and TPE is scheduled every other day with some exceptions when multiple procedures are performed.

Complications

The most common complication is citrate toxicity. Citrate is the most commonly used anticoagulant

TABLE 14.1

Diseases in Which Therapeutic Apheresis Is Accepted as First-Line Therapy, According to American Society for Apheresis Guidelines

Procedure		Diseases
TPE	Neurologic disease	Acute inflammatory demyelinating polyradiculoneuropathy/Guillain-Barré syndrome
		Age-related macular degeneration
		Chronic inflammatory demyelinating polyradiculoneuropathy
		Myasthenia gravis
		N-methyl-D-aspartate receptor antibody encephalitis
		Paraproteinemic demyelinating neuropathies/chronic acquired demyelinating polyneuropathies
		Progressive multifocal leukoencephalopathy associated with natalizumab
	Hematologic disease	Hyperviscosity in monoclonal gammopathies
		Thrombotic microangiopathy, factor H autoantibodies associated
		Thrombotic microangiopathy, ticlopidine associated
		Thrombotic thrombocytopenic purpura
	Kidney disease	ANCA-associated rapidly progressive glomerulonephritis
		Antiglomerular basement membrane disease (Goodpasture syndrome)
		Recurrent focal segmental glomerulosclerosis in transplanted kidney
		ABO-compatible renal transplantation, antibody-mediated rejection/desensitization with living donor
		ABO-incompatible renal transplantation, desensitization with living donor
	Liver disease	Acute liver failure
		Living donor liver transplantation; ABO desensitization
		Wilson disease, fulminant
RBC Ex		Stroke and stroke prophylaxis in sickle cell disease
Erythrocytapheresis		Hereditary hemochromatosis
		Polycythemia vera; erythrocytosis
LDL apheresis		Homozygous familial hypercholesterolemia
ECP		Cutaneous T-cell lymphoma; mycosis fungoides; Sezary syndrome

ANCA, anti-neutrophil cytoplasmic antibody; *ECP*, extracorporeal photopheresis; *LDL*, low-density lipoprotein; *RBC*, red blood cell; *RBC Ex*, RBC exchange; *TPE*, therapeutic plasma exchange.
From Schwartz J, Padmanabhan A, Aqui N, et al. Guidelines on the use of therapeutic apheresis in clinical practice-evidence-based approach from the Writing Committee of the American Society for apheresis: the seventh special issue. *J Clin Apher.* 2016;31(3):149–162; with permission.

during TPE. Citrate ion chelates free ionized calcium and is metabolized into bicarbonate in the liver, therefore serum ionized calcium decreases during the procedure. Decreased ionized calcium can cause excitability of nerve cell membranes leading to spontaneous depolarization. As a result, patients may experience oral tingling, numbness, nausea, and light headedness and electrocardiogram changes in more severe cases. If plasma is used as a replacement fluid in daily TPE or higher volume of blood is processed per procedure, citrate used for TPE in addition to citrate in plasma can cause metabolic alkalosis.[3] Other complications are allergic reaction or infection, mostly when replacement fluid is donor plasma; vasovagal reaction; decrease in hemoglobin; vascular access issues; and cardiac arrhythmias. When the patient is on angiotensin-converting enzyme inhibitors for the treatment of hypertension, increased bradykinin can cause hypotension, flushing, dyspnea, and bradycardia. Removal of proteins other than the target protein can be an issue; for example, removal of coagulation factors and fibrinogen leads to coagulopathy in the setting of multiple consecutive procedures, removal of protein-bound medications requires reevaluation of the medication dosage, or removal of immunoglobulins may require immunoglobulin infusion. Mortality is rare, however, it has been reported due to hemorrhage after central venous line insertion or systemic infection.[4]

Indications

TPE is mainly used to decrease antibodies, pathologic protein, or pathologic substance, and is infrequently used to remove protein-bound medications.

Neurologic diseases

The most frequently encountered neurologic disease that has been treated by TPE is myasthenia gravis (MG). Additional autoantibodies to other neuromuscular junction proteins other than antiacetylcholine receptor (AchR) antibodies have been identified, such as antibodies to muscle-specific kinase (MuSK),[5] muscle proteins titian or ryanodine,[6] lipoprotein receptor–related protein 4,[7] neural agrin, and CoIQ, which is a part of the acetylcholinesterase complex.[8] At present, laboratory tests are available to detect only AchR antibodies and MuSK antibodies. MG symptoms caused by these two antibodies are somewhat different depending on which one is present; however, the efficacy of TPE has been proved for patients with both antibodies and maintenance TPE is also reported to be effective on MuSK MG.[9,10]

Although TPE is reported to work for acute inflammatory demyelinating polyradiculoneuropathy (AIDP, Guillain-Barré syndrome) and chronic inflammatory demyelinating polyradiculoneuropathy, intravenous immunoglobulin (IVIG) has also been effective for AIDP; therefore TPE is usually applied only for patients who did not respond to IVIG well.

The efficacy of TPE treatment for multiple sclerosis (MS), neuromyelitis optica (NMO), and neuromyelitis optica spectrum disorders (NMOSD) is still controversial. Currently, TPE is considered beneficial for patients with steroid-refractory MS in the acute phase as a second-line treatment,[11,12] but not in the chronic phase. Aquaporin 4 antibody also called NMO-IgG is found to be more than 90% specific for NMO, and TPE is reported to be beneficial as a rescue therapy in acute corticosteroid-refractory exacerbations.[13–15] TPE has also been reported to be beneficial in some patients with NMOSD without NMO-IgG; however, low titer of NMO-IgG may not be detectable with current techniques.[16]

TPE has been applied to some types of encephalitis or encephalopathy caused by antibodies as a second-line treatment. N-methyl-D-aspartate receptor antibody encephalitis has been newly listed in the ASFA guidelines as a category I disease.[2]

Hematologic diseases

TPE is the first-line treatment for thrombotic thrombocytopenic purpura. By using plasma as a replacement fluid, TPE can replenish decreased von Willebrand factor–cleaving protease (ADAMTS13) in addition to removal of ADAMTS13 inhibitors. TPE is performed daily for this reason during the acute phase until the level of inhibitor is decreased and platelet count recovers, but complications caused by the removal of other plasma proteins are minimized by using plasma as replacement fluid.

Hyperviscosity caused by monoclonal gammopathies, especially Waldenström macroglobulinemia, is another condition that is encountered relatively often. TPE reduced plasma viscosity by removing IgM, and patients often experience symptomatic improvement quickly.

Atypical hemolytic uremic syndrome (aHUS) is a condition caused by a dysfunctional complement system leading to thrombotic microangiopathy.[17] A majority of cases of aHUS are caused by genetic mutations, and anticomplement medications are currently the first-line treatment. However, although aHUS diagnosis among thrombotic microangiopathies is still uncertain, limited TPE use in this disease has led to some patients seeing mild recovery of their platelet counts most likely due to the presence of complement factors in donor plasma used as replacement fluid.

For cryoglobulinemia, which is usually caused by IgM, TPE is often applied in the acute phase with severe hemolysis or other symptoms. Also, some reports have shown that TPE is effective in preventing the recurrence of pancreatitis by reducing triglycerides. LDL apheresis is not designed to reduce triglycerides, therefore TPE can be performed for hypertriglyceridemia.[18]

Renal diseases

Although TPE is the first-line treatment for some antibody-mediated renal diseases, the best response in patients is observed after several procedures followed by immunosuppression. Human leukocyte antigen (HLA) or other antibodies, which may cause antibody-mediated rejection, can be removed by TPE often followed by IVIG. Some types of HLA antibodies are reported to be difficult to remove, but TPE treatment is reported to stabilize renal function.[19] For ABO-incompatible renal transplantation, TPE removes IgG isoagglutinins as well.[20]

The cause of focal segmental glomerulosclerosis (FSGS) is still not fully understood; however, multiple pathologic proteins in the blood are suggested to cause FSGS and can be removed by TPE. A recent meta-analysis showed that 71% of the patients achieved full or partial remission after treatment with TPE.[21]

Liver diseases

TPE has been applied for some conditions such as fulminant liver failure caused by acetaminophen, viral hepatitis, and Wilson disease, and for desensitization for ABO-incompatible liver transplantation. For Wilson disease, a few reports have shown removal of copper by TPE. However, the biggest role of TPE is to restore hemostasis by providing coagulation factors when plasma is used as the replacement fluid and to remove activated clotting factors or fibrinogen so that the patient can survive through transplantation.

RED CELL EXCHANGE

Procedure

The patient's RBCs are removed by the apheresis device and replaced by donor RBCs in RBC Ex. Target hematocrit (Hct) and fraction of RBC cell remaining (the percentage of the patient's RBC that remains in the patient after the procedure) are set depending on the patient's disease and condition. The amount of RBC needed for the procedure is calculated with the patient's weight, height, and preprocedure Hct.

More recently, newer apheresis devices allow the performance of isovolemic RBC Ex. This procedure decreases a patient's RBC by replacing a predetermined percentage with normal saline or albumin followed by standard RBC Ex with donor RBCs. In this way, the patient's exposure to donor RBC may be reduced and there is a lower risk of iron overload.[22]

For pediatric patients, RBC priming with either donor RBC or reconstituted whole blood may be used when the extracorporeal volume in the circuit is large relative to the patient's total blood volume to avoid hypotensive reactions or anemia during the procedure. Alternatively, manual whole blood exchange using reconstituted whole blood may also be used in patients with body weight less than 10–20 kg instead of automated RBC Ex.

Complications

The most common complication of RBC Ex is citrate toxicity, as stated for TPE, and allergic reactions to plasma proteins in donor RBC units. In addition, transfusion transmitted disease and sensitization are big concerns for many patients with sickle cell disease receiving monthly RBC Ex due to exposures to several RBC units per procedure. Phenotypically matched RBCs are often used for patients who are receiving frequent or maintenance RBC Ex to prevent future RBC alloimmunization.

Indications

RBC Ex is performed mainly for patients with hemoglobinopathies and is infrequently used as an adjunctive therapy for malaria, babesiosis, and erythropoietic porphyria.

RBC Ex is most frequently performed for prophylaxis in patients with homozygous sickle cell disease and is normally scheduled every 4–8 weeks. The procedure is also performed emergently in patients presenting with symptoms of stroke, acute chest syndrome, priapism, multiorgan failure, and splenic/hepatic sequestration. When a patient who has already made RBC alloantibodies needs RBC Ex emergently, it is important to assess if the RBC Ex should be performed with compatible but nonphenotypically matched RBC units, leaving the risk of new RBC antibody production, or if the procedure should be delayed until phenotypically matched RBC units are obtained. It must be emphasized that the more RBC alloantibodies a patient has, the more will it be difficult to find a sufficient number of compatible RBC units.

Patients with heterozygous sickle cell disease, such as sickle cell/Hgb C disease or sickle cell/thalassemia, have for the most part less severe and less frequent pain crises. However, some of these patients may have benefits from prophylactic RBC Ex.

LEUKOCYTAPHERESIS

Procedure

Therapeutic cell depletion includes leukocytapheresis and thrombocytapheresis. In the former, the patient's WBCs are removed by the apheresis device and the remaining blood components are returned to the patient without replacement fluid. The fluid balance at the end of leukocytapheresis is usually equal or even positive because of fluid infusion during priming of the tubes for the procedure and presence of anticoagulant (and calcium supplement) in normal saline; therefore replacement fluid is not necessary. Depending on which WBCs are increased in the patient, mononuclear cell (mainly lymphocytes) depletion or polymorphonuclear cell (mainly granulocytes/blasts) depletion can be performed.

Complications

Complications are similar to those of other procedures mentioned in this chapter such as citrate toxicity or vascular access issues. The leukocytapheresis-specific complication is proximity cell removal. When lymphocytes are targeted for removal, platelets that are in the closest cell layer may also be removed. When granulocytes are targeted for removal, RBCs that are in the closest cell layer may be removed as well. In patients with hyperleukocytosis, Hgb is usually low and RBC transfusion is often required immediately after the procedure. RBC transfusion is usually reserved until after the procedure to avoid a further increase in blood viscosity, which may aggravate a patient's symptoms. RBC transfusion during the procedure is not recommended in general because it causes interface change and careful frequent adjustment of the procedure is required.

Indications

Clinical evidence has shown that leukocytapheresis does not improve long-term survival but reduces early mortality.[23,24] The risks of tumor lysis syndrome and leukostasis increase when the WBC count is >100 × 10^9/L in acute myeloid leukemia (AML), infrequently in chronic myelomonocytic leukemia, and when the WBC count is >400 × 10^9/L in acute lymphoblastic leukemia (ALL). Therefore when patients have more than the aforementioned number of blasts, leukocytapheresis is often used to lower the risk. Due to the smaller size of lymphoid blasts compared with myeloid blasts, ALL has a higher threshold of WBC number with a high risk for leukostasis. Single leukocytapheresis can reduce the WBC count by 30%–60%; however, this percent reduction will be much lower when the preprocedure WBC count is <100 × 10^9/L. However, leukocytapheresis should be performed in patients with AML with monocytosis even if their WBC count is <100 × 10^9/L and reduction rate is minimal because of the nature of the disease course, which can be more severe than other types of AML. Leukocytapheresis is often applied while laboratory or imaging tests are being performed to establish a definitive diagnosis to decide the treatment

plan or immediately before chemotherapy is started to prevent chemotherapy-induced tumor lysis. However, a recent review concluded that early initiation of chemotherapy, hydroxyurea, and supportive care are much more important than leukocytapheresis in patients with hyperleukocytosis without leukostasis.[25]

LOW-DENSITY LIPOPROTEIN APHERESIS
Procedure

Currently, LDL apheresis is the only therapeutic apheresis that uses immunoadsorption technology in the United States. This technology allows the removal of only targeted substance(s) without removing other proteins in the plasma; therefore replacement fluid is not needed. The patient's blood is separated into plasma and cells using a cell separator, and the plasma passes through the adsorption column. The beads in the column contain an adsorber or are coupled to antibodies in the matrix that allows for specific pathogenic substances to be removed by binding to the adsorber. Depending on the type of adsorber, lipids, IgG, IgM, IgA, IgE, fibrinogen, isoagglutinins, anti-C1q antibodies, anti-phospholipids, or anti-double-stranded DNA antibodies can be removed. However, current devices using this technique failed to prove efficacy in some autoimmune diseases in the United States. Frequency of the procedure in patients with hyperlipidemia is usually every 2 weeks.

A device that uses heparin-induced extracorporeal LDL precipitation technique is also available in the United States. This technique uses lipid precipitation by adding acidic acetate solution to separate plasma.

Complications

The complications are similar to those of TPE. However, flow rate is around 75 mL/min, which is slower than that of typical TPE for adults. Therefore vasovagal reactions and cardiac complications may be less frequent than TPE. The most common complications are dizziness, unclassified pain, hypo/hypertension, and vomiting.[26,27] Because current LDL apheresis devices are set up to use heparin as an anticoagulant, the procedure is contraindicated in patients who cannot receive heparin.[28]

Indications

LDL apheresis has been performed in patients with hyperlipidemia, especially but not limited to those homozygous for familial hypercholesterolemia. A previous report has shown a reduction of total cholesterol and LDL in homozygotes by 42.5% and 53.0%, respectively, after 18 weeks of

LDL apheresis treatments, and in heterozygotes by 31.3% and 41.2%, respectively.[29] Another report has shown reduction of LDL after 4 years of LDL apheresis treatments in homozygotes and heterozygotes by 26.7% and 4.5%, respectively.[27] The procedure has also been shown to decrease triglycerides; however, these are not meant to be removed by LDL apheresis. Therefore TPE is usually performed to remove triglycerides.

Recently, LDL apheresis has been applied to primary FSGS and recurrent FSGS after renal transplantation. Secondary hyperlipidemia has been implicated in the progression of FSGS, and some lipid-lowering therapies have been proposed as treatment, including LDL apheresis. These reports are mainly case studies[30–32]; however, the higher efficacy of LDL apheresis compared with TPE has not been demonstrated and long-term efficacy of LDL apheresis is unknown at this time.

Other indications such as peripheral vascular diseases, Refsum disease, and sudden sensorineural hearing loss have been treated by LDL apheresis with some good results.[2,33,34]

HEMATOPOIETIC PROGENITOR CELL COLLECTION
Procedure
HPC collection is not a therapeutic procedure in itself; however, the collected apheresis products are used to treat patients. Autologous and allogeneic peripheral blood progenitor cell collections are becoming a standard source for stem cells to be used in bone marrow transplantations after the safety of the procedure, proved viability of the collected HPCs, and development of protocols using cytotoxic chemotherapy followed by granulocyte colony-stimulating factor (G-CSF) or granulocyte-macrophage–colony stimulating factor (GM-CSF) and plerixafor leading to a high HPC mobilization were established. The procedure is the same as mononuclear cell depletion used for leukocytapheresis; however, a lower collection flow rate is used for HPC collections. Target cell $CD34^+$ cell dose for one bone marrow transplant is usually $2.0–3.0 \times 10^6$ cells/kg with a minimum required dose of $2.0–2.5 \times 10^6$ cells/kg for a 95% probability of achieving granulocyte and platelet recovery in <3 weeks.[35] Two to three procedures may be performed and 10–15 L of blood processed per procedure are required to achieve this $CD34^+$ goal.

Peripheral blood progenitor cells have been found to be superior to bone marrow–harvested cells with regard to engraftment, quality of life, and cost; however, there are no differences in transplantation-related mortality and disease-free survival rates between the two methods.[36]

Complications
Complications are similar to those of leukocytapheresis; however, patients may experience other complications due to G-CSF, GM-CSF, or other medications in preparation for the procedure, such as bone pain, generalized fatigue, nausea, diarrhea, and headache. Although a patient's WBC is higher than the reference range due to G-CSF preconditioning, it is usually $<100 \times 10^9$/L, and removal of platelets and also RBCs can occur with collection. In these cases, platelet or RBC transfusions may be needed before or after a procedure. Sudden increases of WBC count by G-CSF/GM-CSF can also lead to splenomegaly, and spontaneous splenic rupture has been reported.[37] In addition, prevention of central line–associated infection is particularly important because of the nature of the patient's disease state and requirement for blood components.

Indications
Autologous HPC collections are performed for patients with hematologic malignancies, frequently for multiple myeloma, Hodgkin lymphoma, non–Hodgkin lymphoma, or more recently, for patients with sickle cell disease, whereas allogeneic transplants can be done in the setting of AML. In addition to hematologic diseases, HPC transplants have been tried in other diseases such as retinal disease, Parkinson disease, Huntington disease, spinal cord injury, myocardial infarction, type I diabetes mellitus, and pediatric tumors such as neuroblastoma, medulloblastoma, or osteosarcoma.

Lymphocytes can also be collected and infused from the same HPC donor for recipients who show signs of bone marrow graft failure for rescue. Additionally, treatments using manipulated T cells, natural killer cells, and mesenchymal stem cell are also under investigation. Therapy using autologous T cells manipulated ex vivo to make them reactive to specific neoplastic antigens and returned to the patients are being investigated for B-cell/pre-B-cell ALL, chronic lymphocytic leukemia, and glioblastoma. Cells for these therapies are also collected from peripheral blood.

EXTRACORPOREAL PHOTOPHERESIS
Procedure
ECP is different from the other procedures described in this chapter in that it does not remove any cells. In ECP, mononuclear cells are separated by the apheresis device and exposed to ultraviolet-A (UVA) light after addition

of 8-methoxypsoralen (8-MOP) and then returned to the patient with the rest of blood components. The mechanism of action of ECP is not fully understood; however, the combination of 8-MOP and UVA may lead to apoptosis of treated monocytes.[38] The main target cells of ECP are T cells.

Complications

Due to the inactivation of T cells, infectious complications such as pneumonia or sepsis are the biggest concern of using ECP. Other complications include nausea, diarrhea, anemia, thrombocytopenia, tremors, mental status changes, and progressive graft-versus-host disease (GVHD). In addition, there is a risk of mortality since one patient died from multiorgan failure secondary to infection 86 days after enrollment in a study.[38]

Indications

ECP has been used to treat GVHD and T-cell-associated diseases such as cutaneous T-cell lymphoma (mycosis fungoides, Sezary syndrome) or T-cell-mediated allograft transplant rejections. In a report on the effect of 12 weeks of ECP treatment (3 times/week) on post–bone marrow transplant patients with steroid-refractory chronic GVHD, a reduction of more than 50% in corticosteroid dose was achieved in 25% of patients with chronic GVHD who received ECP (ECP group) compared with 12.8% in the group not receiving ECP (control group).[38] Cutaneous lesions also improved in the ECP group versus control group by 14.5% versus 8.5%, eye symptoms improved by 30% versus 7%, oral symptoms improved by 53% versus 27%, and joint symptoms improved by 22% versus 12%, respectively.

ECP has been used to treat other conditions such as psoriasis, pemphigus vulgaris, atopic dermatitis, and some autoimmune diseases, such as scleroderma, Crohn disease, MS, nephrogenic fibrosing dermopathy, and rheumatoid arthritis; however, the efficacy of ECP for these diseases has not been proven.[2,39]

SUMMARY

Only common therapeutic apheresis procedures and their applicable diseases are explained in this chapter; however, the indications of therapeutic apheresis have been expanding. More than 30 more diseases are listed in the ASFA guidelines in 2016 compared with 2007, and more diseases are expected to be added in the coming years. Therapeutic apheresis could be tried for diseases with unknown apheresis efficacy if there is an appropriate biological rationale that therapeutic apheresis may be beneficial to the patient. However, possible complications of apheresis should not be ignored in the setting of a patient's clinical condition, even though apheresis is a relatively safe procedure.

In the future of therapeutic apheresis, devices using other techniques, such as immunoadsorption techniques, may become options in diseases in which a defined pathogenic mediator is to be removed selectively. However, protocols and methods using these technologies in Europe or Asia may have to be modified for practical use in the United States.

REFERENCES

1. Schwab PJ, Fahey JL. Treatment of Waldenstrom's macroglobulinemia by plasmapheresis. *N Engl J Med.* 1960;263:574–579.
2. Schwartz J, Padmanabhan A, Aqui N, et al. Guidelines on the use of therapeutic apheresis in clinical practice-evidence-based approach from the Writing Committee of the American Society for apheresis: the seventh special issue. *J Clin Apher.* 2016;31(3):149–162.
3. Nagai Y, Itabashi M, Mizutani M, et al. A case report of uncompensated alkalosis induced by daily plasmapheresis in a patient with thrombotic thrombocytopenic purpura. *Ther Apher Dial.* 2008;12(1):86–90.
4. Rizvi MA, Vesely SK, George JN, et al. Complications of plasma exchange in 71 consecutive patients treated for clinically suspected thrombotic thrombocytopenic purpura-hemolytic-uremic syndrome. *Transfusion.* 2000; 40(8):896–901.
5. Hoch W, McConville J, Helms S, Newsom-Davis J, Melms A, Vincent A. Auto-antibodies to the receptor tyrosine kinase MuSK in patients with myasthenia gravis without acetylcholine receptor antibodies. *Nat Med.* 2001;7(3):365–368.
6. Romi F, Gilhus NE, Aarli JA. Myasthenia gravis: clinical, immunological, and therapeutic advances. *Acta Neurol Scand.* 2005;111(2):134–141.
7. Higuchi O, Hamuro J, Motomura M, Yamanashi Y. Auto-antibodies to low-density lipoprotein receptor-related protein 4 in myasthenia gravis. *Ann Neurol.* 2011;69(2): 418–422.
8. Cossins J, Belaya K, Zoltowska K, et al. The search for new antigenic targets in myasthenia gravis. *Ann N Y Acad Sci.* 2012;1275:123–128.
9. Yamada C, Pham HP, Wu Y, et al. Report of the ASFA apheresis registry on muscle specific kinase antibody positive myasthenia gravis. *J Clin Apher.* 2017;32(1):5–11.
10. Yamada C, Teener JW, Davenport RD, Cooling L. Maintenance plasma exchange treatment for muscle specific kinase antibody positive myasthenia gravis patients. *J Clin Apher.* 2015;30(5):314–319.
11. Weinshenker BG. Plasma exchange for severe attacks of inflammatory demyelinating diseases of the central nervous system. *J Clin Apher.* 2001;16(1):39–42.

12. Keegan M, Konig F, McClelland R, et al. Relation between humoral pathological changes in multiple sclerosis and response to therapeutic plasma exchange. *Lancet.* 2005;366(9485):579–582.

13. Wingerchuk DM, Weinshenker BG. Neuromyelitis optica. *Curr Treat Options Neurol.* 2005;7(3):173–182.

14. Watanabe S, Nakashima I, Misu T, et al. Therapeutic efficacy of plasma exchange in NMO-IgG-positive patients with neuromyelitis optica. *Mult Scler.* 2007;13(1):128–132.

15. Keegan M, Pineda AA, McClelland RL, Darby CH, Rodriguez M, Weinshenker BG. Plasma exchange for severe attacks of CNS demyelination: predictors of response. *Neurology.* 2002;58(1):143–146.

16. Weinshenker BG, Wingerchuk DM. Neuromyelitis spectrum disorders. *Mayo Clin Proc.* 2017;92(4):663–679.

17. Tsai HM. A mechanistic approach to the diagnosis and management of atypical hemolytic uremic syndrome. *Transfus Med Rev.* 2014;28(4):187–197.

18. Joglekar K, Brannick B, Kadaria D, Sodhi A. Therapeutic plasmapheresis for hypertriglyceridemia-associated acute pancreatitis: case series and review of the literature. *Ther Adv Endocrinol Metab.* 2017;8(4):59–65.

19. Yamada C, Ramon DS, Cascalho M, et al. Efficacy of plasmapheresis on donor-specific antibody reduction by HLA specificity in post-kidney transplant recipients. *Transfusion.* 2015;55(4):727–35.

20. Sivakumaran P, Vo AA, Villicana R, et al. Therapeutic plasma exchange for desensitization prior to transplantation in ABO-incompatible renal allografts. *J Clin Apher.* 2009;24(4):155–160.

21. Kashgary A, Sontrop JM, Li L, et al. The role of plasma exchange in treating post-transplant focal segmental glomerulosclerosis: a systematic review and meta-analysis of 77 case-reports and case-series. *BMC Nephrol.* 2016;17(1):104.

22. Sarode R, Ballas SK, Garcia A, et al. Red blood cell exchange: 2015 American Society for Apheresis consensus conference on the management of patients with sickle cell disease. *J Clin Apher.* 2016. http://dx.doi.org/10.1002/jca.21511.

23. Giles FJ, Shen Y, Kantarjian HM, et al. Leukapheresis reduces early mortality in patients with acute myeloid leukemia with high white cell counts but does not improve long-term survival. *Leuk Lymphoma.* 2001;42(1–2):67–73.

24. Bug G, Anargyrou K, Tonn T, et al. Impact of leukapheresis on early death rate in adult acute myeloid leukemia presenting with hyperleukocytosis. *Transfusion.* 2007;47(10):1843–1850.

25. Ganzel C, Becker J, Mintz PD, Lazarus HM, Rowe JM. Hyperleukocytosis, leukostasis and leukapheresis: practice management. *Blood Rev.* 2012;26(3):117–122.

26. Koziolek MJ, Hennig U, Zapf A, et al. Retrospective analysis of long-term lipid apheresis at a single center. *Ther Apher Dial.* 2010;14(2):143–152.

27. Gordon BR, Kelsey SF, Dau PC, et al. Long-term effects of low-density lipoprotein apheresis using an automated dextran sulfate cellulose adsorption system. Liposorber Study Group. *Am J Cardiol.* 1998;81(4):407–411.

28. Bhoj VG, Sachais BS. Lipoprotein apheresis. *Curr Atheroscler Rep.* 2015;17(7):39.

29. Gordon BR, Kelsey SF, Bilheimer DW, et al. Treatment of refractory familial hypercholesterolemia by low-density lipoprotein apheresis using an automated dextran sulfate cellulose adsorption system. The Liposorber Study Group. *Am J Cardiol.* 1992;70(11):1010–1016.

30. Hattori M, Chikamoto H, Akioka Y, et al. A combined low-density lipoprotein apheresis and prednisone therapy for steroid-resistant primary focal segmental glomerulosclerosis in children. *Am J Kidney Dis.* 2003;42(6):1121–1130.

31. Kawasaki Y, Suzuki S, Matsumoto A, et al. Long-term efficacy of low-density lipoprotein apheresis for focal and segmental glomerulosclerosis. *Pediatr Nephrol.* 2007;22(6):889–892.

32. Masutani K, Katafuchi R, Ikeda H, et al. Recurrent nephrotic syndrome after living-related renal transplantation resistant to plasma exchange: report of two cases. *Clin Transpl.* 2005;19(suppl 14):59–64.

33. Leebmann J, Roeseler E, Julius U, et al. Lipoprotein apheresis in patients with maximally tolerated lipid-lowering therapy, lipoprotein(a)-hyperlipoproteinemia, and progressive cardiovascular disease: prospective observational multicenter study. *Circulation.* 2013;128(24):2567–2576.

34. Matsuzaki M, Hiramori K, Imaizumi T, et al. Intravascular ultrasound evaluation of coronary plaque regression by low density lipoprotein-apheresis in familial hypercholesterolemia: the low density lipoprotein-apheresis coronary morphology and reserve trial (LACMART). *J Am Coll Cardiol.* 2002;40(2):220–227.

35. Weaver CH, Hazelton B, Birch R, et al. An analysis of engraftment kinetics as a function of the CD34 content of peripheral blood progenitor cell collections in 692 patients after the administration of myeloablative chemotherapy. *Blood.* 1995;86(10):3961–3969.

36. Vellenga E, van Agthoven M, Croockewit AJ, et al. Autologous peripheral blood stem cell transplantation in patients with relapsed lymphoma results in accelerated haematopoietic reconstitution, improved quality of life and cost reduction compared with bone marrow transplantation: the Hovon 22 study. *Br J Haematol.* 2001;114(2):319–326.

37. Veerappan R, Morrison M, Williams S, Variakojis D. Splenic rupture in a patient with plasma cell myeloma following G-CSF/GM-CSF administration for stem cell transplantation and review of the literature. *Bone Marrow Transpl.* 2007;40(4):361–364.

38. Flowers ME, Apperley JF, van Besien K, et al. A multicenter prospective phase 2 randomized study of extracorporeal photopheresis for treatment of chronic graft-versus-host disease. *Blood.* 2008;112(7):2667–2674.

39. Marques MB, Adamski J. Extracorporeal photopheresis: technique, established and novel indications. *J Clin Apher.* 2014;29(4):228–234.

CHAPTER 15

New Concepts in Transfusion Medicine

ROBERT W. MAITTA, MD, PHD

DEVELOPMENT OF IN VITRO/EX VIVO BLOOD CELLS

Probably one idea above all has become the holy grail in Transfusion Medicine, that is, how to produce blood that is safe and potentially compatible with the largest number of potential recipients? Although this may sound unrealistic or not based on solid science, the truth is that recent developments in molecular and cellular engineering may have made this a possibility not worth discarding into the realm of the mystical. During the last ten years researchers across the globe have developed new approaches to manipulate and reprogram hematopoietic progenitor cells at different times during their developmental stages to generate mature erythrocytes and in some cases engineer them to lack expression of a particular red cell antigen. This approach alone could prove instrumental to develop cells that can be used in patients in the future; furthermore, these laboratory-derived cells have a clear benefit, that is, they represent a constant supply of cells that are free of bacterial contamination as well as potentially infectious agents.

It is beyond the scope of this chapter to discuss the techniques used in developing these cells in the laboratory, but a few are worth mentioning. The use of lentiviral vectors has changed the way genes can be inserted or silenced during stem cell differentiation. Such technique has allowed attenuated vectors based on human immunodeficiency virus-1 to be used to either overexpress red cell antigens such as Kidd antigens or silence their expression by disrupting their coding regions.[1] Considering that this is one of the most hemolytic known red cell antibodies that tend to be evanescent, it is quite significant. It may not be a stretch to see the possible applications of these findings to develop either reagent cells that overexpress Kidd antigens in sufficient amount to detect these evanescent antibodies at very low concentration or cells that lack Kidd antigens for transfusion support. Both these applications can potentially benefit a great number of patients and help address clear testing and patient transfusion needs.

Before discussing the possibilities one has to begin by listing the difficulties along the way to make the possibility of manufacturing red cells a reality. First, at the center of developing laboratory-derived cells is the selection of an optimal source of progenitor cells that can be used to generate sufficient numbers of red cells. This by itself is not trivial, and a significant number of research groups have described different cell lines that hold promise as sources of mature erythrocytes. Second, even if a cell type is selected, it remains to be determined if a wide enough diverse pool of progenitor cells can be selected or generated that can elicit the largest number of potential combinations of red cell antigens with the desired phenotypic characteristics. One solution to this conundrum may represent the readily available number of stem cells from cord blood, which, as reported, can be expanded ex vivo by up to 10^7-fold leading to the generation of sufficient erythroblasts that eventually enucleate and differentiate into mature erythrocytes.[2] A different source of cells can be in the form of immortalized human erythroid progenitor cells/erythroblasts, which have been shown to develop into mature erythrocytes and provide a continued supply of mature red cells.[3,4] The third difficulty to be overcome is a quantitative one. The limiting factor in manufacturing cells in the laboratory is the technical difficulties of generating red cells in sufficient numbers (2.5×10^{12} or more) to make it logistically and financially feasible in a volume that is small enough to be used for transfusion.[5] Cells in the 10^{13} range have been generated from a single unit of cord blood stem cells, far exceeding what would be needed for a unit of red cells,[6] and an even greater number of red blood cell (RBC) units have been generated from a single cord donation.[7] These reports truly represent breakthroughs that if applied to a diverse pool of stem cells may yield cells that can be used for transfusion. Pluripotent stem cells, however, need not only be of hematopoietic origin. Other tissue sources of stem cells such as fibroblasts and mesenchymal cells have also been used to generate RBCs.[8] This approach has led to the formation of mature RBCs with full tetrameric hemoglobin from fibroblast-derived human pluripotent stem cells.[9] All these advances emphasize that it is possible to generate RBCs in the laboratory, and these advances likely will continue to improve as technology progresses and larger number of cells can be generated in a controlled environment.

Development of laboratory-derived RBCs is an important milestone, but it will not mean much unless it can be used for transfusion support. Reports outlining results of transfusion of these laboratory-derived cells into both animal models and limited human use have indicated that the in vivo survival of these cells was comparable to that of native RBCs without apparent adverse events.[10] Furthermore, close analysis of the metabolic footprint of cells generated in the laboratory in relationship to native cells have shown more than 90% similarity with differences only in some metabolites that are unrelated to RBC function.[11] These results have been corroborated showing that laboratory-derived RBCs are not physiologically different from native ones.[4] Taken together these results indicate that the generation of RBCs in the laboratory is a tangible reality that holds promise in the development of physiologically viable cells that can be used for transfusion support.

RED BLOOD CELLS IN THE SETTING OF HEMOGLOBINOPATHIES

In sickle cell disease treatment, the ultimate goal is to prevent sickling of a patient's erythrocytes to prevent crises ant their complications. In the last two years it has been reported that correction of the mutated hemoglobin gene using the Clustered Regularly Interspaced Short Palindromic Repeats (CRISPR)–associated protein 9 (Cas9) system in stem cells derived from patients with sickle cell disease led to the formation of normal β-globin and red cells that no longer sickle.[12,13] Furthermore, a report this year described a patient with sickle cell disease who was disease free 15 months after having undergone an autologous hematopoietic stem cell transplantation with cells that were transduced with an antisickling β-hemoglobin gene on a lentiviral vector.[14] In the setting of β-thalassemia, use of the CRISPR/Cas9 system has allowed for replacement of the defective hemoglobin leading to normal hemoglobin expression.[15] These reports are the reason for cautious excitement and optimism because considering the potential complications of these severe chronic diseases, the fact that gene therapy can potentially lead to disease remission and potentially be curative means that in the future care for these patients may be

simplified and potentially be a historical success story that will serve as foundation for the treatment of other diseases.

LABORATORY-DERIVED PLATELETS

Platelet units are some of the most expensive blood components with one of the shortest shelf lives. Technologies that could allow for the development of platelets for patient transfusion support are needed because these, as explained in the previous chapter, are becoming increasingly more difficult to obtain due to the shrinking donor pool. Additionally, developing platelets in the laboratory could also allow for the generation of recipient-specific platelets, leading to reduction of alloimmunization rates. As it is the case with RBCs, there has been a concerted effort over the last few years to develop platelets in the laboratory. Recent data have indicated that a very large number of megakaryocytes can be generated from pluripotent stem cells using forward programming, a technique in which cell differentiation is driven by transducing stem cells with megakaryocyte-dependent transcription factors using a lentiviral vector in the absence of outside stimuli such as cytokines or cocultured stromal cells.[16] This approach has led to the formation of up to 2×10^5 megakaryocytes per stem cell.[16] This technology is different from the more traditional one of inducing megakaryocytic lineages and platelet formation by providing a combination of cytokines and growth factors that favor their development, also known as directed differentiation.[17,18] Each megakaryocyte has the potential of releasing between 10 and 20 large platelet precursors, which in turn can develop in circulation into mature platelets.[19] Regardless of the methodology, considering the number of cells that could be propagated from a single stem cell, the large number of megakaryocytes derived can then be used to generate platelets in sufficient numbers, which could then be used for transfusion.

Once megakaryocytes are generated in sufficient numbers, the next logical question is can functional platelets be derived from such cells? The answer is they can be derived. Data indicate that platelets developed in the laboratory show no ultrastructural or morphological differences when compared to native platelets.[20] Functionally, these platelets respond to thrombin stimuli, they form microaggregates and stable clots, and in a mouse model, they lead to thrombi formation at sites of injury.[20] Similarly, they have been observed using in vivo imaging technology to adhere to sites of injury under normal flow conditions.[21] Platelets generated in the laboratory also have been reported to have surface markers similar to those found on fresh donated platelets.[22] Because both morphologically and physiologically laboratory-derived platelets are apparently no different from native platelets, it may not be long before they can be used in transfusions.

Separately, studies have shown that megakaryocytes generated in the laboratory can also generate platelets in vivo safely when infused into patients with malignancies undergoing stem cell transplantation without noticeable adverse events.[23,24] However, animal studies indicate that this approach may lead to megakaryocytes at times not returning to the bone marrow but instead becoming trapped in the lung sinusoids of mice from where they can still generate platelets.[25] Embryonic stem cells also possess the ability of generating cystic-like structures that provide an environment in vitro that enhances megakaryocytic development, which subsequently leads to platelet formation.[26] These reports point to alternative potential mechanisms that can be used to develop functional platelets from laboratory-derived megakaryocytes.

From these promising studies it can be logically inferred that if platelets can be generated in the laboratory, then it may be possible to manipulate stem cells or platelet precursors to induce differentiation of mature platelets that lack specific antigens for increasing their potential utilization. This could involve selective suppression of human leukocyte antigen (HLA) expression, which would mean that platelets generated in the laboratory could potentially lead to lower alloimmunization rates and perhaps limit or eliminate this as a cause of platelet refractoriness. Such an approach targeting HLA has reported that by knocking out the gene encoding β2-microglobulin, formation of the major histocompatibility complex Class I/HLA is abrogated leading to the generation of functional platelets devoid of these receptors.[17] Another approach with similar results utilized lentivirus-mediated disruption of β2-microglobulin in CD34+ hematopoietic progenitor cells to silence HLA Class I expression, which resulted in greater than 85% decreased expression of these receptors on functional platelets that did not differ in their response to in vitro stimuli when compared with blood-derived platelets.[27] Platelets generated from precursor stem cells in which β2-microglobulin expression (HLA) has been silenced have been shown to be unaffected by HLA antibody–mediated cellular cytotoxicity and by lymphocytotoxicity and are able to survive and remain functional both in vitro and in vivo.[28] In addition, in mouse models of platelet refractoriness, HLA-silenced platelets failed to be cleared and megakaryocytes were not lysed by passively administered circulating antibodies.[28,29] These platelets are also physiologically indistinguishable from native platelets in their response to adenosine diphosphate and thrombin.[29] Considering that one of the main limiting factors of platelet transfusions is the increased risk of platelet refractoriness with greater platelet transfusion exposure, these results hold promise and may bring closer to reality the idea of generating universal platelets.

In clinical settings other platelet antigens may lead to thrombocytopenic presentations that require specific platelet units for a given recipient. Unlike HLA, human platelet alloantigens (HPA) can lead to disease and require prompt procurement of platelets negative for the offending antigen. Etiologies such as neonatal alloimmune thrombocytopenia and posttransfusion purpura occur in response to platelet-specific antigens. In the large majority of cases, lack of HPA-1a leads to an antibody response that opsonizes platelets leading to their enhanced clearance from circulation. Therefore just as in the case of silencing HLA, laboratory-derived platelets have the potential to aid in transfusion support of these patients if expression of these receptors can be decreased. The use of CRISPR/Cas9 technology has allowed for the development of laboratory-derived platelets that encode the HPA-1b antigen.[30] These platelets can potentially be used in patients alloimmunized by HPA-1a leading to reduced complications of the aforementioned etiologies. For more on this topic I refer the reader to the chapters describing transfusions in pediatric settings and transfusion complications.

NEW TESTING APPROACHES

Blood banks have answered the call and moved to testing methodologies that are accurate and can provide prompt results. The use of automated platforms has revolutionized how antibodies are identified and has resulted in significant decreases in the turnaround times to screen for the presence of alloantibodies. However, there is also a need to further optimize existing systems and to develop new technologies such that results can reach clinicians sooner and lead to faster allocation of compatible units for patients in need of transfusion. Recently, a report described a new methodology to carry out both forward and back typing on patient samples using paper dye system (chromogen). which contains immobilized alloantibodies that can detect ABO and up to five Rhesus antigens and depending on the chromogenic change can provide an ABO type in ~30 s once the colorimetric reaction is measured by an appropriate analyzer.[31] Additionally, it can test sample plasma without centrifugation, leading to further reduction in the time needed to do an ABO and Rh test.[31]

There is also broad agreement that in many clinical settings O-negative RBC units may be unnecessarily transfused to patients who do not require them. Up to this point, the controversy lies in how to determine who should receive the few and precious O-negative units available. In obstetric patients an argument can be made that when discordant RhD testing occurs, the patient being worked up should undergo genotypic testing to determine if results are due to a lower expression of the D antigen (weak D).[32] Using this approach, patients who test D-positive genotypically will not require O-negative units leading to preservation of these units for truly D-negative patients. However, this still does not address the significant number of units still used in acute settings such as emergency department when patients with no prior visits to that hospital arrive in need for transfusion. Future technologies will need to be streamlined to provide rapid and accurate results in this clinical setting.

PLATELET UNITS' SHELF LIFE

One of the hot topics in Transfusion Medicine is the current discussion of extending platelets' shelf lives from 5 to 7 days. In the setting of decreasing number of platelet units being able to extend the shelf life of units beyond the 5 days currently in use by most centers across the country is desirable. One of the challenges of implementing such change is that with longer shelf life the risk of bacterial growth/secondary to contamination increases due to platelet units' room temperature storage. Furthermore, even if the shelf life is extended to 7 days there may be some degree of apprehension to use them for patients' transfusions in some clinical settings, and this also needs to be addressed before they can be widely implemented across the country.

Medical centers that have implemented 7-day platelets have reported a much lower number of outdated platelets, which has resulted in significant institutional financial savings.[33] However, the decision to store platelets longer cannot just be measured as a budgetary item. The pressing question is if these platelet units are physiologically comparable to platelets stored for 5 days. Functionally, there appears to be a quantitative decline in platelet recovery

and function when units' shelf life is extended to 7 days.[34,35] From this it can be inferred that extending the shelf life of platelet units requires storing platelets in an environment suitable for longer storage in which fewer physiologic changes occur, which makes them comparable to platelets stored for shorter time periods. This is an area of active investigation. However, platelet turnover while in storage is expected because platelets, regardless of the environment, will reach their maximum life span and constantly die both in vivo and while in storage. Of interest, there are data indicating that this quantitative decline in platelet counts while in the bag could be more significant if not for the presence of larger, younger immature platelets that may still form mature platelets during storage.[34]

Recently, the Food and Drug Administration (FDA) published its draft guidance outlining the steps needed to be taken to improve platelet safety if platelets' shelf life is extended to 7 days.[36] Why is this guidance needed? The simple answer is to minimize the risk of bacterial contamination and, if this does occur, to have systems in place that can detect these units and remove them from the inventory. Recent data indicate that the number of contaminated platelets may be larger than previously thought and that the number of transfusion reactions resulting from these compromised units may go underreported. New figures from active surveillance indicate that 1/2500 platelet units may be bacterially contaminated and up to 1/10,000 platelet recipients may develop a septic reaction.[37] As a result, the FDA has recommended that additional testing (culture based) be done closer to the end of a platelet unit's shelf life, either day 4 or 5, to address the new active surveillance data. Furthermore, this new draft guidance indicates that the pathogen reduction technology INTERCEPT™ Blood System is the only such technology approved to reduce potential infectious agents in platelets.[36] Additionally, it recommends that to extend the shelf life of platelets to 7 days proper manufacturing registration by hospitals releasing such platelets is required. Moving forward, as blood collection centers and hospitals move toward these 7-day platelets, such change may make practitioners nervous and they may question if such platelets are safe to transfuse. This is a valid concern that has not gone unnoticed by the FDA and others, and this is one of the driving forces behind the proposed guidance. However, it must be stated that those hospitals that have implemented the use of 7-day platelets have done so in a smooth transition that more importantly has not resulted in a higher incidence of adverse events from these platelets.[38]

A brief discussion of the proposed pathogen reduction system is warranted at this point. The INTERCEPT™ Blood System works by using a type of psoralen (amotosalen), a photoactive compound that targets nucleic acids, that becomes active in the presence of ultraviolet A and cross-links these nucleic acids preventing replication/or leading to inactivation of viruses, bacteria, and parasites that could be present in a platelet unit.[39] A prospective study of more than 19,000 platelet transfusions using this system showed that these platelets do not lead to a greater propensity of adverse events compared with conventional platelet units.[40] A closer look of the INTERCEPT system, however, does reveal some caveats. A review of the literature indicates that use of pathogen-reduced platelets using this system could lead to a greater risk of bleeding complications, which could require greater number of transfusions to achieve a desired platelet target of either $>10 \times 10^9$/L or $>20 \times 10^9$/L.[41] Similarly, meta-analyses of trials reporting the use of these pathogen-reduced platelets indicate that they appear to be as safe as conventional platelets but that these treated platelet units tend to give lower count increments and are associated with greater need to transfuse and greater risk of non-life-threatening bleeding.[42] However, lack of count increments may also be the result of the clinical state of transfusion recipients because in some settings platelet count increments have been reported.[43] Nevertheless, this system may prove instrumental to blood banking as a whole, not only by reducing the presence of pathogens in platelet units but also by expanding its use in the near future to include RBCs and whole blood donations as well.[44] However, use of such pathogen reduction system must occur soon after the blood component is collected because any delays may result in significant bacterial contamination due to suboptimal inactivation.[45] Taken together, the aforementioned results indicate that 7-day platelets are likely to become a reality soon and their use will require a renewed effort by transfusion medicine physicians to make every effort to ease up clinicians' concerns. Likewise, clinicians will need to feel comfortable with their use and feel reassured that these platelets will undergo rigorous testing before being issued to patients.

APHERESIS

This is a field closely embedded and linked to the transfusion medicine community because physicians in this group are by far the most likely to oversee apheresis procedures. The single most important concept over the last twenty years is the strong support toward clinical practices supported by the strongest evidence possible. With this in mind, societies such as the American Society for Apheresis (ASFA), publish guidelines updated every few years that go over the most recent relevant disease-specific clinical literature to update apheresis treatment recommendations for a large number of disease presentations.[46] At times, even when no ASFA updates are due recommendations are still made by apheresis experts when new data become available.[47] In the setting of therapeutic plasma exchange (TPE) it can be said that most of the diseases that have pathology mediated by antibody-mediated dysregulation tend to respond to procedures. However, the advent of monoclonal antibody immunotherapies and use of intravenous immunoglobulin have reduced the need for TPE in some indications.

For etiologies such as thrombotic thrombocytopenic purpura (TTP) TPE represents a first-line treatment that has led to a profound decrease in the mortality rates historically associated with this disease. At presentation, patients with TTP present with a clinical picture that may resemble several other etiologies that are not responsive to TPE, but deficiency of the metalloprotease ADAMTS13 has been shown to be pathognomonic of its diagnosis and when deficient it represents a good marker to predict who will benefit from TPE.[48] It is these overlapping features that make it difficult at times to differentiate TTP from other microangiopathic hemolytic anemia (MAHA) etiologies.[49] Therefore laboratory parameters that can be used to aid in the early recognition and differentiation of TTP from other MAHA presentations are needed. In this setting, recent data suggest that measuring platelet production dynamic changes may aid in understanding a patient's thrombocytopenic presentation. In particular, changes in immature platelet counts early in a patient's presentation may not only indicate TTP but also help rule out those presentations that are likely not TTP and therefore not benefit from TPE.[50] How would this work? When a patient presents with thrombocytopenia and MAHA, testing of the patient's complete blood count for the newest platelets formed (immature and significantly larger than mature ones) yields information of the real-time bone marrow status of the patient. If the disease has affected production at the bone marrow, the immature count would be low. In the setting of TTP, production of these new larger platelets is limited and significantly lower than in those without TTP. More importantly, upon initiation of TPE, only those patients with ADAMTS13 deficiency respond with a marked increase in their immature platelet production. Once patients recover from TTP and platelet count normalizes, it is accompanied by a corresponding return to baseline of immature platelet counts in a negative feedback manner. These results hold promise that platelet negative feedback and immature platelet dynamics may aid in working up these patients.

Other reports indicate that immature platelet measurements may also aid diagnostically in the setting of idiopathic thrombocytopenic purpura.[51] Use of such early platelet production markers will likely benefit patients in their presentation; however, further research looking at how to best utilize such measurements will be needed not only in the setting of these diseases but also in the setting of other thrombocytopenic etiologies.

SUMMARY

Transfusion Medicine is changing and so is the way we see and use blood components. As results from new basic discoveries become available, the field will need to adapt as they move from the bench to the clinical setting. Similarly, the field will need to work with clinicians as new evidence-based guidance becomes available in how to best provide transfusion support to specific patient populations. All medical disciplines will benefit from the new era of medical discovery currently taking place. No longer a utopia, we are marching toward an age in which blood will be the safest it has ever been and this may involve its manufacture from the stem cell stage to mature blood element in a laboratory setting.

REFERENCES

1. Bagnis C, Chapel S, Chiaroni J, Bailly P. A genetic strategy to control expression of human blood group antigens in red blood cells generated in vitro. *Transfusion.* 2009;49(5):967–976.
2. Huang X, Shah S, Wang J, et al. Extensive ex vivo expansion of functional human erythroid precursors established from umbilical cord blood cells by defined factors. *Mol Ther.* 2014;22(2):451–463.
3. Kurita R, Suda N, Sudo K, et al. Establishment of immortalized human erythroid progenitor cell lines able to produce enucleated red blood cells. *PLoS One.* 2013;8(3):e59890.
4. Trakarnsanga K, Griffiths RE, Wilson MC, et al. An immortalized adult human erythroid line facilitates sustainable and scalable generation of functional red cells. *Nat Commun.* 2017;8:14750.
5. Migliaccio AR, Whitsett C, Papayannopoulou T, Sadelain M. The potential of stem cells as an in vitro source of red blood cells for transfusion. *Cell Stem Cell.* 2012;10(2):115–119.
6. Fujimi A, Matsunaga T, Kobune M, et al. Ex vivo large-scale generation of human red blood cells from cord blood CD34+ cells by co-culturing with macrophages. *Int J Hematol.* 2008;87(4):339–350.
7. Timmins NE, Athanasas S, Gunther M, Buntine P, Nielsen LK. Ultra-high-yield manufacture of red blood cells from hematopoietic stem cells. *Tissue Eng Part C Methods.* 2011;17(11):1131–1137.
8. Chang KH, Huang A, Hirata RK, Wang PR, Russell DW, Papayannopoulou T. Globin phenotype of erythroid cells derived from human induced pluripotent stem cells. *Blood.* 2010;115(12):2553–2554.
9. Lapillonne H, Kobari L, Mazurier C, et al. Red blood cell generation from human induced pluripotent stem cells: perspectives for transfusion medicine. *Haematologica.* 2010; 95(10):1651–1659.
10. Giarratana MC, Rouard H, Dumont A, et al. Proof of principle for transfusion of in vitro-generated red blood cells. *Blood.* 2011;118(19):5071–5079.
11. Darghouth D, Giarratana MC, Oliveira L, et al. Bio-engineered and native red blood cells from cord blood exhibit the same metabolomic profile. *Haematologica.* 2016;101(6):e220–e222.
12. DeWitt MA, Magis W, Bray NL, et al. Selection-free genome editing of the sickle mutation in human adult hematopoietic stem/progenitor cells. *Sci Transl Med.* 2016;8(360): 360ra134.
13. Huang X, Wang Y, Yan W, et al. Production of gene-corrected adult beta globin protein in human erythrocytes differentiated from patient iPSCs after genome editing of the sickle point mutation. *Stem Cells.* 2015; 33(5):1470–1479.
14. Ribeil JA, Hacein-Bey-Abina S, Payen E, et al. Gene therapy in a patient with sickle cell disease. *N Engl J Med.* 2017;376(9):848–855.
15. Xie F, Ye L, Chang JC, et al. Seamless gene correction of beta-thalassemia mutations in patient-specific iPSCs using CRISPR/Cas9 and piggyBac. *Genome Res.* 2014;24(9): 1526–1533.
16. Moreau T, Evans AL, Vasquez L, et al. Large-scale production of megakaryocytes from human pluripotent stem cells by chemically defined forward programming. *Nat Commun.* 2016;7:11208.
17. Feng Q, Shabrani N, Thon JN, et al. Scalable generation of universal platelets from human induced pluripotent stem cells. *Stem Cell Rep.* 2014;3(5):817–831.
18. Pick M. Generation of megakaryocytes and platelets from human pluripotent stem cells. *Methods Mol Biol.* 2016;1307:371–378.
19. Machlus KR, Italiano Jr JE. The incredible journey: from megakaryocyte development to platelet formation. *J Cell Biol.* 2013;201(6):785–796.
20. Lu SJ, Li F, Yin H, et al. Platelets generated from human embryonic stem cells are functional in vitro and in the microcirculation of living mice. *Cell Res.* 2011;21(3): 530–545.

21. Nishimura S, Manabe I, Nagasaki M, et al. In vivo imaging visualizes discoid platelet aggregations without endothelium disruption and implicates contribution of inflammatory cytokine and integrin signaling. *Blood.* 2012;119(8):e45–e56.
22. Takayama N, Eto K. Pluripotent stem cells reveal the developmental biology of human megakaryocytes and provide a source of platelets for clinical application. *Cell Mol Life Sci.* 2012;69(20):3419–3428.
23. Bertolini F, Battaglia M, Pedrazzoli P, et al. Megakaryocytic progenitors can be generated ex vivo and safely administered to autologous peripheral blood progenitor cell transplant recipients. *Blood.* 1997;89(8): 2679–2688.
24. Xi J, Zhu H, Liu D, et al. Infusion of megakaryocytic progenitor products generated from cord blood hematopoietic stem/progenitor cells: results of the phase 1 study. *PLoS One.* 2013;8(2):e54941.
25. Fuentes R, Wang Y, Hirsch J, et al. Infusion of mature megakaryocytes into mice yields functional platelets. *J Clin Invest.* 2010;120(11):3917–3922.
26. Takayama N, Nishikii H, Usui J, et al. Generation of functional platelets from human embryonic stem cells in vitro via ES-sacs, VEGF-promoted structures that concentrate hematopoietic progenitors. *Blood.* 2008;111(11): 5298–5306.
27. Figueiredo C, Goudeva L, Horn PA, Eiz-Vesper B, Blaszczyk R, Seltsam A. Generation of HLA-deficient platelets from hematopoietic progenitor cells. *Transfusion.* 2010;50(8): 1690–1701.
28. Gras C, Schulze K, Goudeva L, Guzman CA, Blaszczyk R, Figueiredo C. HLA-universal platelet transfusions prevent platelet refractoriness in a mouse model. *Hum Gene Ther.* 2013;24(12):1018–1028.
29. Figueiredo C, Blaszczyk R. Genetically engineered blood pharming: generation of HLA-universal platelets derived from CD34+ progenitor cells. *J Stem Cells.* 2014;9(3):149–161.
30. Zhang N, Zhi H, Curtis BR, et al. CRISPR/Cas9-mediated conversion of human platelet alloantigen allotypes. *Blood.* 2016;127(6):675–680.
31. Zhang H, Qiu X, Zou Y, et al. A dye-assisted paper-based point-of-care assay for fast and reliable blood grouping. *Sci Transl Med.* 2017;9(381).
32. Sandler SG, Flegel WA, Westhoff CM, et al. It's time to phase in RHD genotyping for patients with a serologic weak D phenotype. College of American Pathologists Transfusion Medicine Resource Committee Work Group. *Transfusion.* 2015;55(3):680–689.
33. Hay SN, Immel CC, McClannan LS, Brecher ME. The introduction of 7-day platelets: a university hospital experience. *J Clin Apher.* 2007;22(5):283–286.
34. Hong H, Xiao W, Maitta RW. Steady increment of immature platelet fraction is suppressed by irradiation in single-donor platelet components during storage. *PLoS One.* 2014;9(1):e85465.
35. Dumont LJ, AuBuchon JP, Whitley P, et al. Seven-day storage of single-donor platelets: recovery and survival in an autologous transfusion study. *Transfusion.* 2002;42(7): 847–854.
36. US Food and Drug Administration. Bacterial Risk Control Strategies for Blood Collection Establishments and Transfusion Services to Enhance the Safety and Availability of Platelets for Transfusion 2016. http://www.fda.gov/Biolo gicsBloodVaccines/GuidanceComplianceRegulatoryInfor mation/Guidances/default.htm.
37. Hong H, Xiao W, Lazarus HM, Good CE, Maitta RW, Jacobs MR. Detection of septic transfusion reactions to platelet transfusions by active and passive surveillance. *Blood.* 2016;127(4):496–502.
38. Dunbar NM, Dumont LJ, Szczepiorkowski ZM. How do we implement Day 6 and Day 7 platelets at a hospital-based transfusion service? *Transfusion.* 2016;56(6):1262–1266.
39. Wollowitz S. Fundamentals of the psoralen-based Helinx technology for inactivation of infectious pathogens and leukocytes in platelets and plasma. *Semin Hematol.* 2001;38(4 suppl 11):4–11.
40. Knutson F, Osselaer J, Pierelli L, et al. A prospective, active haemovigilance study with combined cohort analysis of 19,175 transfusions of platelet components prepared with amotosalen-UVA photochemical treatment. *Vox Sang.* 2015;109(4):343–352.
41. Vamvakas EC. Meta-analysis of the studies of bleeding complications of platelets pathogen-reduced with the Intercept system. *Vox Sang.* 2012;102(4):302–316.
42. Butler C, Doree C, Estcourt LJ, et al. Pathogen-reduced platelets for the prevention of bleeding. *Cochrane Database Syst Rev.* 2013;(3): CD009072.
43. Infanti L, Stebler C, Job S, et al. Pathogen-inactivation of platelet components with the INTERCEPT Blood System: a cohort study. *Transfus Apher Sci.* 2011;45(2):175–181.
44. Drew VJ, Barro L, Seghatchian J, Burnouf T. Towards pathogen inactivation of red blood cells and whole blood targeting viral DNA/RNA: design, technologies, and future prospects for developing countries. *Blood Transfus.* 2017:1–11.
45. Schmidt M, Hourfar MK, Sireis W, et al. Evaluation of the effectiveness of a pathogen inactivation technology against clinically relevant transfusion-transmitted bacterial strains. *Transfusion.* 2015;55(9):2104–2112.
46. Schwartz J, Padmanabhan A, Aqui N, et al. Guidelines on the use of therapeutic apheresis in clinical practice-evidence-based approach from the Writing Committee of the American Society for Apheresis: the seventh special issue. *J Clin Apher.* 2016;31(3):149–162.
47. Pham HP, Schwartz J. New apheresis indications in hematological disorders. *Curr Opin Hematol.* 2016;23(6):581–587.
48. Bendapudi PK, Li A, Hamdan A, et al. Impact of severe ADAMTS13 deficiency on clinical presentation and outcomes in patients with thrombotic microangiopathies: the experience of the Harvard TMA Research Collaborative. *Br J Haematol.* 2015;171(5):836–844.

49. Bittencourt CE, Ha JP, Maitta RW. Re-examination of 30-day survival and relapse rates in patients with thrombotic thrombocytopenic purpura-hemolytic uremic syndrome. *PLoS One*. 2015;10(5): e0127744.

50. Hong H, Xiao W, Stempak LM, Sandhaus LM, Maitta RW. Absolute immature platelet count dynamics in diagnosing and monitoring the clinical course of thrombotic thrombocytopenic purpura. *Transfusion*. 2015;55(4):756–765.

51. Greene LA, Chen S, Seery C, Imahiyerobo AM, Bussel JB. Beyond the platelet count: immature platelet fraction and thromboelastometry correlate with bleeding in patients with immune thrombocytopenia. *Br J Haematol*. 2014;166(4):592–600.

CHAPTER 16

Challenges Facing Transfusion Practices

ROBERT W. MAITTA, MD, PHD

BLOOD SUPPLY

The discussion of challenges to transfusion practices cannot avoid the large albino mammal in the room, specifically the blood supply. To those in the field it has become all too clear that quantitative changes to current donations are a matter of concern as the number of blood shortages from suppliers have increased over the last decade. What used to be a rare difficulty now has become a routine occurrence that has led to many Transfusion Medicine services across the country to come up with contingency plans to maintain basic operations while providing blood components support to patients requiring them without interruptions. In most instances, these shortages may occur without the clinicians caring for patients being aware of these instances, which speaks volumes of the extraordinary work that specialists in the field carry out behind the scenes to minimize the effect of these shortages on patient care. This problem has been progressive and unchanged because the trend does not appear to improve in the future. More importantly, many of these shortages involve the inventory of Rh-negative red cell units, AB plasma, and recently platelets, which in most clinical settings represent the components most likely to be transfused during emergencies. In light of this new reality, changes to clinical practice may need to be accomplished in a short time to guarantee the long-term viability of the blood supply. Furthermore, this has to be taken as part of a comprehensive institutional-wide effort in which clinical departments using blood components in significant numbers, blood banks, hospital administration, and in many settings ethics departments may need to come to a consensus of how to address such shortages if they become serious and long lasting. This is no easy task, but it is one that owing to current realities needs to be addressed to maintain an effective delivery system that still provides blood components to patients in need of transfusion support.

The current state of the blood supply brings to bear an important question, what is best to do at times of shortages and how to manage them? Depending on whom you ask, a Transfusion Medicine physician or a clinician, the answer may be markedly different; however, both sides need to seek common ground to meet patients' needs. First and foremost, there must be free and unambiguous communication with clinical departments about shortages. This is not a matter of debate. This communication must be initiated by Directors of Transfusion Medicine services/Blood Banks to determine necessary subsequent steps that need to be taken. Failure to communicate may lead to distrust, misunderstanding, and a sense of uneasiness, which could be solved if there are candid and prompt conversations that involve those services in most need of blood components.[1] This will not only prioritize transfusions to those most likely to require them leading to better clinical outcomes but also lead to an active and productive partnership with clinical departments, which will address future shortages when they occur. Nevertheless, the burden of this undertaking cannot fall just on Transfusion Medicine services; this is a two-way approach that will require from clinicians a deep reassessment of what needs to be accomplished, and eliminate or limit transfusions that in some settings may not be immediately necessary (prophylaxis).

How Severe Is the Problem?

As mentioned earlier, blood component shortages are not foreign to the lexicon of Transfusion Medicine specialists, but clinicians caring for critically ill patients, those performing surgeries, or emergency room physicians may be unaware of these events. In the United States it has been reported that of the entire population, approximately 40% can donate blood but only 5% of this group actually does.[2] Over the years a number of surveys have reported on the health of the blood supply. The US Department of Health and Human Services (DHHS) has carried out such surveys, and their

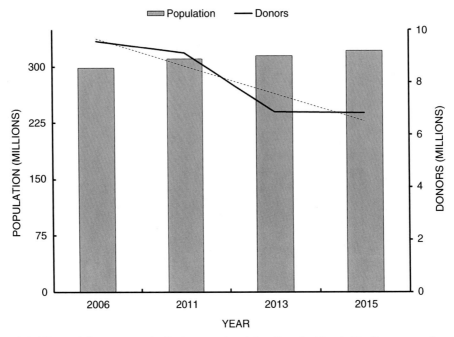

FIG. 16.1 US population compared with donor pool and donations for blood utilization surveys from 2006 to 2015. *Bars* represent US population (Y axis) in a given year according to US Census Bureau figures with corresponding number of donors for that year (Z axis). *Black solid line* represents actual number of donors and *dashed line* represents blood donor trend. (Data from US Department of Health, Human Services. *The 2007 National Blood Collection and Utilization Survey Report.* Available at: http://www.nhs.gov/ash/bloodsa fety/2007nbcus_survey.pdf; US Department of Health, Human Services. *The 2011 National Blood Collection and Utilization Survey Report.* Available at: http://www.nhs.gov/ash/bloodsafety/2011nbcus-survey.pdf; Whitaker B, Rajbhandary S, Kleinman S, Harris A, Kamani N. Trends in United States blood collection and transfusion: results from the 2013 AABB blood collection, utilization, and patient blood management survey. *Transfusion.* 2016;56(9):2173–2183; Ellingson KD, Sapiano MRP, Haass KA, et al. Continued decline in blood collection and transfusion in the United States-2015. *Transfusion.* 2017;57(suppl 2):1588–1598; Sapiano MRP, Savinkina AA, Ellingson KD, et al. Supplemental findings from the national blood collection and utilization surveys, 2013 and 2015. *Transfusion.* 2017;57(suppl 2):1599–1624.)

reports indicate that back in 2006 the apparent decline in collections may have had its beginning.[3] Taking into consideration population growth in the United States it could be expected that the number of donors should increase as the population increases because more individuals join the ranks of those able to donate; however, this has not been the case. Estimates indicate that the US population in 2006 was 298.4 million, increasing to 310.5, 315, and 321 million in 2011, 2013, and 2015, respectively (Fig. 16.1).[4] Therefore those able to donate have increased from 119.4 million in 2006 to 128.6 million in 2015. Nevertheless, these population increases have not translated into an expanding donor pool, something that becomes evident when donor trends over the same decade are compared with those during the prior one. It is this careful analysis

that clearly points to an unchanging downturn in the number of blood donations and components available across the country.

Additional surveys by organizations such as American Association of Blood Banks (AABB) of hospitals and blood collection facilities have reported on the same data over the last few years, and comparison with the data gathered by the DHHS brings into focus the current state of donations. As indicated in Table 16.1, in the last year of the 20th century the number of RBC units collected in the United States was 13,876,000, which were mostly procured from allogeneic volunteer donors.[5] This number seems large and adequate when taking into consideration that 12,389,000 of these units (89.3% of the total) were transfused. Just 2 years later, the number of units collected increased

TABLE 16.1
RBC Donations, Number of Donations and Donors, and RBC and Platelet Usage in US Blood Centers and Hospitals

Year	RBC Units	Number of Donors	Autologous RBC	Allogeneic RBC	Transfused RBC Units	Platelets Transfused
1999[5]	13,876,000		651,000	13,109,000	12,389,000	9,052,000
2001[6]	15,320,000		619,000	14,259,000	13,898,000	10,196,000
2006[3]	16,174,000	9,553,000	335,000	15,688,000	14,461,000	10,388,000
2011[7]	15,721,000	9,100,000	116,800	13,400,000	13,785,000	2,169,000
2013[8]	13,590,000	6,847,000	55,000	11,679,000	13,181,000	2,448,000[a]
2015[9,10]	12,591,000	6,812,000	23,000	11,264,000	11,349,000	2,436,000[a]

RBC, red blood cell.
Donation totals as reported in the US Department of Health and Human Services survey and to AABB in the years indicated.
[a]This number represents platelets distributed to hospitals.

significantly largely in part to the outpouring of support from donors in response to the September 2001 tragedy. RBC units at that time increased to 15,320,000, with the increase coming from both higher number of first-time allogeneic donors and repeat donors; however, this occurred in a background of higher number of units transfused, which was 13,898,000 (90.7% of the total). This is over 1,500,000 more than the number transfused in 1999.[6] In 2007 DHHS published a bulletin that indicated a shift in blood donations versus utilization according to 2006 data. This report indicated that at this time 16,174,000 RBC units were collected in the United States. This number of collected RBC units is significantly higher than in 2001; however, 14,461,000 (89.4% of total) were transfused, a number that is almost 600,000 more than in 2001 and over 2,100,000 more than in 1999, which mostly nullified the increase in units collected.[3] More importantly, the 2007 survey for the first time provided the number of donors for these units, which was 9,553,000, so that each donor on average donated 1.7 units that year. Close analysis of donating demographics showed that in the 18- to 65-year age group the RBC collection rate was 84.1 units per 1000 US donor population (Fig. 16.2). By 2011, this number had decreased significantly so that in this age group the number of units was 76.2 per 1000 US donor population, which explains the almost 500,000 donors lost this year compared with 2006 when only 4.5% of the US population of donation age actually donated.[7] This trend became more significant based on the 2013 data published by AABB. In this year, the number of donors decreased significantly further to 6,847,000, which is 28% and 25% lower compared with donor numbers in 2006 and 2011, respectively

(Fig. 16.1).[8] The mean number of units per donor in 2013 was 2.0 up from 1.7 in 2006. Likewise, the number of units per 1000 donors decreased even further to 65.5 units per 1000 US donor population in 2013. The 2015 data indicate that 12,591,000 units were collected in the country. This number of units is 1 million lower than what was collected in 2013, and this corresponded to a significant reduction in the number of RBC collections to 60.4 units per 1000 donor population (Fig. 16.2).[9] Furthermore, the downtrend in the number of donors continues in 2015, although it is less dramatic than in prior reports because 35,000 fewer donors were reported compared with 2013.[10] However, this occurred in a background of significantly fewer RBC units transfused during the same time period.[9] All of these statistics provide a stern reality of blood availability in the country and stress the need for adaptability by hospitals and clinicians in the use of blood components when strictly necessary and to adhere to conservative transfusion practices. Of interest, the trend of less dependency on autologous donations/transfusions is apparent by the marked decrease in the number of collections from 1999 when they were over 600,000 to 2015 when only 23,000 units were collected. This implies that there is a greater confidence among other factors in the safety of the donated allogeneic blood supply.

Platelet transfusions also increased from 1999 to 2006 when the number of apheresis and prestored pooled platelets increased from just over 9 million to 10,388,000. In subsequent years, the number of platelets collected has also decreased but this occurred in the setting of fewer units transfused as shown in Table 16.1; however, the number of platelets transfused may not be complete as listed because in the last two surveys a

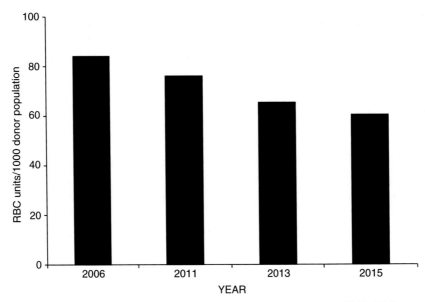

FIG. 16.2 Number of donations per 1000 donor population for the survey years 2006–15. *Bars* represent actual numbers as reported in each survey for that year, indicating downtrend of donations over the last decade. (Data from US Department of Health, Human Services. *The 2007 National Blood Collection and Utilization Survey Report*. Available at: http://www.nhs.gov/ash/bloodsafety/2007nbcus_survey.pdf; US Department of Health, Human Services. *The 2011 National Blood Collection and Utilization Survey Report*. Available at: http://www.nhs.gov/ash/bloodsafety/2011nbcus-survey.pdf; Whitaker B, Rajbhandary S, Kleinman S, Harris A, Kamani N. Trends in United States blood collection and transfusion: results from the 2013 AABB blood collection, utilization, and patient blood management survey. *Transfusion*. 2016;56(9):2173–2183; Ellingson KD, Sapiano MRP, Haass KA, et al. Continued decline in blood collection and transfusion in the United States-2015. *Transfusion*. 2017;57(suppl 2):1588–1598; Sapiano MRP, Savinkina AA, Ellingson KD, et al. Supplemental findings from the national blood collection and utilization surveys, 2013 and 2015. *Transfusion*. 2017;57(suppl 2):1599–1624.)

number of hospitals failed to respond to the surveys. It is safe to say that platelet transfusions have been more or less at a level equivalent to collections.

Demographic and Ethnic Differences Between Blood Donors and Recipient Patient Populations

The demographics of the current donor pool in the United States have remained constant for the last forty years, and it has been characterized by approximately 90% Caucasian donors and 10% from other ethnic groups.[11] Not surprisingly, these proportions are not exempt from US population shifts as shown by recent data indicating that the number of Caucasian donors, although still the majority, have started to decrease in the last decade when 80% of RBC units were collected from this donor group.[12] This by itself would not be a matter of concern if not for the reality that specific patient populations different from most of the donor pool tend to be more dependent on transfusions to

avoid health crises. Lack of participation from other donor populations, including those from minority backgrounds, is particularly accentuated in large metropolitan areas where outreach donation programs have been met with limited success despite broad appeals.[13] This has represented one of the major challenges to addressing the blood transfusion needs of patients such as those with sickle cell disease (SCD), because the substantial majority of these patients are of African descent. Their transfusion requirements are often driven by lack of expression of certain red cell antigens, such as Rh, Kell, Duffy, and MNSs, in a significant number of patients from this ethnic group, which are more highly expressed in Caucasians.[14] In theory, if there were a larger proportion of African Americans in the donor pool, there would be a greater likelihood of finding units with greater degree of antigen compatibility, leading to reduced exposures of immunologically naive recipients to potential red cell alloantigens. Therefore, the makeup of the current donor pool makes it more difficult to readily find a large number of compatible donors, especially for those patients who are already alloimmunized to red cell antigens. To yield support for a more diverse donor pool, it has been reported that in societies where donors are more ethnically similar to recipients the formation of alloantibodies to red blood cells is significantly reduced,[15,16] and in countries where most donors are multiethnic (those who descend from mixed ethnic backgrounds) the rates of alloimmunization also tend to be significantly lower.[17] This later finding may be explained by the higher likelihood of finding compatible units in countries with donors of mixed backgrounds. As mentioned earlier, despite an intense campaign to recruit a more diverse donor pool, the fact remains that these approaches have not led to an increased participation of donors from minority backgrounds. To bring this point home, approaches established by blood collection centers in major American metropolitan cities with a large proportion of African American and Hispanic/Latino populations have fallen short of their stated targets to significantly increase the number of donors from these ethnic groups.[18] The reasons behind this reduced participation are likely multifactorial, but it makes finding solutions paramount to develop a comprehensive roadmap to encourage blood donations from these populations, which take into account apprehensions that donors from these groups may have to donate.

Nevertheless, what drives red blood cell alloimmunization is likely greater exposure to red blood transfusions over time.[19] Therefore finding, adding, and keeping more minority donors may not fully address concerns for red cell alloimmunization because this can still occur as shown by alloimmunization encountered when donations from Rh-matched minority donors are used,[20] which is not that different from the red cell alloimmunization rate described when units for patients with SCD are matched for a greater number of antigens using a mostly Caucasian donor pool.[21] In some instances, exposures to a greater number of RBC units may resolve an acute presentation but in the long term can lead to greater difficulty of finding compatible blood once alloantibodies form while not always benefiting patients. In the United States, there is a greater number of RBC units transfused (44 units/1000 population) compared with 33/1000 population in the United Kingdom and 22/1000 population in Canada.[22] This overreliance on RBC transfusions perhaps driven by inconsistent transfusion thresholds may begin to explain the higher alloimmunization rates found in the United States.[17] This is something not unique to a specific chronically transfused patient population

undergoing long-term transfusion because it has been reported that patients with myeloid neoplasms given chemotherapy are alloimmunized at higher rates than other patients, which is dependent on exposure to a greater number of RBC units.[23] Therefore, conservative transfusion approaches may have an added benefit, which is to decrease potential RBC alloimmunization. This is discussed in greater detail in a following section.

The number of patients with SCD significantly affects the proportion of units that are needed to treat these patients at times of crises. According to recent reports, as many as 10% of patients with SCD are currently on chronic red cell exchanges (erythrocytapheresis) to avoid sickle cell complications, such as cerebrovascular accidents and acute chest, among others.[24] Of interest, it has been reported that, in pediatric patients erythrocytapheresis may lead to fewer red cell alloantibodies compared with those receiving simple transfusions.[25] Similar findings, although with much higher alloimmunization rates, have been described in adults undergoing erythrocytapheresis compared with patients receiving simple transfusions.[26] This may be counterintuitive when one considers that these patients are exposed to a greater number of RBC units during automated procedures. This can be explained by the dynamics of erythrocytapheresis because during an exchange there is a constant removal of RBC, and in the second part of the exchange those cells transfused earlier in the procedure are removed, limiting their presence in the body thus decreasing the risk of exposure because the overall antigen load for a given unit would be lower. In the case of adult patients, because they would have been exposed to many more transfusions/exchanges in their lifetime alloimmunization rates would be expected to be higher.

It has been recommended that these automated procedures be performed in patients with SCD to prevent disease complications and to minimize those brought about by higher iron loads in the setting of simple transfusions. This is the current practice model, and erythrocytapheresis tends to be performed at larger medical centers because these are located in large urban areas where the greater number of patients with SCD tends to reside. This has resulted in cities bearing the load of logistically addressing these patients' transfusion needs while taking on the profound financial stress of treating this disease. This is clearly shown to be significant when the number of hospitalizations and overall cost to treat patients with SCD during times of disease crises are analyzed.[19] As the number of donations diminishes, long-term exchange programs may need to adjust their targets so that they remain viable while still tackling patients' treatment needs.

To improve the care of patients with SCD, an expert panel has made specific recommendations to provide transfusion support for these patients based on available scientific and clinical evidence.[27] Management focuses on preventive measures and recommendations for the use of hydroxyurea whenever possible and maintaining a sickle hemoglobin target of 30% or less. However, this expert panel acknowledged that these recommendations were based on evidence that is mostly of low quality. Meta-analyses of available data in children with SCD also indicate that the available data are low quality but do point out that children with initially minimal transfusion history seem to benefit more from long-term transfusions to prevent sickle cell–associated complications.[28] When transfusions are given to this patient population, antigen-negative units for Rh and Kell may need to be preferentially given to limit red cell alloimmunization. Some groups have proposed giving phenotypically matched/similar units to these patients to limit alloimmunization.[21] However, phenotyping units may not represent, in some instances, the best way to address Rh polymorphisms that can be found in these patients, and some have proposed instead giving genotypically matched units because phenotyping may be unable to discern when such antigen polymorphisms exist.[29] Data to support this approach have been reported in patients with SCD with Rh variants.[30] There is one major caveat in this recommendation: to achieve this an adequate donor pool with sufficient donors who can be tested to find suitable units is needed.[31] In addition, to make sound clinical decisions much better studies are needed to provide adequate evidence that addresses transfusion needs not only in the acute setting but also in the management of chronic sickle cell complications.[32] As a result, the jury is still out in how to optimize matching of units for these patients in light of current donations.

BLOOD USAGE AND MANAGEMENT

The underlying message of the narrative thus far cannot be separated from its obvious next step, to carefully review blood component usage in clinical settings. It has been reported that hospitals that developed and implemented a system to help transfusion decisions in a background of physician education that includes conservative transfusion practices have led to better blood component utilization.[33] In regard to platelets, implementation of an institutionally generated transfusion system established to optimize their use led to fewer units being discarded as a result of outdating and met its intended goal of better platelet transfusion

management.[34] The implication is that education represents the single most important foundation in developing such a system. Education can be effective in significantly reducing the number of RBC units transfused at large referral medical centers.[35] The question that needs to be answered next is, what is required to establish such a program? Undoubtedly, this likely has to be institutionally driven because the needs from one institution may differ from those of another. What is clear is that this needs to be an ongoing effort that regularly intervenes to reeducate physicians when new evidence becomes available to lead to an effective use of blood components. Furthermore, when hospitals encourage fewer RBC transfusions in response to a hemoglobin trigger of seven, blood utilization is markedly improved, leading to a marked reduction in the number of units transfused.[36] In this context, Transfusion Medicine physicians can be instrumental in coordinating with clinical departments education programs that address the practices of specific clinical services and when needed help develop management programs that take into consideration the needs of their patients. This may also be a forum to exchange ideas with clinicians of how to best tackle times when blood availability is an issue and can extend that to those periods when other components, such as platelets, are in short supply.

Liberal Versus Restrictive Transfusion Practices

This has been a matter of debate for years and it is unlikely to be settled in the minds of some practitioners. The support for a more conservative transfusion management of patients was first established in a large multicenter, randomized, controlled clinical trial that analyzed euvolemic critically ill patients showing that using fewer RBC units was not inferior but actually better to a more liberal transfusion strategy.[37] More recent meta-analyses of available studies have shown that hemostasis also is not improved by targeting a higher hemoglobin threshold because there was no difference in the risk of thrombotic or bleeding events when liberal RBC transfusion was compared with restrictive transfusions.[38] Extending these observations to patients with sepsis has also failed to show differences in outcomes when liberal and restrictive transfusions are compared.[39,40] Similarly, patients with cardiovascular disease do not appear to respond any differently when restrictive or liberal transfusion approaches are used.[41] In the setting of myocardial infarction, there also may be higher mortality when liberal transfusion practices are used.[42,43] In addition, intubated patients do not spend more time mechanically ventilated when restrictive transfusions are used compared with a more liberal approach.[44] Likewise, transfusion practices that address a particular patient population, such as those undergoing cardiac surgery, can be developed and lead to improved clinical outcomes, and fewer RBC and even plasma component utilization.[45] However, these studies address requirements of adult patients, which are not the same as those of younger pediatric patients because more restrictive transfusion approaches in premature infants may not prove to be beneficial.[46] Taken together, all of the above data indicate that a judicious and perhaps less ambitious use of blood components may lead to better outcomes for a significant number of patient populations.

Fresh Versus Older RBC Units

This is perhaps one of the hot topics in clinicians' minds. Considering that blood is a precious asset to hospitals, clinicians have to feel comfortable using available units, which at times may not always be the freshest. The most current meta-analyses of trials reporting outcomes using fresher versus older RBC units indicate that, when one compares their effectiveness, there seems to be no difference in patient outcomes,[47–49] especially when randomized controlled trials are analyzed.[49] Paradoxically, there are data to suggest that there may be a higher incidence of infections when fresher units are used.[48] The latter is something that may be due to bacteria, which compromised the unit at the time of collection but may become less viable as the unit is stored for longer time periods at low temperatures. Nevertheless, it can be inferred that outcomes may also be dependent on the recipient population under study.[50] In premature or low-birth-weight infants the use of blood greater than 7 days old did not result in outcomes different from those in children receiving fresh blood.[51] This may be contrary to what is believed among pediatricians, but this study focused on RBC units not near their outdate but instead on those on average a week older than those considered fresh. Further research is required in this field, but there may be insufficient to no data to establish the inferiority of older units compared with fresh ones.[52] Therefore linking storage times of RBC units to outcomes in a given patient population likely may not be sufficient to establish their degree of effectiveness.

EMERGING INFECTIONS AND BLOOD SAFETY

Although this has been discussed with different emphasis in other chapters, it is worth to put infectious agents at the forefront of current and future potential challenges to blood collections and blood safety. It must be restated that blood components are safer than they have ever been because current testing methodology and thorough donor screenings have led to a significant decrease in the number of discarded units and donations that may potentially transmit infectious agents. However, despite these successes it has become evident over the last thirty years that infectious agents have led to major challenges to blood collection services and by default blood banks to provide safe blood to patients. This is brought into focus by a disclaimer, which is part of every conversation when obtaining consent from a patient before transfusion. No matter how safe the blood is there is always a remote possibility that infectious transmission can occur. Long asymptomatic incubation periods and new infectious agents that can cause disease now seem to be discovered with more frequency. Along these lines, over the last few decades, viruses such as human immunodeficiency virus (HIV), West Nile virus, Chikungunya virus, and more recently Zika virus (ZIKV), among others have led to a flurry of concern for increasing blood safety through development of new tests because these infectious agents can be transmitted via blood transfusions. Importantly, there have been successes in the fight to maintain a safer blood supply. HIV and hepatitis B and hepatitis C viruses are good examples because transmission from these viral agents via transfusion is very low.

The latest health crisis affecting blood collection facilities and by default hospitals is ZIKV infections and potential transmission by blood products. Therefore, it can be used as a model of the potential difficulties that emerging infections can cause to the blood supply chain. The rapid propagation of the ZIKV over the last couple of years has dominated not only news media but also reports from governmental agencies such as the US Centers for Disease Control (CDC) and the European Center for Disease Prevention and Control, which have described in detail the seriousness of the spread of this new infectious agent and refer the reader to their respective websites for the most up–to-date ZIKV information. Complications caused by this virus have been described, which include infections in- utero that lead to microcephaly and brain disorders in newborns to even death,[53,54] and in adults, infections may lead to Guillain-Barré syndrome and death.[55,56] The ZIKV outbreak in French Polynesia, through broad testing of blood donors, showed that asymptomatic donors (3% of all donations) had ZIKV detected by polymerase chain reaction.[57] This possibility made the scientific and blood transfusion communities pay attention in light of the reports describing the potential complications that this infection can cause. Reports from Brazil,[58] and later reaffirmed by the CDC, have made it clear that this infection can be transmitted via transfusion.[59] Therefore a large undertaking was put in place to potentially catch donors exposed to the virus before donation. This is not an easy task, because the geographical region where ZIKV has been found covers most of the countries south of the United States and all of the Caribbean from its origin in Africa in the earlier part of the 20th century.[60] Second, the asymptomatic incubation period is rather long, and in some cases no noticeable symptoms may be apparent to the person exposed to the virus. Third, the mosquito(es) responsible for transmitting the infection are already found in most of the continental United States. As a result, the possibility of infection by ZIKV has not been taken lightly by US health agencies and led to the extreme recommendation of suspending blood collections in the US territory of Puerto Rico owing to the alarming number of cases found in the island.[59] Of interest, the ZIKV isolate found in Brazil is more closely related to the Asian strain described 50 years ago.[61] However, other strains have been identified in the Americas and likely exchange of genetic material is at the heart of the current foci of infections reported across the continent. Tests that have been developed and are currently in trials to determine their effectiveness will likely begin in the near future to relieve the pressure off blood centers and blood banks across the country.

CULTURE CHANGE

Since blood components first began to be used, they have been used with a particular function in mind. RBC transfusions were given to improve the oxygen-carrying capacity in those unable to rapidly increase production owing to sudden losses or chronic diseases, and in the case of platelets transfusions were used to prevent, reduce, or minimize bleeding. Today we know this is an oversimplification of the function of blood cells. The better utilization of blood components is a subject that clinicians and blood bankers tend to agree upon; however, they differ in the mechanisms to achieve the desired reduction in blood usage. As mentioned earlier, the United States transfuses more blood per 1000 patients than any other country. This overreliance on transfusions is at the core of the higher rates of alloimmunization seen in the country and it is dependent at times on practices that may not follow current transfusion guidelines set forth by different expert groups. What can be done to overcome this dependency? The starting point is to change the way clinicians see blood. Specifically, there has to be a conscientious change to

the medical culture driving transfusion. What is meant by culture? Medical practice is in part bound to physicians' prior experiences that are passed on from one generation while training the next. If the approach to transfusion is based on this model, then the use of blood this way is seen as the norm by those who train later. Based on this, it can be envisioned that to increase the level of awareness of proper blood usage, physicians may need to be retrained using the most current clinical evidence. This is in theory being taught by academic centers. However, this is not a static process but one that needs to remain constantly changing as new evidence becomes available.

Culture changes can be successful, but they are processes that once set in motion may take years of reeducation to see practice adjustments. Reports indicating that better management of blood components through lower transfusion triggers, staff education using evidence-based guidelines, blood conservation/salvage, and increases in the cost of procuring blood components has resulted in significant decreases in usage,[62] which can be substantial even if limited to reducing the number of units per transfusion.[63] In the long term once such programs are established, continued reductions in blood utilization are still seen in surgical practice years after their implementation; however, in other non-surgical settings as the number of older adults requiring transfusions continues to grow this will require blood management programs that take into account medical practice in these environments.[64] Institutional cultural challenges are evident when comparisons between hospitals within the same healthcare network show that the institutional practice and surgeon's expertise have the greatest effect in the number of blood components used.[65] This could be due in part to a hospital's ability to address the needs of complex procedures. Those that routinely perform very complex surgical procedures likely have on staff surgeons with greater expertise conserving blood and may use fewer components compared with institutions where the same procedures are performed with less frequency. Nevertheless, differences cannot be explained by this alone. It is understood that, in the setting of emergency procedures and/or massive transfusion protocols, blood conservation is the least concern in the minds of physicians. However, in settings where certain surgical procedures are planned, careful planning assessing surgical risk, optimizing patients' potential anemia, anticipation of bleeding complications, intraoperative blood conservation, and conservative transfusion guidelines can result in a hospital cultural change that leads to fewer transfusions.[66]

SUMMARY

Challenges facing transfusion practices are diverse and likely require close collaboration among practitioners and Transfusion Medicine physicians to adapt to a blood supply that is unlikely to expand. This requires adherence to guidelines based on the strongest clinical evidence in the setting of conservative transfusion practices. Likewise, technologies and processes that prioritize blood conservation must be undertaken. Patient outcomes are at the center of clinical decision making, but this has to take into consideration the nongrowing availability of blood components. New infectious agents will emerge, but the development of appropriate detection testing is becoming more streamlined and will continue improving in the years ahead. We must agree that a viable blood supply is a diverse blood supply, and this will have the greatest impact in reducing alloimmunization rates once such a diverse donor pool is achieved. However, this will only improve in a background of fewer or limited exposures to blood.

REFERENCES

1. McCarthy LJ. How do I manage a blood shortage in a transfusion service? *Transfusion.* 2007;47(5):760–762.
2. James AB, Hillyer CD, Shaz BH. Demographic differences in estimated blood donor eligibility prevalence in the United States. *Transfusion.* 2012;52(5):1050–1061.
3. US Department of Health and Human Services. *The 2007 National Blood Collection and Utilization Survey Report.* Available at: http://www.nhs.gov/ash/bloodsafety/2007nbcus_survey.pdf.
4. United States Census Bureau. *United States and World Population Clock.* Available at: https://www.census.gov/popclock/.
5. Sullivan MT, Wallace EL. Blood collection and transfusion in the United States in 1999. *Transfusion.* 2005;45(2):141–148.
6. Sullivan MT, Cotten R, Read EJ, Wallace EL. Blood collection and transfusion in the United States in 2001. *Transfusion.* 2007;47(3):385–394.
7. US Department of Health and Human Services. *The 2011 National Blood Collection and Utlization Survey Report.* Available at: http://www.nhs.gov/ash/bloodsafety/2011nbcus-survey.pdf.
8. Whitaker B, Rajbhandary S, Kleinman S, Harris A, Kamani N. Trends in United States blood collection and transfusion: results from the 2013 AABB blood collection, utilization, and patient blood management survey. *Transfusion.* 2016;56(9):2173–2183.
9. Ellingson KD, Sapiano MRP, Haass KA, et al. Continued decline in blood collection and transfusion in the United States - 2015. *Transfusion.* 2017;57(suppl 2):1588–1598.
10. Sapiano MRP, Savinkina AA, Ellingson KD, et al. Supplemental findings from the national blood collection and utilization surveys, 2013 and 2015. *Transfusion.* 2017;57(suppl 2):1599–1624.
11. Vichinsky EP, Earles A, Johnson RA, Hoag MS, Williams A, Lubin B. Alloimmunization in sickle cell anemia and transfusion of racially unmatched blood. *N Engl J Med.* 1990;322(23):1617–1621.
12. Yazer MH, Delaney M, Germain M, et al. Trends in US minority red blood cell unit donations. *Transfusion.* 2017;57(5):1226–1234.
13. Shaz BH, James AB, Hillyer KL, Schreiber GB, Hillyer CD. Demographic patterns of blood donors and donations in a large metropolitan area. *J Natl Med Assoc.* 2011;103(4):351–357.
14. Chou ST, Liem RI, Thompson AA. Challenges of alloimmunization in patients with haemoglobinopathies. *Br J Haematol.* 2012;159(4):394–404.
15. Olujohungbe A, Hambleton I, Stephens L, Serjeant B, Serjeant G. Red cell antibodies in patients with homozygous sickle cell disease: a comparison of patients in Jamaica and the United Kingdom. *Br J Haematol.* 2001;113(3):661–665.
16. Natukunda B, Schonewille H, Ndugwa C, Brand A. Red blood cell alloimmunization in sickle cell disease patients in Uganda. *Transfusion.* 2010;50(1):20–25.
17. Zheng Y, Maitta RW. Alloimmunisation rates of sickle cell disease patients in the United States differ from those in other geographical regions. *Transfus Med.* 2016;26(3):225–230.
18. Frye V, Caltabiano M, Kessler DA, et al. Evaluating a program to increase blood donation among racial and ethnic minority communities in New York City. *Transfusion.* 2014;54(12):3061–3067.
19. Brousseau DC, Panepinto JA, Nimmer M, Hoffmann RG. The number of people with sickle-cell disease in the United States: national and state estimates. *Am J Hematol.* 2010;85(1):77–78.
20. Chou ST, Jackson T, Vege S, Smith-Whitley K, Friedman DF, Westhoff CM. High prevalence of red blood cell alloimmunization in sickle cell disease despite transfusion from Rh-matched minority donors. *Blood.* 2013;122(6):1062–1071.
21. Lasalle-Williams M, Nuss R, Le T, et al. Extended red blood cell antigen matching for transfusions in sickle cell disease: a review of a 14-year experience from a single center (CME). *Transfusion.* 2011;51(8):1732–1739.
22. Murphy MF, Yazer MH. Measuring and monitoring blood utilization. *Transfusion.* 2013;53(12):3025–3028.
23. Leisch M, Weiss L, Lindlbauer N, et al. Red blood cell alloimmunization in 184 patients with myeloid neoplasms treated with azacitidine – a retrospective single center experience. *Leuk Res.* 2017;59:12–19.
24. Kelly S, Quirolo K, Marsh A, Neumayr L, Garcia A, Custer B. Erythrocytapheresis for chronic transfusion therapy in sickle cell disease: survey of current practices and review of the literature. *Transfusion.* 2016;56(11):2877–2888.
25. Wahl SK, Garcia A, Hagar W, Gildengorin G, Quirolo K, Vichinsky E. Lower alloimmunization rates in pediatric sickle cell patients on chronic erythrocytapheresis compared to chronic simple transfusions. *Transfusion.* 2012;52(12):2671–2676.

26. Michot JM, Driss F, Guitton C, et al. Immunohematologic tolerance of chronic transfusion exchanges with erythrocytapheresis in sickle cell disease. *Transfusion*. 2015;55(2):357–363.

27. Yawn BP, Buchanan GR, Afenyi-Annan AN, et al. Management of sickle cell disease: summary of the 2014 evidence-based report by expert panel members. *JAMA*. 2014;312(10):1033–1048.

28. Estcourt LJ, Fortin PM, Hopewell S, Trivella M, Wang WC. Blood transfusion for preventing primary and secondary stroke in people with sickle cell disease. *Cochrane Database Syst Rev*. 2017;1:CD003146.

29. Casas J, Friedman DF, Jackson T, Vege S, Westhoff CM, Chou ST. Changing practice: red blood cell typing by molecular methods for patients with sickle cell disease. *Transfusion*. 2015;55(6 Pt 2):1388–1393.

30. da Costa DC, Pellegrino Jr J, Guelsin GA, Ribeiro KA, Gilli SC, Castilho L. Molecular matching of red blood cells is superior to serological matching in sickle cell disease patients. *Rev Bras Hematol Hemoter*. 2013;35(1):35–38.

31. Ribeiro KR, Guarnieri MH, da Costa DC, Costa FF, Pellegrino Jr J, Castilho L. DNA array analysis for red blood cell antigens facilitates the transfusion support with antigen-matched blood in patients with sickle cell disease. *Vox Sang*. 2009;97(2):147–152.

32. Savage WJ, Buchanan GR, Yawn BP, et al. Evidence gaps in the management of sickle cell disease: a summary of needed research. *Am J Hematol*. 2015;90(4):273–275.

33. Butler CE, Noel S, Hibbs SP, et al. Implementation of a clinical decision support system improves compliance with restrictive transfusion policies in hematology patients. *Transfusion*. 2015;55(8):1964–1971.

34. Gomez AT, Quinn JG, Doiron DJ, Watson S, Crocker BD, Cheng CK. Implementation of a novel real-time platelet inventory management system at a multi-site transfusion service. *Transfusion*. 2015;55(9):2070–2075.

35. Zuckerberg GS, Scott AV, Wasey JO, et al. Efficacy of education followed by computerized provider order entry with clinician decision support to reduce red blood cell utilization. *Transfusion*. 2015;55(7):1628–1636.

36. Yang WW, Thakkar RN, Gehrie EA, Chen W, Frank SM. Single-unit transfusions and hemoglobin trigger: relative impact on red cell utilization. *Transfusion*. 2017;57(5):1163–1170.

37. Hebert PC, Wells G, Blajchman MA, et al. A multicenter, randomized, controlled clinical trial of transfusion requirements in critical care. Transfusion requirements in Critical Care Investigators, Canadian Critical Care Trials Group. *N Engl J Med*. 1999;340(6):409–417.

38. Desborough MJR, Colman KS, Prick BW, et al. Effect of restrictive versus liberal red cell transfusion strategies on haemostasis: systematic review and meta-analysis. *Thromb Haemost*. 2017;117(5):889–898.

39. Dupuis C, Sonneville R, Adrie C, et al. Impact of transfusion on patients with sepsis admitted in intensive care unit: a systematic review and meta-analysis. *Ann Intensive Care*. 2017;7(1):5.

40. Rygard SL, Holst LB, Wetterslev J, et al. Higher vs. lower haemoglobin threshold for transfusion in septic shock: subgroup analyses of the TRISS trial. *Acta Anaesthesiol Scand*. 2017;61(2):166–175.

41. Hebert PC, Yetisir E, Martin C, et al. Is a low transfusion threshold safe in critically ill patients with cardiovascular diseases? *Crit Care Med*. 2001;29(2):227–234.

42. Chatterjee S, Wetterslev J, Sharma A, Lichstein E, Mukherjee D. Association of blood transfusion with increased mortality in myocardial infarction: a meta-analysis and diversity-adjusted study sequential analysis. *JAMA Intern Med*. 2013;173(2):132–139.

43. Nikolsky E, Mehran R, Sadeghi HM, et al. Prognostic impact of blood transfusion after primary angioplasty for acute myocardial infarction: analysis from the CADILLAC (Controlled Abciximab and Device Investigation to Lower Late Angioplasty Complications) trial. *JACC Cardiovasc Interv*. 2009;2(7):624–632.

44. Hebert PC, Blajchman MA, Cook DJ, et al. Do blood transfusions improve outcomes related to mechanical ventilation? *Chest*. 2001;119(6):1850–1857.

45. Bilecen S, de Groot JA, Kalkman CJ, Spanjersberg AJ, Moons KG, Nierich AP. Effectiveness of a cardiac surgery-specific transfusion protocol. *Transfusion*. 2014;54(3):708–716.

46. Bell EF, Strauss RG, Widness JA, et al. Randomized trial of liberal versus restrictive guidelines for red blood cell transfusion in preterm infants. *Pediatrics*. 2005;115(6):1685–1691.

47. Chai-Adisaksopha C, Alexander PE, Guyatt G, et al. Mortality outcomes in patients transfused with fresher versus older red blood cells: a meta-analysis. *Vox Sang*. 2017;112(3):268–278.

48. Alexander PE, Barty R, Fei Y, et al. Transfusion of fresher vs older red blood cells in hospitalized patients: a systematic review and meta-analysis. *Blood*. 2016;127(4):400–410.

49. Remy KE, Sun J, Wang D, et al. Transfusion of recently donated (fresh) red blood cells (RBCs) does not improve survival in comparison with current practice, while safety of the oldest stored units is yet to be established: a meta-analysis. *Vox Sang*. 2016;111(1):43–54.

50. Brunskill SJ, Wilkinson KL, Doree C, Trivella M, Stanworth S. Transfusion of fresher versus older red blood cells for all conditions. *Cochrane Database Syst Rev*. 2015;(5):CD010801.

51. Fergusson DA, Hebert P, Hogan DL, et al. Effect of fresh red blood cell transfusions on clinical outcomes in premature, very-low-birth-weight infants: the ARIPI randomized trial. *JAMA*. 2012;308(14):1443–1451.

52. Marti-Carvajal AJ, Simancas-Racines D, Pena-Gonzalez BS. Prolonged storage of packed red blood cells for blood transfusion. *Cochrane Database Syst Rev*. 2015;(7):CD009330.

53. Brasil P, Pereira Jr JP, Moreira ME, et al. Zika virus infection in pregnant women in Rio de Janeiro. *N Engl J Med*. 2016;375(24):2321–2334.

54. Mlakar J, Korva M, Tul N, et al. Zika virus associated with microcephaly. *N Engl J Med*. 2016;374(10):951–958.

55. Cao-Lormeau VM, Blake A, Mons S, et al. Guillain-Barre syndrome outbreak associated with Zika virus infec-

tion in French Polynesia: a case-control study. *Lancet.* 2016;387(10027):1531–1539.

56. Lazarus C, Guichard M, Philippe JM, Paux T, Vallet B. The French experience of the threat posed by Zika virus. *Lancet.* 2016;388(10039):9–11.

57. Musso D, Nhan T, Robin E, et al. Potential for Zika virus transmission through blood transfusion demonstrated during an outbreak in French Polynesia, November 2013 to February 2014. *Euro Surveill.* 2014;19(14).

58. Barjas-Castro ML, Angerami RN, Cunha MS, et al. Probable transfusion-transmitted Zika virus in Brazil. *Transfusion.* 2016;56(7):1684–1688.

59. Vasquez AM, Sapiano MR, Basavaraju SV, Kuehnert MJ, Rivera-Garcia B. Survey of blood collection centers and implementation of guidance for prevention of transfusion-transmitted Zika virus infection–Puerto Rico, 2016. *Morb Mortal Wkly Rep.* 2016;65(14):375–378.

60. Faye O, Freire CC, Iamarino A, et al. Molecular evolution of Zika virus during its emergence in the 20(th) century. *PLoS Negl Trop Dis.* 2014;8(1):e2636.

61. Zanluca C, Melo VC, Mosimann AL, Santos GI, Santos CN, Luz K. First report of autochthonous transmission of Zika virus in Brazil. *Mem Inst Oswaldo Cruz.* 2015;110(4): 569–572.

62. Wallis JP, Wells AW, Chapman CE. Changing indications for red cell transfusion from 2000 to 2004 in the North of England. *Transfus Med.* 2006;16(6):411–417.

63. Oliver JC, Griffin RL, Hannon T, Marques MB. The success of our patient blood management program depended on an institution-wide change in transfusion practices. *Transfusion.* 2014;54(10 Pt 2):2617–2624.

64. Tinegate H, Pendry K, Murphy M, et al. Where do all the red blood cells (RBCs) go? Results of a survey of RBC use in England and North Wales in 2014. *Transfusion.* 2016;56(1): 139–145.

65. Jin R, Zelinka ES, McDonald J, et al. Effect of hospital culture on blood transfusion in cardiac procedures. *Ann Thorac Surg.* 2013;95(4):1269–1274.

66. Sherman CH, Macivor DC. Blood utilization: fostering an effective hospital transfusion culture. *J Clin Anesth.* 2012;24(2):155–163.

Index

Note: 'Page numbers followed by "f" indicate figures, "t" indicate tables and "b" indicate boxes.'

Printed in the United States
By Bookmasters